Delmar's
MATERNAL–INFANT

NURSING
CARE PLANS

Delmar's
MATERNAL–
INFANT

NURSING
CARE PLANS

2nd Edition

KARLA L. LUXNER, RNC, ND

DELMAR
CENGAGE Learning™

Australia • Brazil • Japan • Korea • Mexico • Singapore • Spain • United Kingdom • United States

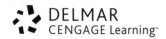
DELMAR
CENGAGE Learning™

Delmar's Maternal–Infant Nursing Care Plans, 2nd edition
by Karla L. Luxner

Vice President, Health Care Business Unit: **William Brottmiller**

Editorial Director: **Cathy L. Esperti**

Acquisitions Editor:
Matthew Filimonov

Senior Developmental Editor:
Elisabeth F. Williams

Marketing Director: **Jennifer McAvey**

Marketing Coordinator:
Karen Summerlin

Editorial Assistant: **Patricia Osborn**

Technology Director: **Laurie K. Davis**

Art/Design Specialist:
Connie Lundberg-Watkins

Production Coordinator: **Bridget Lulay**

Project Editor: **Jennifer Luck**

For product information and technology assistance, contact us at
Professional & Career Group Customer Support, 1-800-648-7450

For permission to use material from this text or product, submit all requests online at **www.cengage.com/permissions**
Further permissions questions can be emailed to
permissionrequest@cengage.com

ExamView® and ExamView Pro® are registered trademarks of FSCreations, Inc. Windows is a registered trademark of the Microsoft Corporation used herein under license. Macintosh and Power Macintosh are registered trademarks of Apple Computer, Inc. Used herein under license.

ISBN-13: 978-0-7668-5993-7

ISBN-10: 0-7668-5993-2

Delmar Cengage Learning
5 Maxwell Drive
Clifton Park, NY 12065-2919
USA

Cengage Learning products are represented in Canada by Nelson Education, Ltd.

For your lifelong learning solutions, visit **delmar.cengage.com**

Visit our corporate website at **www.cengage.com**

Notice to the Reader
Publisher does not warrant or guarantee any of the products described herein or perform any independent analysis in connection with any of the product information contained herein. Publisher does not assume, and expressly disclaims, any obligation to obtain and include information other than that provided to it by the manufacturer. The reader is expressly warned to consider and adopt all safety precautions that might be indicated by the activities described herein and to avoid all potential hazards. By following the instructions contained herein, the reader willingly assumes all risks in connection with such instructions. The publisher makes no representations or warranties of any kind, including but not limited to, the warranties of fitness for particular purpose or merchantability, nor are any such representations implied with respect to the material set forth herein, and the publisher takes no responsibility with respect to such material. The publisher shall not be liable for any special, consequential, or exemplary damages resulting, in whole or part, from the readers' use of, or reliance upon, this material.

Printed in Canada
6 7 8 9 10 12 11 10 9 8

CONTENTS

PREFACE

Pregnancy, childbirth, the puerperium, and the newborn transition to extrauterine life are natural physiologic processes. The healthy mother and her infant usually require little in the way of medical intervention during these life events; they may however, benefit greatly from comprehensive nursing care. Maternal–infant nursing is provided in diverse settings, from homes and schools to clinics, hospitals, and OB Intensive Care Units. Perinatal health promotion and wellness teaching form the foundation of this care and lay the groundwork for healthy families of the future. For the families experiencing a complicated pregnancy or birth, skilled nursing care based on sound scientific knowledge is needed—not instead of, but in addition to health promotion and wellness teaching. Knowledge and respect for cultural variations is essential to modern nursing practice.

CONCEPTUAL APPROACH

The nursing process serves as a learning tool for readers and as a practice and documentation format for clinicians. Based on a thorough assessment, the nurse formulates a specific plan of care for each individual client. The care plans in this book are provided to facilitate that process for readers and practitioners. To that end, each care plan solicits specific client data and prompts the nurse to individualize the interventions, consider cultural relevance, and evaluate the client's individual response. The book provides basic nursing care plans for healthy clients during prenatal, intrapartum, postpartum, and newborn periods through the first six weeks of life. Common perinatal and neonatal complications for each section are then presented with associated care plans. Home visit care plans are included for the prenatal, postpartum, and newborn clients, reflecting current practice.

ORGANIZATION

Delmar's Maternal–Infant Nursing Care Plans, 2nd edition, includes plans that have been developed to reflect comprehensive perinatal nursing care for mothers and their infants. The book is divided into five units: Pregnancy, Intrapartum, Postpartum, Newborn, and Infant: Birth to Six Weeks. Each unit begins with an overview of the general physiologic and psychological changes associated with the period. Additional pertinent information is presented in flowchart format. Care Paths provide an overview of common health care practices.

Perinatal and neonatal complications are briefly described, including risk factors and common medical care if indicated. Important relationships are presented in flowcharts to facilitate understanding of the basis for care. Nursing diagnoses relevant to the complication are cross-referenced when applicable and followed by specific diagnoses common for the condition.

Nursing care begins with a comprehensive review and assessment of each individual client. The data is then analyzed and a specific plan of care developed. The format for each nursing care plan in this book is summarized below.

- Nursing diagnoses as approved by the North American Nursing Diagnosis Association (NANDA) taxonomy (2003–2004); the complete NANDA listing is found in Appendix A (new to this edition).

- Related factors (etiology) for each diagnosis are suggested and the user is prompted to choose the most appropriate for the specific client.

- Defining characteristics for each actual diagnosis are listed with prompts to the user to include specific client data from the nursing assessment.

- Goals are related to the nursing diagnosis and include a time frame for evaluation to be specified by the user.
- Appropriate outcome criteria specific for the client are suggested. In keeping with current practice, this edition includes a Nursing Outcome Classification (NOC) label for each nursing diagnosis. Appendix B offers a complete listing of NOC labels.
- Nursing interventions and rationales are comprehensive. They include pertinent continuous assessments and observations. Common therapeutic actions originating from nursing and those resulting from collaboration with the primary caregiver are suggested with prompts for creativity and individualization. Client and family teaching and psychosocial support are provided with respect for cultural variation and individual needs. Consultation and referral to other caregivers is suggested when indicated.
- Nursing Intervention Classification (NIC) labels are provided in this new edition for each nursing diagnosis. These are inserted after the interventions and rationales to assist the user in becoming familiar with this classification process for nursing interventions. Appendix C provides the complete listing of NIC labels.
- Evaluation of the client's goal and presentation of data related to the outcome criteria is followed by consideration of the next step for the client.

A new, descriptive introductory chapter outlines how to customize care plans for an individual client based on the standardized care plans found in this book.

A CD is included in the back of this book that contains electronic files for all the care plans in the book. Readers can create new care plans, customize care plans, add and delete nursing diagnoses and interventions, and print the plans of care for use in the clinical setting.

ACKNOWLEDGMENTS

I am grateful to my family, students, nurse colleagues, and the many mothers, fathers, grandparents, and babies who have enriched my understanding and shaped my practice. This book is dedicated to the memory of my parents, Arthur and Elizabeth Romaine.

Karla L. Luxner

REVIEWERS

Anne Quinn-Wallace, RN, BA, SCM
Professor of Nursing
Conestoga College
Ontario, Canada

Kathleen S. Bush, RN
Staff Nurse/Freelance Writer
Mount Timpanogos Women's Health Care Center
American Fork, Utah

Jean Tillman, RN, BSN, MSN
Instructor of Nursing
Holyoke Community College
Holyoke, Massachusetts

AN INTRODUCTION TO THE USE OF THE NURSING CARE PLANS

INTRODUCTION

Excellent nursing practice reflects proficient use of the nursing process demonstrated by skillful assessment, diagnosis, planning, outcome identification, intervention, and evaluation. The nursing process provides the framework that directs nursing practice. Nursing care planning is the application of the nursing process to a specific client situation. Written nursing care plans are a means of communication among health care providers, clients, and families. They ensure that care is coordinated to achieve desired health care outcomes.

A thorough assessment is the foundation of the nursing process. The assessment data are then reviewed and organized according to client needs. Nursing diagnoses, derived from the assessment, provide the basis for selection of interventions to achieve outcomes for which the nurse is accountable (NANDA, 2003). "Now, as never before, today's nurse must make more complex professional decisions, determine what things to do and what things not to do for which clients. Priorities are critical: often the nurse must make hard choices between what is essential and what is merely beneficial" (Barnum, 1999). The primary purpose of the nursing diagnostic processes applied by nurses is to design a plan of care for and in conjunction with the client that results in the prevention, reduction, or resolution of the client's health problem (Harkreader, 2004).

In the current multidisciplinary health care environment, nurses are positioned for a high level of accountability. The nurse is required to make many independent decisions and to coordinate the various disciplines working together and sharing responsibility for client outcome achievement. This environment affords nursing an opportunity to define its boundaries and to use the nursing process to coordinate care across disciplines. Nurses need to develop strong assessment skills, organize the data obtained to prioritize client needs, predict achievable, measurable client outcomes, and tailor interventions for the individual client. This text is designed to assist the user in that process.

NURSING CARE PLANS AND INDIVIDUAL CLIENT CARE NEEDS

This book is intended to facilitate the care planning process for nurses working with maternal-infant clients based on recognized nursing standards. Each of the nursing diagnoses is from NANDA's Taxonomy II (NANDA, 2003). The outcome criteria include the appropriate Nursing Outcome Classification (NOC) as well as prompts to assist the user in developing individualized outcomes. This text also contains suggested Nursing Intervention Classifications (NIC) for each nursing diagnosis in addition to suggested comprehensive and individualized interventions for each diagnosis.

Each section begins with essential introductory information about the condition and the current medical management when appropriate. A thorough assessment of the client is essential to developing a plan of care. The user is prompted to insert specific client data into the care plan at strategic points in each diagnosis. The user is offered a variety of common and additional nursing diagnoses for each condition including:

1. The etiology (related to) for each diagnosis using specific client data obtained in the assessment.

2. Possible defining characteristics, with prompts for individualization, which support the diagnosis.

3. A client goal related to the nursing diagnosis with a prompt to identify an appropriate time frame for evaluation of the outcomes.

4. Measurable outcome criteria requiring the use of specific client data and individualized parameters.

5. Comprehensive and detailed nursing interventions with guidance to individualize care for the specific client.

6. Rationales for the nursing interventions to demonstrate evidence-based practice.

7. Evaluation based on individual client information. The user is prompted to evaluate goal achievement and present the specific client data called for in the outcome criteria.

The nursing care plans provided in this text are intended to serve as a framework on which to design individualized client care reflecting current nursing standards of care. The user must first obtain comprehensive, reliable, and detailed assessment information for the particular client using all available sources. The initial assessment data should then be interpreted and organized into categories reflecting prioritized client needs. Frequently, after reflecting on the initial assessment, the nurse will find that additional focused assessment data must be obtained before care can be planned. Appropriate nursing diagnoses are then selected and prioritized. Individual client data are the defining characteristics that support the choice of nursing diagnosis. A specific goal and the necessary outcome criteria that will be used to identify when the goal has been met should be based on the defining characteristics. Outcome criteria reflect the individual client's capabilities and expectations. The nurse then selects a comprehensive array of interventions to provide current evidence-based client care directed toward the outcomes and resolution of the problem. Interventions should also be prioritized and may include additional ongoing assessments, therapeutic nursing activities, collaborative interventions, client and family teaching, and referrals. Current standards of care for maternal-infant nursing practice have been incorporated throughout the text. Every effort has been made to prompt the user to insert individual client data and to specify the parameters of care as the care plan is developed. Thoughtful use of this text will guide the user to develop comprehensive individualized care plans based on current scientific knowledge and evidence for best practices.

The process for planning individualized care involves the same steps as the nursing process.

1. Collect assessment data from all available sources including the client, the family, other providers, and the chart. Chart data may include: nurse's notes or flow sheets; laboratory, diagnostic, or surgical reports; progress notes from dietary, rehab, or physical therapy; the physician's history and physical, and progress notes. Assess the client's current status through the interview, observation, and physical examination. After studying the health record and obtaining assessment data, organize the information into prioritized problem or client need categories.

2. Identify viable nursing diagnoses and potential client risks suggested by the categories of assessment data. Review the appropriate chapter in this text and review the nursing diagnoses provided for the condition. Choose the diagnoses that fit the specific client. The diagnostic process is individualized by identifying "related to" factors and "defining characteristics" that flow from the comprehensive client assessment. For example, "Acute pain related to surgical incision" is supported by the client data, "verbalizes pain at a 9 on the scale of 0–10." The client's own words and pain rating support the diagnosis and guide the nurse to choose an outcome criteria of "verbalizes pain as less than 9 on a scale of 1–10" and interventions that must include assessment of pain using a scale of 1–10.

3. Plan to identify and meet client goals using specific outcomes as evidence. The goal pertains to the diagnosis and moves the client toward resolution of the problem within a reasonable time frame. The outcome criteria included in the text indicate options to measure goal attainment and encourage specific qualifiers such as when, how much, and individual client variables to be added to individualize the plan. "Client will experience decreased pain within 24 hours" is a clear goal with an achievable target time. "Verbalizes pain as 5 or less on a scale of 1–10" would be a measurable outcome that, if based on the particular client situation and capabilities, individualizes the plan and indicates goal attainment.

4. Design interventions to meet the goal and resolve the nursing diagnosis. Choose interventions pertinent to the client that are consistent with the medical orders. Ongoing assessment of the client's pain perception, positioning, teaching the client to ask for medication before pain becomes severe, and the administration of pain medications, specifying the drug, dose, route, and times as ordered, are examples of both independent

and collaborative nursing interventions, which would achieve the outcome, attain the goal, and resolve the "Acute Pain" diagnosis.

5. Evaluate the effectiveness of the plan. By setting a client goal and specific observable outcomes, the plan communicates the need for ongoing evaluation and updating. Evaluation of the outcome criteria at the specified time will either indicate resolution of the problem or the need to continue or revise the care plan.

CRITICAL THINKING, THE NURSING PROCESS, AND CARE PLAN DEVELOPMENT

Critical thinking and decision-making skills are used to identify nursing diagnoses. Critical thinking entails purposeful, goal-directed thinking and analysis of information. The nurse uses critical thinking to make clinical judgments based on evidence. The nurse synthesizes the information collected in the assessment and then makes judgments about how to put the information together to form nursing diagnoses. The format of this book encourages the nurse to review the client history and obtain thorough assessment data that are significant for a particular condition. The nurse is then prompted to insert relevant assessment findings as appropriate to formulate an individualized nursing care plan.

The following case study illustrates how to apply individual client data to a care plan in this book.

ADOLESCENT PREGNANCY CASE STUDY

A 15-year-old primigravida is referred to the prenatal clinic by her pediatrician. She is at 24 weeks gestation. The client is single and lives at home with her mother, father, and younger brother, age 13. Her father works full time at the post office. The mother takes on part-time work as a cleaning woman when she is able to obtain work. Her father has a drinking problem but refuses to get help. The client had considered abortion but decided she wanted to keep the baby so that she could have someone to care about her. She plans to finish high school and go to college but does not think her parents will help with this now. She states she would like to get married one day and have more children. She is looking forward to having the baby and says, "it will be a lot of fun." She is no longer in contact with the baby's father but he is aware of the pregnancy.

Her age at menarche was 11.5 years. Height is 62 inches and current weight is 105 pounds. Her fundus measures 22 cm. The fetal heart tones are heard in the LUQ at 156 beats per minute. She has not gained any weight with this pregnancy. She reports that her usual diet consists of: nothing for breakfast; a diet soda and slice of pizza or sandwich for lunch; a candy bar snack mid-afternoon; dinner at home consists of some meat, a vegetable she does not usually eat, a starch, and soda or milk. She denies alcohol or illicit drug use but she does smoke one pack of cigarettes per day.

NURSING DIAGNOSIS #1

Ineffective Health Maintenance

Related to: Unplanned adolescent pregnancy.

Defining Characteristics: Delayed seeking care: first prenatal visit at 24 weeks; poor dietary intake during pregnancy: inadequate nutrients resulting in no weight gain at 24 weeks. Smokes 1PPD.

Goal: Client will change behaviors to maintain health by next prenatal visit.

Outcome Criteria:

✔ Client will identify three current unhealthy behaviors.

✔ Client will verbalize plan to stop smoking, eat a balanced diet for pregnancy, and obtain regular prenatal care.

NOC: *Health-Promoting Behavior*

INTERVENTIONS

Develop a trusting relationship with client, remain nonjudgmental, and demonstrate empathy by allowing time for interaction and the expression of feelings about pregnancy.

Assess underlying reasons for unhealthy behaviors, discuss impact on growing fetus, and encourage her to adapt self-care to meet her own and the baby's needs.

Explain the physiologic risks associated with lack of prenatal care, poor nutrition, and smoking during pregnancy: anemia, preterm birth, low birth weight, mental retardation, fetal or neonatal death, and maternal complications.

Assist client to plan healthy behavior changes: stop smoking, change dietary habits to obtain necessary nutrients during pregnancy, and obtain prenatal care. Collaborate with the physician to obtain nicotine patches if needed to help decrease addiction.

(continues)

INTERVENTIONS

Praise client for planning and attempting to change behaviors. Reinforce positive steps and support her when she has a setback.

Assist client to obtain needed resources from WIC and the health department's adolescent pregnancy program.

Refer client to appropriate supportive services, (specify smoking cessation programs, substance abuse, resource mothers programs, etc.)

NIC: *Support System Enhancement*

NURSING DIAGNOSIS #2
Delayed Growth and Development

Related to: Interruption of the normal psychosocial development of adolescence and detachment from parents.

Defining Characteristics: Client is 15 years old, 62 inches, and 105 lb at 24 weeks gestation. Parents are nonsupportive. Client appears unrealistic about the demands of motherhood: she decided to keep the baby to have someone to care for her and thinks a baby will be "fun."

Goal: Client will demonstrate adequate growth and age-appropriate psychosocial development while accomplishing the development tasks of pregnancy.

Outcome Criteria:

✔ Client will gain 25–35 lb during pregnancy, verbalize plans to complete high school education, and acknowledge that she will need help to care for the baby appropriately.

NOC: *Child Development: Adolescence*

INTERVENTIONS:

Assess client's physical growth at each prenatal visit. Encourage her to include a family member in prenatal visits to support her needs.

Reinforce nutrition teaching relating it to the client's growth needs as well as the fetus. Teach client to take daily iron supplements as ordered.

Assist the client and family member to realistically discuss the effect of pregnancy on her education and future plans for a career.

Encourage client to finish basic schooling and make realistic plans for the future including childcare.

Discuss body image issues and correct misconceptions, evaluating her expectations, perceptions, and feelings about her body.

Assist client to assess relationships with parents and peers, and plan ways to improve these.

Teach client and family member about the developmental tasks of adolescence and the tasks of pregnancy.

Make referrals as indicated to the school counselor, social services, and financial assistance.

NIC: *Self-Responsibility Facilitation*

CLINICAL PATHWAYS: A METHOD OF ACHIEVING OUTCOMES ACROSS THE CONTINUUM OF CARE

Health care consumers expect affordable care and optimal outcomes. Third-party providers scrutinize client outcomes to validate the need for expensive health care services. Health care organizations report outcomes to state, federal, and independent agencies to verify practice standards and attract consumers and providers. The demand for the most effective and cost-efficient manner of restoring clients to health has led to collaborative responsibility for client care demonstrated by the clinical pathway. Clinical pathways, also known as "care maps," are care management tools that outline the expected clinical course and outcomes for a specific client type (Kelly-Heidenthal, 2003). The manner in which a pathway is constructed is usually agency-specific but typically it follows the client's length of stay on a day-by-day basis for the specific disease process or surgical intervention. Clinical pathways are a clinical tool that organizes, directs, and times the major care activities and interventions of the entire multidisciplinary team for a particular diagnosis or procedure. Their design is intended to minimize delays, maximize appropriate resource utilization, and promote high-quality care. "The clinical pathway describes a blended plan of care constructed by all providers, considering the subject together" (Barnum, 1999).

Clinical pathways identify standard client outcomes against which the efficiency of care may be measured. The pathway guides the care team along a sequence of interdisciplinary interventions that incorporate standardized aspects such as client and family teaching, nutrition, medications, activities, diagnostic studies, and treatments. The tool is developed collaboratively by all health team members and includes predictable and established time frames, usually by delineating each hospital day as an event requiring new intervention along a continuum. A care map provides consistency of client care activities. Clinical pathways also, because of their standardization of practice, allow for measuring performance improvement within an agency and between similar agencies over time.

Clinical pathways can only guide rather than dictate the course of care for an individual. They do not take into account additional client problems that may affect the client's recovery. Therefore, the process of incorporating clinical pathways is the same

as in individualizing care plans. The nurse must include the individualized client needs in conjunction with the standard clinical pathway. When the client's needs vary from the expected outcome time frame, the nurse must reassess, report, and manage the variance to meet the client's needs. The manner of reporting variances is agency-specific. Not all clients' care can be organized into a clinical pathway model. For more complex client care situations an individualized care plan applying the various nursing diagnoses in this text, is more appropriate.

Well-designed nursing care plans and/or care maps move the client from one level of care on the health continuum to another. These tools help the nurse to monitor and guide the progress of the client through a particular health condition including preventive and restorative phases and end-of-life care. Care planning organizes and coordinates client care according to relevant standards, promotes consistency and communication between caregivers, and incorporates the problem-solving process which integrates responsiveness to client needs and cost-efficiency.

UNIT 1
PREGNANCY

CHAPTER 1.0

HEALTHY PREGNANCY

Pregnancy is a normal physiologic process. The goal of health care during pregnancy is to promote and maintain the health of the mother and fetus. Risk assessment, problem identification and intervention, and health teaching are important aspects of prenatal care.

PHYSICAL CHANGES

The placental hormones influence changes in maternal physiology during pregnancy. These hormones maintain pregnancy and promote an optimal environment for the growing fetus.

- Physiologic changes include a 50% increase in blood volume, an increased sensitivity to CO_2 and a need for higher insulin production.
- Mechanical changes result from the growing uterus and include pressure on the bladder during the first and third trimesters, a shifting center of gravity, and stretching of uterine ligaments.

LAB VALUE CHANGES

	NON-PREGNANT	PREGNANT
Hgb (g/dL)	12–16	11–13
Hct (%)	36–48	33–39
BUN (mg/dL)	10–16	7–10
Albumin (g/dL)	4.3	3.5
WBC (mm³)	4000–11000	5000–15000

PSYCHOLOGICAL CHANGES

Developmental issues and possibly hormone levels influence changes in maternal emotions and out-look. Ambivalence is common during the first trimester. Maternal psychological tasks of pregnancy may include:

- Acceptance of the fact of pregnancy (first trimester)
- Acknowledgment of the fetus as a separate being (second trimester)
- Preparation for birth and motherhood (third trimester)

FETAL GROWTH AND DEVELOPMENT

Fetal growth and development are monitored at each prenatal visit. The gestational age of the fetus is calculated from the mother's last normal menstrual period. A full-term pregnancy is 40 weeks (plus or minus 2 weeks) from the LNMP.

- During the first trimester all organ systems develop and the fetus is most vulnerable to teratogens.
- The fetal heart rate (FHT) can be heard with a Doppler from 8–12 weeks. Normal FHTs are from 110–160 beats per minutes.
- Fetal movement ("quickening") is usually noticed by the mother from 16–20 weeks.
- Lanugo is fine hair, which covers the fetus from about 20 weeks until the third trimester when it thins and disappears.
- Vernix caseosa is a thick cheesy secretion that covers and protects the fetal skin from about 26 weeks. This disappears by term except in body creases.
- Viability depends on maturation of the respiratory and neurological systems. A fetus born as early as 24 weeks may survive but will require intensive care.

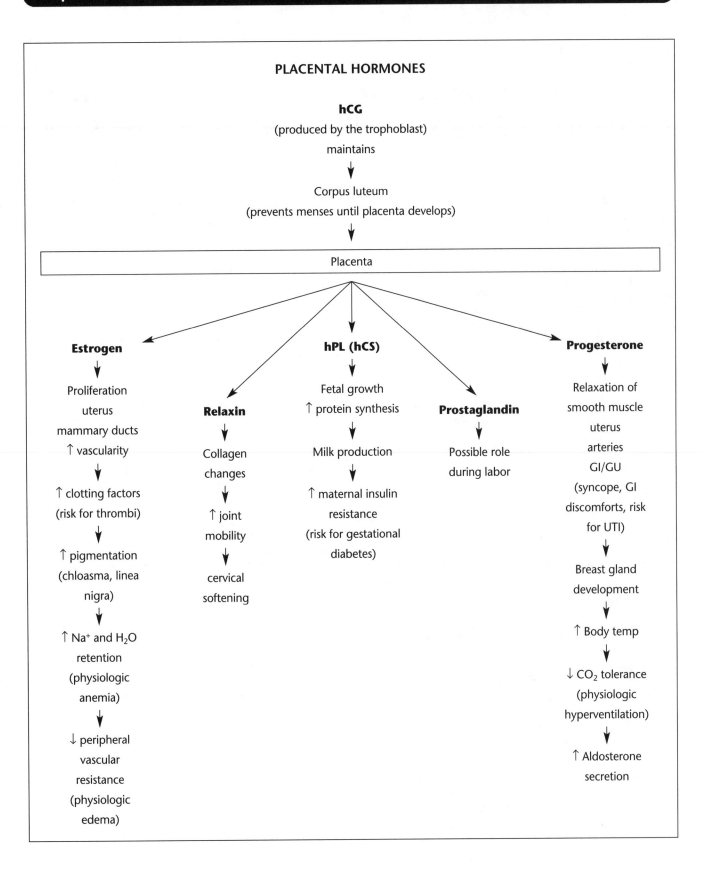

PLACENTAL HORMONES

hCG
(produced by the trophoblast)
maintains

Corpus luteum
(prevents menses until placenta develops)

Placenta

Estrogen

Proliferation
uterus
mammary ducts
↑ vascularity

↑ clotting factors
(risk for thrombi)

↑ pigmentation
(chloasma, linea
nigra)

↑ Na⁺ and H₂O
retention
(physiologic
anemia)

↓ peripheral
vascular
resistance
(physiologic
edema)

Relaxin

Collagen
changes

↑ joint
mobility

cervical
softening

hPL (hCS)

Fetal growth
↑ protein synthesis

Milk production

↑ maternal insulin
resistance
(risk for gestational
diabetes)

Prostaglandin

Possible role
during labor

Progesterone

Relaxation of
smooth muscle
uterus
arteries
GI/GU
(syncope, GI
discomforts, risk
for UTI)

Breast gland
development

↑ Body temp

↓ CO₂ tolerance
(physiologic
hyperventilation)

↑ Aldosterone
secretion

CHAPTER 1.1

BASIC CARE PLAN: HEALTHY PREGNANCY

The nursing care plan is based on a thorough nursing history, assessment, and review of medical and laboratory findings. Specific client-related data should be inserted wherever possible and within parentheses.

NURSING DIAGNOSES

HEALTH-SEEKING BEHAVIORS: PRENATAL CARE

Related to: Client's desire for a healthy pregnancy and newborn.

Defining Characteristics: Client makes and keeps prenatal care appointment (date). Client states (specify: e.g., "I think that I am pregnant; I want to have a healthy baby"). List appropriate subjective/objective data.

Goal: Client will obtain prenatal care by: (date/time to evaluate)

Outcome Criteria

✔ Client will keep all prenatal appointments.
✔ Client will call the health care provider for any concerns related to pregnancy.

NOC: *Knowledge: Health Promotion*

INTERVENTIONS	RATIONALES
Establish rapport: ensure privacy, listen attentively, and allow adequate time to address client's concerns.	Client will feel comfortable in the care setting and be willing to share concerns.
Assess reason for seeking care, remain nonjudgmental, use open-ended questions, and observe nonverbal clues.	Client concerns are the basis of nursing care. Therapeutic techniques help the nurse obtain the most information.
Assess knowledge level of pregnancy and prenatal care (previous OB hx).	Assessment provides data for development of an individualized teaching plan.

INTERVENTIONS	RATIONALES
Assess client concerns related to pregnancy/prenatal care (e.g., cultural expectations; emotional, family, financial concerns).	Socioeconomic concerns may interfere with the ability to obtain care. Issues may interfere with compliance.
Observe interaction with significant other, if present.	Observation provides information about social support.
Describe the components of prenatal care with rationales (schedule of care, fetal assessments, lab tests, etc.).	Understanding what to expect allays fear and promotes compliance.
Provide emotional support during invasive or painful procedures.	Most women dislike pelvic exams. Nursing support can decrease discomfort by promoting relaxation.
Modify plan of care based on client requests/needs (e.g., female care provider, teaching session rather than literature for illiterate clients).	Individualizing the routines of prenatal care shows respect for the client's unique needs and concerns.
Provide the name and phone number (specify) for client to call with any questions.	Often questions will arise outside of appointments. Client will feel comfortable with a person to contact.
Provide written or video information about pregnancy.	Written information is available to the client in her home.
Refer client as needed (WIC, social services, etc.).	Ensures client will obtain needed assistance.

NIC: *Self-Modification Assistance*

Evaluation

(Date/time of evaluation of goal)

(Has goal been met? not met? partially met?)

(Has client kept all prenatal appointments? Give data.)

(Has client called with concerns? Give data.)

(Revisions to care plan? D/C care plan? Continue care plan?)

IMBALANCED NUTRITION: LESS THAN BODY REQUIREMENTS

Related to: Increased demands of pregnancy, inability to obtain/ingest/utilize adequate nutrients.

Defining Characteristics: Specify: (Client's reported daily intake versus requirements for this pregnancy, reported nausea and vomiting, pica), (EGA, Ht, Wt, Hgb and Hct, serum albumin, blood glucose, condition of skin, hair, nails, teeth); list appropriate subjective and objective data.

Goal: Client will ingest adequate nutrients during pregnancy for maternal and fetal needs (date/time to evaluate).

Outcome Criteria

✔ Client reports eating a balanced diet based on the Food Guide Pyramid modified for pregnancy (or prescribed diet).

✔ Client takes prenatal vitamins and iron as prescribed (specify).

✔ Client gains 25 to 35 pounds during pregnancy (2–5 pounds first 12 weeks, 1 pound/week thereafter), ↑ for multiple gestation).

NOC: *Nutritional Status: Nutrient Intake*

INTERVENTIONS	RATIONALES
Assess current food intake; 24 hour diet recall; pica; and appetite changes (at each prenatal visit).	Assessment provides baseline data. Pica is the ingestion of nonfood substances (dirt, starch, ice, etc.).
Assess for nausea and vomiting (amount, times).	Assessment provides information about the client's ability to ingest and absorb nutrients.
Assess skin (texture, turgor), hair, eyes, mouth, nails for signs of adequate nutrition.	Assessment provides information about general nutrition status. Skin should be smooth and elastic, hair shiny, nails smooth, pink, and not brittle.
Assess weight at each visit and compare with previous weight and expected gains. Remain nonjudgmental about weight gain.	Assessment provides information about weight gain and the pattern of gain. Shows respect for client and helps allay fears related to weight gain.
Assist client to compare her usual diet with the Food Guide Pyramid recommendations for pregnancy.	Involving the client in assessment and planning encourages compliance.

INTERVENTIONS	RATIONALES
Praise positive eating habits and discuss the relationship with optimal fetal growth and development.	Praise reinforces healthy eating. Understanding the fetal needs provides incentive for obtaining optimum nutrition.
Assist client to plan a nutritious diet using the Food Guide Pyramid modified for pregnancy taking into account personal and cultural preferences and financial ability (specify: diabetic, vegetarian, kosher, etc.).	Promotes compliance by recognizing individual variations and includes client in planning.
Teach client to avoid highly processed foods or those with many artificial additives (clients with PKU need to avoid phenylalanine).	Unprocessed, natural foods contain the most nutrients. Additives may adversely affect the fetus (high phenylalanine levels may cause mental retardation in the fetus of PKU moms).
Reinforce need for prenatal vitamins and iron if prescribed (specify).	Provides additional nutrients that may be difficult to obtain by diet alone.
Reinforce positive nutrition habits at each prenatal visit.	Reinforcement motivates the client to maintain a healthy diet during pregnancy.
Refer to dietitian, as needed (e.g., diabetes mellitus, strict vegetarian).	Referral provides additional information and support for clients with special dietary needs.

NIC: *Nutrition Management*

Evaluation

(Date/time of evaluation of goal)

(Has goal been met? not met? partially met?)

(Does client report eating a balanced diet based on the Food Guide Pyramid modified for pregnancy?)

(Does client take prenatal vitamins and iron as prescribed?)

(What is client weight gain?)

(Revisions to care plan? D/C? Continue?)

RISK FOR INJURY: MATERNAL/FETAL

Related to: Exposure to teratogens, complications of pregnancy, physical imbalance or trauma.

Defining Characteristics: None, as this is a potential diagnosis.

Goal: Client and her fetus will not experience any injury during pregnancy.

Outcome Criteria

✔ Client denies any known exposure to teratogens.

✔ Client denies experiencing any danger signs of pregnancy (specify).

✔ Client's BP remains <140/90, reflexes same as baseline (specify), urine negative for protein.

✔ FHTs remain between 110–160; growth is appropriate for EGA.

NOC: *Risk Control*

INTERVENTIONS	RATIONALES
Assess maternal risk for exposure to teratogens (at first prenatal visit): environmental toxins, infections, alcohol, medications/drugs, employment, or pets.	Assessment provides information about client risk factors. The fetus is at highest risk from teratogens during the first 12 weeks when organogenesis takes place.
Assess wt gain, BP, reflexes, edema; dip urine for protein and glucose (at each visit) and compare to baseline data. Assess immunity to rubella (history, immunization).	Signs and symptoms of PIH include an increase in BP of 30/15 mm Hg or more, sudden ↑ in wt, edema, and proteinuria. Gestational diabetes may cause consistent glycosuria; rubella is a known teratogen.
Assess fetal well-being at each visit. Ask about fetal movement, listen to FHT for a full minute, measure fundal height, and compare to EGA.	Complications of pregnancy may affect the fetus by interfering with placental function. The stressed fetus may have ↓ movements or ↓ fundal height. Size–dates discrepancies may indicate IUGR.
Perform, or assist with, other fetal assessments as indicated or ordered (specify: CVS, amniocentesis, NST, ultrasound, CST, biophysical profile, etc.).	Testing provides information about fetus. The fetus may exhibit signs of distress such as decreased FHR variability or late decelerations.
Teach client to avoid exposure to teratogens during pregnancy: medications/drugs not prescribed by the physician, including OTC meds; radiation (including X-rays); cat litter or raw meat; viral infections (rubella); prolonged exposure to heat (hot tubs, saunas); alcohol.	Client may be unaware of risks associated with commonplace exposures. Provides needed information to help prevent harm to the fetus.

INTERVENTIONS	RATIONALES
Teach good body mechanics and appropriate exercise: not to lie flat on back; wear sensible shoes; keep back straight and feet apart when bending/lifting; usually may engage in nonweight-bearing exercises (e.g., swimming, cycling); avoid over-heating.	Avoids maternal or fetal injury while allowing the client to continue to participate in appropriate exercise during pregnancy.
Teach client to wear both lap and shoulder seat belts; lap belt should be worn low.	The mother and fetus are at highest risk of injury from being thrown from the car in an accident.
Discuss safe sex practices with client and significant other if available (e.g., risks of STD/HIV, proper use of condoms); address any concerns the couple may have about sex during pregnancy.	Client may not know how to protect herself and the fetus. Client and significant other may have concerns about sexuality during pregnancy.
Teach good hygiene practices: hand washing, wiping front to back after using the toilet, daily bathing.	Good hygiene prevents the spread of microorganisms, prevents fecal contamination of vagina/urethra.
Teach warning signs that client should report: severe nausea and vomiting, s/s of infection, vaginal bleeding/watery discharge, severe headache, visual disturbances, epigastric pain, severe abdominal pain, s/s of preterm labor, marked changes in fetal movement.	These are s/s of serious complications of pregnancy: hyperemesis gravidarum, placenta previa, placental abruption, pregnancy-induced hypertension, PROM, preterm labor, fetal distress. Early identification ensures prompt treatment.
Provide written or visual reinforcement of teaching topics and verify understanding.	Written or video reinforcement enables client to review teaching at home. Verification allows for clarification and ensures understanding.

NIC: *Surveillance: Safety*

Evaluation

Date/time of evaluation of goal

Has goal been met? not met? partially met?

Does client deny any warning signs?

What is BP? reflexes? urine protein?

What are FHTs? Is fetal growth appropriate for EGA?

Revisions to Care Plan? D/C? Continue?

ACUTE PAIN

Related to: Physiologic changes of pregnancy.

Defining Characteristics: Specify: (client's report of backache, leg cramps, and so forth. Client should rate on a scale of 1 to 10. Appropriate objective data: grimacing, etc.).

Goal: Client will experience less pain related to pregnancy (date/time goal to be evaluated).

Outcome Criteria

✔ Client reports a decrease in pain to less than specify on a scale of 1 to 10.

✔ Client does not show objective signs of discomfort grimacing, etc.; specify what client had been indicating.

NOC: *Pain Control*

INTERVENTIONS	RATIONALES
Assess client for discomfort at each prenatal visit. Observe for nonverbal signs such as grimacing, guarding, and so forth. Ask client if she has any discomfort.	Client may think discomfort is normal during pregnancy, or may not wish to complain. Some cultures do not approve of showing discomfort.
Ask client to rate the discomfort on a scale of 1 to 10 with 1 being the least and 10 the most.	A rating scale helps the nurse to measure the effectiveness of interventions.
Assess what the client usually does to alleviate the discomfort and how effective that has been.	Provides information about the methods already tried by the client to alleviate discomfort.
Explain the physiologic basis for each discomfort the client identifies and suggest possible interventions for each discomfort.	Understanding the physiologic basis helps to allay fear, an emotion that may increase the discomfort.
(Fatigue/fainting: Teach client to obtain 7–8 hours of sleep at night and plan for a rest or nap during the day. Teach to rise slowly when changing position and if she feels faint to sit and lower her head. Instruct to eat small frequent meals. Monitor labs for anemia. ↓ blood glucose or anemia may cause fatigue/ fainting.)	Fatigue may be caused by hormone changes in first trimester and ↑ demands during last trimester. Postural hypotension may be related to venous pooling in the lower extremities from general vascular relaxation.
(Urinary frequency: Teach client to void frequently, not to "hold	May be caused by pressure on the bladder from the enlarging

INTERVENTIONS	RATIONALES
it." Teach Kegal exercises and signs/symptoms of UTI to report: pain, burning, and urgency in addition to frequency.)	uterus—more common during first and last trimesters. UTIs may cause preterm labor and need to be identified and treated early.
(Vaginal discharge (leukorrhea): Assess for infection, STDs; teach client to wear cotton underwear and bathe daily. May wear peri pad if changed frequently.)	Hyperplasia and ↑ vaginal and cervical secretions are the result of hormone changes. Good hygiene may prevent infection.
(Leg cramps: Assess calcium intake. Teach clients to extend her leg and dorsiflex the foot of the affected leg to relieve cramp. Evaluate for DVT if indicated.)	Cramps may be related to possible calcium imbalance or uterine pressure.
(Heart burn (gastroesophageal reflux): Teach client to eat small frequent meals, avoid fatty foods and flat positioning. Instruct to take antacids as prescribed [specify: e.g., Maalox].)	Progesterone causes ↓ motility and relaxes the cardiac sphincter. Increased uterine pressure causes gastro-esophageal reflux. Antacids neutralize gastric acid.
(Varicose veins: Teach client to change positions frequently, rest with legs elevated, engage in regular exercise and wear support hose without garters.)	Decreased peripheral vascular resistance, ↑ blood volume, and uterine pressure may cause venous stasis leading to ↑ varicose veins and risk for thrombus formation.
(Backache: Needs to be differentiated from preterm labor. Assess for contractions; teach good body mechanics and pelvic rock exercise. Teach client to wear low sturdy shoes and rest with feet elevated.)	Preterm labor is often felt as lower back pain. In the third trimester the center of gravity shifts which puts added stress on lower back muscles.
(Braxton–Hicks contractions: Teach client to differentiate from labor; usually painless, don't ↑ in intensity over time, may decrease if activity changes (walking or resting). Suggest client practice breathing techniques with B–H contractions.	The uterus contracts throughout pregnancy. Labor contractions usually ↑ over time, becoming more uncomfortable no matter what the client does. Client may feel reassured about labor if she practices with Braxton–Hicks contractions.
Notify caregiver for unusual symptoms or severe discomfort.	Unusual or severe discomfort may indicate a complication.

NIC: *Pain Management*

Evaluation

(Date/time of evaluation of goal)

(Has goal been met? not met? partially met?)

(What does client report the intensity of discomfort to be on a scale of 1 to 10?)

(Describe objective signs of discomfort or change in them [e.g., client is smiling and no longer grimacing?])

(Revisions to care plan? D/C care plan? Continue care plan?)

NAUSEA

Related to: Irritation of the gastrointestinal system during pregnancy

Defining Characteristics: Client reports (specify e.g. "nausea", "feeling sick", "throwing-up in the morning")

Goal: Client will experience less nausea by (specify date/time to evaluate)

Outcome Criteria

✔ (Specify: Client reports less nausea; Client denies any nausea.)

NOC: *Comfort Level*

INTERVENTIONS	RATIONALES
Assess the client's nausea: onset, duration, frequency and contributing factors.	Assessment provides baseline data on which to formulate the plan of care.
Obtain information on usual dietary practices and foods commonly eaten.	Particular foods may be more offensive during pregnancy.
Suggest eating dry crackers or hard candy before getting slowly out of bed in the morning.	An empty stomach, low blood sugar, and sudden movement may contribute to feelings of nausea.
Encourage the client to eat small, frequent meals spread out	Keeping the stomach neither empty nor too full may help

INTERVENTIONS	RATIONALES
through the day rather than fewer, large meals.	relieve nausea.
Provide client with a list of foods that may not cause nausea (specify: e.g., lemonade, carbonated beverages, salty foods, peppermint tea, etc.). Suggest that the client avoid greasy or spicy foods as long as nausea persists.	Anecdotal evidence suggests that greasy or spicy foods increase the likelihood of nausea.
Inform the client about other nontraditional methods of reducing nausea such as acupressure bracelets, meditation.	Pressure on the wrist at acupressure points has been reported to decrease nausea.
Reassure the client that nausea in pregnancy is usually limited to the first trimester.	Nausea and vomiting are associated with high hCG levels in early pregnancy and usually resolve by the second trimester.
Provide teaching (specify) about anti-emetic medications (specify drug, dose route, and times).	Specify action of drug prescribed.
Caution client to maintain fluid intake and to report signs of dehydration (severely decreased urine output, dry mouth) or severe nausea and vomiting to her care provider.	Dehydration or ketoacidosis may cause teratogenic harm to the developing embryo-fetus.

NIC: *Nausea Management*

Evaluation

(Date/time of evaluation of goal)

(Was goal met? Not met? Partially met?)

(Does client report less nausea or does client deny any nausea?)

TABLE 1.1   Prenatal Care Path

WEEK	INTERVIEW	PHYSICAL EXAM	TESTS	TEACHING	REFERRAL	OTHER
1st Visit	Chief c/o Med/OB hx Psychosocial Religious Cultural concerns & resources Risk assessment	Ht, Wt, BP, TPR, reflexes Physical exam Fundal ht. & FHT if indicated Pelvic exam, adequacy, size/ dates	CBC, ABO, Rh, VDRL, Rubella titer, Antibody titer, (HBsAg) (HIV), UA, Pap, GC, Chlamydia (u/s)	Normal pregnancy, Nutrition, Substance abuse, Fetal growth & development, Relief of common discomfort, Danger signs	Social Services, WIC	PNV, iron
12	Client concerns	Wt., vital signs, FHT, fundal ht.	Urine dip for protein & glucose	As needed	As needed	
16			MsAFP			
20	Quickening?		Urine dip ultrasound prn			
24	Client concerns & discomforts			Home visit		
28			Hgb. 1hr. GTT, Rh/antibody titer if Rh neg	S/S PTL		RhoGAM prn
32			Urine dip		Childbirth Education VBAC classes prn	
34				Home visit childbirth ed.		
36			cultures: GC, Chlamydia, GBS			Chart to L&D
38 to del.		Pelvic exam if indicated				

CHAPTER 1.2

BASIC CARE PLAN: PRENATAL HOME VISIT

Prenatal home visits provide information about the client's home environment and family support system. Additional benefits are client convenience and comfort, which facilitate learning.

COMMON NURSING DIAGNOSES

 See BASIC CARE PLAN: HEALTHY PREGNANCY

ADDITIONAL NURSING DIAGNOSES

 HOME MAINTENANCE: IMPAIRED

Related to: (Specify: inadequate finances, lack of understanding, insufficient support systems, etc.)

Defining Characteristics: Specify: (Client states she can't maintain the home—home is dirty, infested, overcrowded, etc. Home has no plumbing, heat, window screens, etc. Client states she can't afford basic hygiene needs; has inadequate support systems to help with finances and maintenance, etc.).

Goal: Client will maintain a safe, clean, and growth-promoting home environment by (date/time to evaluate).

Outcome Criteria

✔ Client will identify hygienic needs in the home (specify).

✔ Client will obtain financial assistance to maintain home (specify).

✔ Client will develop a plan to improve home maintenance support system (specify).

NOC: *Family Functioning*

INTERVENTIONS	RATIONALES
Assess client's understanding of the need for a clean, safe, growth-promoting environment for herself and her family.	Assessment provides information about the client's understanding of basic home maintenance needs.
Assess home environment for water supply, plumbing, air quality, heating, screens, cleanliness, food preparation area, and bathing facilities.	Assessment provides information about the safety and cleanliness of the home environment for the client and family.
Assess client's plans for newborn care area (separate room, area of other room, crib, bassinet, etc.).	Assessment provides information about the client's knowledge of infant needs and her plans to meet them.
Assist client to identify needed changes in the home (specify: safety issues, cleanliness, basic services, etc.).	Process involves the client in the plan to improve home maintenance.
Provide teaching about factors the client doesn't identify (specify).	Provides information about basic home maintenance needs.
Inform client of community services and agencies that may offer support in meeting basic home maintenance needs (specify).	Teaching provides information about available resources.
Assist the client to develop a plan to improve and maintain a clean, safe, and growth-promoting home (specify).	Assistance promotes self-esteem and encourages the client to maintain a healthy environment.
Make referrals as needed to help client implement plan (specify: Social services, WIC, community agencies, etc.).	Referrals provide additional financial or resource assistance to client.

NIC: *Home Maintenance Assistance*

Evaluation

(Date/time of evaluation of goal)

(Has goal been met? not met? partially met?)

(Has client identified hygienic needs? Specify.)

(Has client obtained financial assistance? Specify.)

(Has client developed a plan to improve support systems? Specify.)

(Revisions to care plan? D/C care plan? Continue care plan?)

READINESS FOR ENHANCED FAMILY COPING

Related to: Family adaptation and preparation for birth of new member of family.

Defining Characteristics: Family members describe impact of pregnancy in enhancing growth (specify: e.g., sibling states "I'm going to be a big brother and help take care of the baby!", etc.). Family members are involved in prenatal visits and preparations for baby (specify: e.g., husband attends childbirth classes, Grandma plans to babysit, etc.).

Goal: Family will continue to adapt and cope effectively during pregnancy by (date/time to evaluate).

Outcome Criteria

✔ Family will express positive feelings about the pregnancy.

✔ Family will be involved in prenatal care and preparations for the new baby (other specifics as appropriate).

NOC: *Family Normalization*

INTERVENTIONS	RATIONALES
Assess family structure and encourage participation in home visit as appropriate (specify according to ages of children).	Client may be part of a non-traditional family. Participation during the prenatal period helps the family to bond with the new baby.
Assess family members' responses to the pregnancy: verbal and nonverbal.	Family members may need assistance to identify feelings and thoughts about the new baby.
Provide information about changes the family may experience due to the pregnancy and birth (specify for each family member).	Information provides anticipatory guidance to help the family adjust to changes they will experience.

INTERVENTIONS	RATIONALES
Provide age-appropriate (specify) information to siblings of new baby: pictures, books, stories, and so forth.	Enhances the child's self-esteem to be included in the home visit with age-appropriate methods.
Identify and praise effective coping mechanisms used by the family (specify).	Identification and praise provides positive reinforcement to the family and helps identify skills they already possess.
Refer family members to appropriate childbirth education classes (specify: sibling, grandparent, and VBAC classes, etc.).	Childbirth education provides additional information about the childbearing process for different age groups.

NIC: *Developmental Enhancement*

Evaluation

(Date/time of evaluation of goal)

(Has goal been met? not met? partially met?)

(Does family express positive feelings about the pregnancy?)

(Is family involved in prenatal care and preparations for the new baby?)

(Revisions to care plan? D/C care plan? Continue care plan?)

DEFICIENT KNOWLEDGE: PREPARATION FOR LABOR AND BIRTH OF NEWBORN

Related to: (Specify: first pregnancy, first VBAC, etc.)

Defining Characteristics: Client expresses a lack of knowledge about preparing for labor and birth of newborn (specify). Client expresses erroneous ideas about labor and birth of newborn (specify).

Goal: Client will obtain knowledge about preparation for labor and birth of newborn (date/time to evaluate).

Outcome Criteria

✔ Client is able to describe what happens during normal labor and vaginal delivery.

✔ Client and significant other prepare a birth plan.

NOC: *Knowledge: Labor and Delivery*

INTERVENTIONS	RATIONALES
Assess client and significant other's perceptions about what happens during childbirth.	Assessment provides information about the client's learning needs and possible fears.
Teach client and significant other about the stages and phases of labor using visual aids: 1st stage: contractions, effacement and dilatation, 3 phases (latent, active, transition); 2nd stage: contractions, pushing, birth; 3rd stage: contractions, placenta delivery.	Understanding the physiology of labor and birth decreases fear and interrupts the fear → tension → pain syndrome. Decreases the perception of discomfort and assists the client and significant other to become active participants in the birth. Visual aids enhance verbal and written instruction.
Teach client and significant other to differentiate true from false labor: true labor contractions get more intense and closer together over time, are unaffected by position or activity changes.	Teaching provides needed information about when labor has begun.
Inform client when to come to hospital: when her water breaks, when contractions are 5 minutes apart for primigravida or regular for a multipara (per caregiver's preference).	Provides necessary information. Clients should be seen after membranes rupture to r/o a prolapsed cord. Clients will be more comfortable at home until active labor.
Teach methods to cope with discomfort (specify: breathing/ relaxation techniques, back rub, whirlpool, birthing ball, etc.).	Teaching provides information so client and significant other can choose the most effective methods to cope with discomfort.
Describe specific pharmacological pain relief methods that may be available to client (specify: IV analgesia, epidural, intrathecal, local, etc.).	Description provides information to the client before she is in pain. This allows client participation in decision making for pain relief methods prior to onset of labor.
Inform client and significant other of the routine admission orders for her health care provider (specify: prep, enema, IV, blood work, etc.).	Information about what to expect when client is admitted to the hospital helps decrease anxiety.

INTERVENTIONS	RATIONALES
Inform client and significant other that they will need to make decisions at the time of delivery: whether or not to have circumcision for a boy baby, and on a method of feeding their baby (breast, bottle, and combination). Discuss the benefits of breast-feeding.	Information provides an opportunity for anticipatory guidance related to considerations about circumcision and the benefits of breast-feeding.
Verify client and significant other's understanding of information presented.	Verification insures that client and significant other have accurate information about labor and birth.
Assist client and significant other to make a birth plan based on the information provided. Instruct the client to share the plan with her provider and the hospital staff on admission (send plan to L&D prior to admission if very different from routine care).	A birth plan empowers the client to become a participant in the birth of her baby. It ensures that all participants understand the client's wishes.
Refer client to written information, childbirth education classes, and/or her health care provider as indicated for additional information.	Referral provides more information to interested clients.

NIC: *Teaching: Individual*

Evaluation

(Date/time of evaluation of goal)

(Has goal been met? not met? partially met?)

(Does client describe what occurs during normal labor and delivery?)

(Has client made a birth plan?)

(Revisions to care plan? D/C care plan? Continue care plan?)

CHAPTER 1.3

ADOLESCENT PREGNANCY

The pregnant teenager is at risk for physical, psychological, and socioeconomic complications. Early prenatal care that is sensitive to the needs of adolescents can decrease these risks and help the adolescent gain control of her future.

PHYSIOLOGIC RISKS

- Poor dietary habits, anemia, substance abuse (including cigarettes), STDs
- Preterm birth, low birth-weight (LBW) infant
- Pregnancy-induced hypertension (PIH)
- Cephalopelvic disproportion (CPD) leading to cesarean delivery (greater risk if under 15 years old)

PSYCHOLOGICAL ISSUES

- Striving for identity formation and independence; authority figures may be seen as a threat to autonomy—may have difficulty asking for help
- Concerned about confidentiality—may use denial as a major coping mechanism
- Strong peer influence—may fear isolation and rejection; pregnancy may be seen as a "rite of passage" or cultural norm
- Concerned with body image: often idealistic regarding pregnancy, relationships, and motherhood; preoccupied with self
- May engage in risk-taking behaviors; feels invulnerable; may be impulsive and unpredictable at times

SOCIOECONOMIC ISSUES

- Many adolescent mothers drop out of school and never complete their basic education
- Lack of education leads to decreased career options, low-paying jobs, poverty and dependence on the welfare system

- High divorce rates for adolescent marriages reflect their difficulty in establishing stable families; the grandmother may end up caring for the infant.
- Children of adolescent mothers are at risk for developmental delays, neglect, and child abuse as well as adolescent pregnancy themselves

COMMON NURSING DIAGNOSES

 See BASIC CARE PLAN: HEALTHY PREGNANCY

 See BASIC CARE PLAN: PRENATAL HOME VISIT

ADDITIONAL NURSING DIAGNOSES

 DECISIONAL CONFLICT: PREGNANCY

Related to: Pregnancy options (specify: marriage, single parenting, adoption, termination of pregnancy).

Defining Characteristics: Client verbalizes uncertainty about choices; delays decision making; reports distress (specify: e.g., "I don't know what to do," "My Dad is gonna kill me"; client doesn't seek prenatal care until second trimester, etc.).

Goal: Client will be able to make an informed decision about pregnancy by (date/time to evaluate).

Outcome Criteria

- ✔ Client will list her options as she sees them.
- ✔ Client will describe the advantages and disadvantages of each option.
- ✔ Client will relate her fears and anxieties about each option.
- ✔ Client will make and follow through with a decision.

NOC: *Participation: Health Care Decisions*

INTERVENTIONS	RATIONALES
Assess client's usual method of making decisions (e.g., alone, with help from friends and/or parents, etc.).	Assessment helps client to explore how she usually makes major decisions. Intervention shows respect for client as someone capable of making decisions.
Ask client to describe decisions she has made in the past that she feels good about.	Assessment reinforces self-esteem and the belief that she can make good decisions.
Assist the client to identify factors influencing her decision-making ability at this time. (Specify: e.g., fear of parent or boyfriend's response; value conflict; lack of information about options.)	Client may feel confused and afraid. Identifying the main concerns helps the client to begin the decision-making process.
Encourage client to involve her significant others (specify: parents, boyfriend, etc.) in helping her to explore options.	Social support can positively affect the outcome of adolescent pregnancy.
Assist client to explore her values about pregnancy and to identify those that are most important to her; remain nonjudgmental.	Individual, social, and cultural values and mores are important to the adolescent's growing sense of her own identity.
Assist client to list the possible choices she thinks she has (specify: keeping the baby, marriage, living at home, adoption, termination of pregnancy, etc.).	Listing options is the first step in logical decision making. Only the client can decide which options are possible for her.
For each option, ask client to explore her fears and anxieties as well as the risks of not making a decision.	Fears and anxieties may negatively affect the client's ability to think clearly. Denial is a common coping mechanism.
Assist client to list advantages and disadvantages of each option. Provide accurate information as needed (e.g., open and closed adoption, education options, GED, abortion, etc.).	Exploring advantages and disadvantages based on accurate information helps the client to see which options are most likely to result in a positive outcome.
Encourage and or assist client to seek spiritual advice if this is important to her. Refer to agencies as indicated (teen pregnancy groups, etc.).	Client may have a strong need for spiritual advice and direction.
Encourage client to make a decision regarding pregnancy as soon as possible.	Encouragement reinforces the client's right to make her own decisions.

NIC: *Decision-Making Support*

Evaluation

(Date/time of evaluation of goal)

(Has goal been met? not met? partially met?)

(Has client listed her options? Has client described advantages and disadvantages of each option? Has client related her fears and anxieties? Has client made a decision and is she following through?)

(Revisions to care plan? D/C care plan? Continue care plan?)

INEFFECTIVE HEALTH MAINTENANCE

Related to: Specify: Lack of ability to make deliberate and thoughtful judgments; lack of material resources; poor coping skills, immaturity

Defining Characteristics: Client reports smoking cigarettes (specify packs/day), drinking, or using other drugs (specify substance and amount). Client reports poor dietary habits (specify ↑ fat diet, skips meals, drinks soda instead of milk, etc.). Client states inaccurate information about sexuality/reproductive needs (specify: e.g., "I don't need to see a doctor, I feel fine").

Goal: Client will change behaviors to maintain health by (date/time to evaluate).

Outcome Criteria

✔ Client will identify current unhealthy behaviors.

✔ Client will verbalize plan to engage in healthy behaviors (specify: stop smoking, avoid alcohol and other drugs, eat a balanced diet for pregnancy, obtain prenatal care, etc.).

NOC: *Health-Promoting Behavior*

INTERVENTIONS	RATIONALES
Develop a trusting relationship with client. Remain nonjudgmental.	Trust is necessary for the client to talk about behaviors that may make her feel guilty.
Assess underlying reasons for unhealthy behaviors: consider poor self-esteem, history of abuse, and so forth.	Assessment provides information about motivation for unhealthy behaviors (may lack knowledge, poverty, addiction, peer pressure, cultural norms, etc.).

INTERVENTIONS	RATIONALES
Explain the physiologic risks associated with the behaviors (specify: anemia, preterm birth, LBW or addicted infant, fetal alcohol syndrome, complications of pregnancy associated with adolescent mothers: PIH, CPD, STDs, etc.).	Client will be informed of the risks to herself and her baby if she doesn't improve her health maintenance behaviors. Early prenatal care has been shown to decrease the physiologic risks.
Assist client to plan healthy behaviors (specify: quit smoking, change dietary habits, obtain prenatal care, etc.).	Client will identify the problem and decide on a plan for change.
Praise client for planning and attempts to change behaviors.	Praise may reinforce attempts to alter behavior.
Assist client to obtain needed resources (specify: WIC, AFDC, social services, etc.).	Poverty may be a factor in poor dietary habits. Lack of transportation may affect ability to obtain prenatal care.
Refer client to appropriate supportive services (specify: smoking cessation program, substance abuse programs, 12-step, peer support groups, resource mothers programs, etc.).	Support programs have been successful in helping clients to overcome addiction and maintain healthy lifestyles. Peer groups and resource mothers programs are effective with adolescents.

NIC: *Support System Enhancement*

Evaluation

(Date/time of evaluation of goal)

(Has goal been met? not met? partially met?)

(Has client identified unhealthy behaviors? Specify.)

(Does client verbalize a plan to change unhealthy behaviors? Specify.)

(Revisions to care plan? D/C care plan? Continue care plan?)

DELAYED GROWTH AND DEVELOPMENT

Related to: Interruption of the normal psychosocial development of adolescence.

Defining Characteristics: Clients younger than 15 have not completed their own skeletal growth (specify: age, ht, wt, and percentile). Client expresses dislike of body image changes (specify). Client reports difficulty in school, with peers, or parent(s) related to the pregnancy and/or plans for the future (specify).

Goal: Client will demonstrate adequate growth and age-appropriate psychosocial development while accomplishing the developmental tasks of pregnancy.

Outcome Criteria

✔ Client will gain appropriate weight for pregnancy and normal physical growth.

✔ Client will make plans to complete at least a high school education.

✔ Client reports satisfactory relationship with parent(s), significant other, and peers.

✔ Client will express acceptance of pregnancy and body changes.

NOC: *Child Development: Adolescence*

INTERVENTIONS	RATIONALES
Assess client's physical growth at each prenatal visit.	Assessment provides information about physical growth.
Reinforce nutrition teaching relating it to the client's growth needs as well as the fetus.	Young adolescents may need more nutrients and calories than usual during pregnancy.
Assess the impact of pregnancy on client's education and future plans for a career.	Teen pregnancy may adversely affect the development of a mature identity.
Discuss body image issues and correct misconceptions (e.g., "I'll never wear a bikini again").	The adolescent may fear mutilation or permanent disfigurement from pregnancy.
Encourage client to finish basic schooling and make realistic plans for the future including childcare.	Lack of education leading to low income becomes a vicious cycle for many teen mothers.
Assist client to assess relationships with parent(s), significant other, and peers, and plan ways to improve these if needed.	Pregnancy may affect relationships. Teens need social interaction in order to develop identity and independence.
Teach client about the developmental tasks of adolescence (Erikson) and the tasks of pregnancy.	Teaching may decrease some confusion from conflicting feelings and desires.
Make referrals as indicated (specify: school counselor, social services and financial assistance, home-tutors, etc.).	Social support will assist the client to become a mature and productive member of society.

NIC: *Self-Responsibility Facilitation*

Evaluation

(Date/time of evaluation of goal)

(Has goal been met? not met? partially met?)

(Has client gained appropriate weight for pregnancy and normal growth? Specify. Does client verbalize a plan to complete her education? Specify. Does client report satisfactory relationships? Specify. Does client verbalize acceptance of pregnancy and body changes? Give quote if possible.)

(Revisions to care plan? D/C care plan? Continue care plan?)

CHAPTER 1.4

HYPEREMESIS GRAVIDARUM

Hyperemesis gravidarum is a rare condition of severe nausea and vomiting which starts in the first 20 weeks of gestation. The vomiting results in weight loss, dehydration, acidosis from starvation, alkalosis from loss of hydrochloric acid, and electrolyte imbalances. The fetus is at risk for IUGR, abnormal development, and death if the condition is not treated.

The cause of hyperemesis is unknown. Theories include psychological as well as physiologic causes. It is diagnosed by its severity (weight loss ≥5% of prepregancy weight) and by ruling out other possible causes such as hydatidiform mole, gastroenteritis, or pancreatitis.

MEDICAL CARE

- Fluid replacement with intravenous therapy: D_5LR or D_5NS with multivitamins and electrolytes
- Antiemetic drug therapy: phenothiazines, antihistamines, 5-HT$_3$ antagonists
- Possible nasogastric feeding once nausea has decreased, or TPN (total parenteral nutrition) may be necessary
- Possible psychiatric consult
- Progressive diet after stabilization

COMMON NURSING DIAGNOSES

See HEALTH SEEKING BEHAVIORS: PRENATAL CARE

Related to: Desire for a healthy pregnancy and newborn.

Defining Characteristics: Client keeps all prenatal appointments. Client complies with plan or care for controlling hyperemesis gravidarum.

See RISK FOR INJURY: MATERNAL/FETAL

Related to: Excessive nausea and vomiting during pregnancy.

See READINESS FOR ENHANCED FAMILY COPING

Related to: Family adaptation and assistance with care of mother experiencing hyperemesis gravidarum.

Defining Characteristics: Family members share in household duties normally done by the client (specify). Family members assist the client to cope with excessive nausea and vomiting.

See ANXIETY

Related to: Fears of maternal and fetal well-being.

Defining Characteristics: Client and family express anxiety about fetal tolerance of excessive nausea and vomiting (specify). Client and family express fear for client's health (specify). Client rates anxiety on a scale of 1 to 10 (specify).

ADDITIONAL NURSING DIAGNOSES

DEFICIENT FLUID VOLUME

Related to: Excessive losses and insufficient intake: nausea and vomiting.

Defining Characteristics: Client reports nausea and vomiting (use quotes, indicate amounts). ↑ serum sodium ↑ urine specific-gravity, and ketones (other labs as available). Insufficient intake (describe amount/24 hours), weight loss (specify), dry mucous membranes, and ↓ skin turgor.

Goal: Client will demonstrate fluid balance by (date/time to evaluate).

Outcome Criteria

✔ Client will have intake equal to output.

✔ Client's mucous membranes will be moist, skin turgor will be elastic.

NOC: *Fluid Balance*

INTERVENTIONS	RATIONALES
Assess intake and output: measure all fluid intake (po, IV, NG, TPN, etc.) and compare to all output (emesis, urine, NG aspirate, diaphoresis, etc.). (Specify timing: e.g., q 1–24 hours depending on dehydration and fluid rates.)	Assessment provides information to determine positive or negative fluid balance. Normal adult intake equals output (usually about 2500 ml in and out in 24 hours).
Assess client's weight on same scale each morning.	Weight changes provide information on severity of losses.
Assess for signs of dehydration: poor skin turgot, dry mucous membranes and skin, ↑ urine specific gravity, ↑ BUN, ↑ Hct, vital sign changes: ↓ BP, ↑ pulse (specify timing).	Fluid moves out of the tissues to replace losses in the vascular space; urine and blood become concentrated, circulating volume ↓, and heart rate ↑ to compensate.
Assess for signs of electrolyte imbalance: muscle weakness, cramps, irritability, irregular heart beat. Monitor electrolyte lab values.	Potassium and magnesium are lost through prolonged vomiting. Potassium plays an important role in the myocardium.
Initiate and maintain IV therapy as ordered (specify: fluids, rate, site, via pump, etc.).	Provides fluid replacement until vomiting is under control (specify how fluid ordered will correct deficit).
Assess IV rate and site for redness, swelling, and tenderness at each visit. Change tubing q 24 hours. (If client is on IV therapy at home, teach client and significant others to maintain IV, run pump, assess site, etc.)	IV infiltration, or infection at the site are possible complications of IV therapy. Clients may benefit from IV therapy at home.
Administer antiemetic medications as ordered (specify: drug, dose, route, and time).	(Specify action of prescribed drug related to nausea and vomiting.)
Monitor for side effects of medications (specify for each drug). Teach client about common or serious side effects to report.	(Specify the problems with each side effect related to the drug and nursing diagnosis.)

INTERVENTIONS	RATIONALES
Suggest to client that lying down in a quiet darkened room may relieve the nausea.	Client may need "permission" to lie down frequently.
Provide information about acupressure as a possible additional therapy.	Many women report a ↓ in nausea and vomiting with acupressure wrist bands.
Provide support and teaching about the risks of dehydration to client and significant others.	The client and significant others will need support to cope with the demands of hyperemesis.

NIC: *Fluid Management*

Evaluation

(Date/time of evaluation of goal)

(Has goal been met? not met? partially met?)

(Specify client's intake and output in cc's/time frame.)

(Describe client's skin turgor and mucous membranes.)

(Revisions to care plan? D/C care plan? Continue care plan?)

 IMBALANCED NUTRITION: LESS THAN BODY REQUIREMENTS

Related to: Inability to ingest or absorb nutrients due to excessive vomiting.

Defining Characteristics: Client reports anorexia and vomiting and is unable to eat (specify amount of food client has been able to keep down/time). Client is not gaining appropriate weight or is losing weight (specify).

Goal: Client will absorb sufficient nutrients for maternal needs and fetal growth by (date/time to evaluate).

Outcome Criteria

✔ Client will ingest and absorb (specify caloric requirements for this client) kcal/day.

✔ Client will gain appropriate weight (specify gain and time frame: e.g., 2–4 pounds in first trimester).

NOC: *Nutritional Status: Food and Fluid Intake*

INTERVENTIONS	RATIONALES
Assess weight and weight gain at each visit.	Provides information about nutritional status.
Assess for physiologic signs of starvation: jaundice, bleeding from mucous membranes, or ketonuria at each visit.	Deficiencies of vitamins C and B-complex, hypothrombinemia, and ketosis may result from insufficient nutrition.
Once acute nausea has passed, begin oral intake as tolerated: clear liquids (broth, juices), potato chips, small meals of any desired foods q 2–3 hours.	Many women report that they can't tolerate water, desire salty foods (chips have ↑ potassium, folic acid, and vitamin C than saltines), feel better if liquids aren't taken with meals.
Suggest herbal teas such as ginger, mint, or chamomile.	Ginger offers relief for some women; herbal teas may be soothing.
If client is to receive TPN, initiate and titrate according to physician's orders and nursing protocols (specify).	TPN can be formulated to provide glucose, lipids, amino acids, electrolytes, minerals, and trace elements.
Monitor blood glucose as ordered. Report levels over 120 mg/dL.	Hyperglycemia may be detrimental to the fetus.
Monitor labs for triglycerides, cholesterol level and liver function.	Excessive fats may cause maternal hyperlipidemia, ↑ cholesterol.
If client is to receive nasogastric feedings, insert tube according to nursing protocols. Ensure proper placement (add specifics), use pump.	Proper placement of feeding tubes prevents aspiration of the feeding solution. A pump ensures correct rate with no boluses of glucose.

INTERVENTIONS	RATIONALES
Initiate feedings of prescribed product (specify) at 50 cc/hour and increase as client tolerates to 75 cc/hr (specify amount to be given/day as ordered).	Infusion rates should be adjusted according to the client's feelings of fullness. After client is comfortable, rate may be ↑ to provide specified amounts.
Teach client to maintain infusion if at home, teach to assess tube placement, may also teach to reinsert tube with assistance of significant other.	Client may need feeding tube for days or weeks until nausea has stopped. Allows client to participate in her care.
Maintain strict I&O while on TPN or NG feedings.	Provides information to avoid overload.
Refer client to Registered Dietitian and/or support groups as needed (specify).	Support groups may offer additional ideas, dietitian can help the client plan an optimum diet.

NIC: *Nutrition Management*

Evaluation

(Date/time of evaluation of goal)

(Has goal been met? not met? partially met?)

(List kcal/day that client is receiving. Compare with those needed for this client.)

(What is client's weight gain/loss? Is this appropriate for goal?)

(Revisions to care plan? D/C care plan? Continue care plan?)

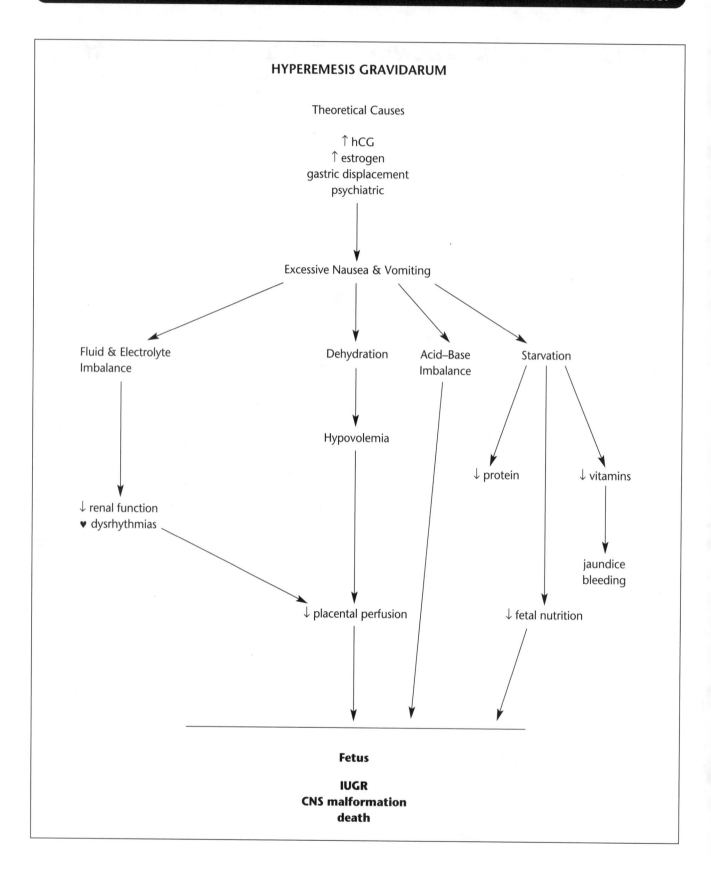

HYPEREMESIS GRAVIDARUM

Theoretical Causes

↑ hCG
↑ estrogen
gastric displacement
psychiatric

Excessive Nausea & Vomiting

Fluid & Electrolyte
Imbalance

Dehydration

Acid–Base
Imbalance

Starvation

Hypovolemia

↓ protein

↓ vitamins

↓ renal function
♥ dysrhythmias

jaundice
bleeding

↓ placental perfusion

↓ fetal nutrition

Fetus

IUGR
CNS malformation
death

CHAPTER 1.5

THREATENED ABORTION

Vaginal bleeding during the first half of pregnancy is considered a sign of a threatened spontaneous abortion. About 20–25% of women will experience some bleeding in early pregnancy. About half of these will eventually abort in a matter of days or even weeks (Cunningham et al., 1997). Uterine cramping and/or low back pain often accompanies this bleeding. The other causes of early spotting or bleeding may be implantation of the trophoblast, cervical lesions, or polyps disturbed by exercise or intercourse. These conditions usually do not cause pain or cramping.

Other serious causes of vaginal bleeding during the first trimester may be ectopic pregnancy or gestational trophoblastic disease. All pregnant women should be taught to report any vaginal bleeding to their health care provider.

MEDICAL CARE

- Sterile speculum exam to r/o dilatation of the cervix (inevitable abortion)
- Bed rest with analgesia if needed
- Hbg and Hct if bleeding heavily, CBC, blood type and screen
- Vaginal ultrasound, serum ß hCG, progesterone levels to assess if conceptus is alive
- Possible D&C if no living conceptus or missed abortion, followed by examination of the tissue for abnormalities
- Rh negative mothers who are not sensitized are given RhoGam after an abortion

COMMON NURSING DIAGNOSES

See ANXIETY

Related to: Possible pregnancy loss.

Defining Characteristics: Client verbalizes fears about pregnancy loss (specify). Client is (specify physical signs of anxiety e.g., crying, pale, tremors, etc.).

See RISK FOR DEFICIENT FLUID VOLUME

Related to: Excessive losses: vaginal bleeding during pregnancy.

ADDITIONAL NURSING DIAGNOSES

RISK FOR INFECTION

Related to: Internal site for organism invasion secondary to vaginal bleeding during pregnancy.

Defining Characteristics: None, as this is a potential diagnosis.

Goal: Client will not experience infectious process by (date/time to evaluate).

Outcome Criteria

- ✔ Client will maintain (specify: oral, tympanic, etc.) temperature <100°F.
- ✔ Vaginal discharge will not be foul smelling.

NOC: *Risk Control*

INTERVENTIONS	RATIONALES
Assess for signs of infection (specify how often: e.g., q 4 hrs): temperature (route), pulse, BP, odor of vaginal discharge, abdominal tenderness.	Provides information about the signs of inflammatory response and infectious processes.
Wash hands thoroughly with warm water, soap, and friction before and after providing client care. Teach client to wash her hands before and after using the bathroom, changing peri pads, and before eating, and so forth.	Effective handwashing removes pathogenic organisms from the hands. Prevents transmission of microorganisms.
Monitor lab values as obtained: CBC, cultures, and so on. Notify caregiver of any abnormal values.	Allows early identification of infectious processes and allows prompt treatment.

(continues)

(continued)

INTERVENTIONS	RATIONALES
Wear clean gloves wen changing peri pads for client.	Protects client and nurse from cross-contamination.
Teach client to change peri pad frequently (specify: at least q 2h or when soiled).	Decreases dark moist environment, which enhances growth of microorganisms.
Teach client to wipe and clean perineum from front to back.	Prevents contamination of vagina with fecal microorganisms.
Administer antibiotics as ordered (specify: drug, dose, route, times for each drug). Monitor for side effects of each drug (specify).	(Specify action of each antibiotic: e.g., destroys bacterial cell walls.)
Teach client to always take whole course of antibiotics as prescribed (specify).	Teaching prevents development of antibiotic resistant bacteria.
Teach client signs of infection to report: fever, abdominal tenderness, foul vaginal discharge.	Provides information the client needs to identify infections early.

NIC: *Infection Protection*

Evaluation

(Date/time of evaluation of goal)

(Has goal been met? not met? partially met?)

(What is client's temp? Is vaginal discharge foul smelling?)

(Revisions to care plan? D/C care plan? Continue care plan?)

ANTICIPATORY GRIEVING

Related to: Threatened abortion; potential for infant with congenital anomalies (specify).

Defining Characteristics: Client and significant other report perceived loss (specify quotes: e.g., "I think I'm going to have a miscarriage," "We're afraid the baby will be damaged," etc.).

Goal: Client and significant other will begin the grieving process.

Outcome Criteria

✔ Client and significant other identify the meaning of the possible loss to them.

✔ Client and significant other are able to express their grief in culturally appropriate ways (specify).

NOC: *Coping*

INTERVENTIONS	RATIONALES
Assess the client and significant other's beliefs about the likelihood of perceived loss.	Assessment provides information and allows clarification.
Provide accurate information (specify: percentages of miscarriage with current condition, viability with these diagnoses, congenital anomalies, etc.).	Client and significant other may be overly anxious caused by being uninformed about current condition or may not realize how serious the situation is.
Assist client and significant other to describe what the perceived loss means to them. Don't offer interpretations such as "You can always have another baby," and so forth.	With an early abortion, the client may feel relieved or devastated. Identifying the meaning of this loss for themselves helps to begin the grief process.
Allow and support the client and significant other's cultural expressions of grieving (specify: anger, crying, screaming, tearing of clothes, etc.).	Different cultures express grief in different ways—the nurse needs to allow and facilitate grief work without being judgmental.
Teach client and significant other about the normal grief process and stages and what they may experience. Provide written materials if literate.	Knowing that depression, insomnia, crying, and anger are normal reactions will help the family to cope with these feelings.
Support client and significant other in the stage they are in and assist with reality-orientation (specify: "I can see that you are angry, this is a normal way to feel," or "I can see that you are still hoping things will turn out OK, I am hoping so too").	Assists the client and significant other to work through the process without feeling disapproval. Presents reality. Anger may be turned on staff who need to recognize that this is normal.
Allow visitors as client wishes.	Client advocacy: may wish no visitors or a large support group.
Explain to client that sedation may delay grief work.	Sedation may cloud the events with which the client must cope.
Ask client and family if there are cultural traditions that they would like to observe. Facilitate as needed.	Provides information and support for the cultural needs of the family.
Offer to contact the client's clergy or the hospital chaplain if indicated.	Religious support may be helpful to some clients.

NIC: *Grief-Work Facilitation: Perinatal Death*

Evaluation

(Date/time of evaluation of goal)

(Has goal been met? not met? partially met?)

(What do client and significant other describe as the meaning of the possible loss? Use quotes. Describe grief reactions the client and significant other express: crying, anger, being stoic, etc. Relate to culture as indicated.)

(Revisions to care plan? D/C care plan? Continue care plan?)

THREATENED ABORTION

Causes

1st trimester: abnormal development (50%)
2nd trimester: maternal infection, chronic diseases, endocrine
defects, autoimmune (antiphospholipid antibodies, HLA)
incompetent cervix, uterine defects,
environmental toxins

↓

Threatened Abortion

vaginal bleeding/spotting before 20 weeks
cervix closed, may or may not have cramping

Inevitable
Abortion
obvious rupture of
membranes,
cervical dilatation,
cramping, bleeding

Continued
Pregnancy
bleeding stops

Missed Abortion
death of the
conceptus
without expulsion

Complete
Abortion
expulsion of the
complete products
of conception;
bleeding and
cramping stop

Incomplete
Abortion
retention of some
tissue, usually the
placenta; bleeding
and cramping
continue; requires
D&C

CHAPTER 1.6

INFECTION

Maternal infection may pose a threat to the pregnancy. Infection may affect the fetus by crossing the placenta or ascending the vagina. During the first trimester, infections may result in spontaneous abortion or fetal developmental defects. Later, infections may cause preterm birth, CNS defects, or neonatal infection and sepsis.

Prevention of infection is the primary goal. Prenatal screening and identification of risk factors, along with client teaching, can lead to early identification and prompt treatment.

MEDICAL CARE

- Rubella vaccination prior to pregnancy
- Screening for TORCH infections, Group B streptococcus, and possibly hepatitis and HIV
- Medications: prophylactic antibiotics, antiviral: zidovudine (AZT), antiinfectives, immune globulins, and so forth
- Fetal screening/ultrasounds to determine effects of infections

COMMON NURSING DIAGNOSES

See ANXIETY

Related to: Effects of prenatal infection on developing fetus.

Defining Characteristics: Client expresses concern about the effects of infection on fetus (specify). Client exhibits physical signs of anxiety (specify: e.g., tension, pallor, insomnia, crying, etc.).

See ANTICIPATORY GRIEVING

Related to: Perceived potential loss of fetus, or developmental defects secondary to infection.

Defining Characteristics: Client exhibits distress about the perceived loss (specify: e.g., crying, sorrow, anger, guilt, anorexia, etc.).

See DECISIONAL CONFLICT

Related to: Continuing pregnancy with diagnosis of (specify: HIV, fetal developmental defects, etc.).

Defining Characteristics: Client expresses conflict about continuing pregnancy (specify: uncertainty, questioning of personal values, etc.). Client delays making a decision.

ADDITIONAL NURSING DIAGNOSES

RISK FOR INFECTION

Related to: Specify conditions that cause risk (e.g., heart disease, HIV positive, IV drug abuser, history of recurrent STDs, etc.).

Defining Characteristics: None, as this is a potential diagnosis.

Goal: Client will not experience infectious processes by (specify data/time to evaluate).

Outcome Criteria

✔ Client reports no symptoms of infection (specify: no fever, malaise, respiratory congestion, diarrhea, urinary burning, etc.).

✔ Client describes steps to avoid infection (specify: handwashing, avoiding people with infections, dirty needles, safe sex practices, etc.).

NOC: *Risk Control*

INTERVENTIONS	RATIONALES
Assess for fever, malaise, anorexia, weakness, fatigue, night sweats, respiratory congestion, diarrhea, urinary burning, skin lesions, joint pain, and swollen lymph nodes.	Assessment provides information about signs and symptoms of active infectious processes and opportunistic infections such as *Pneumocystis carinii* pneumonia, Kaposi's sarcoma, and lymphoma.
Assess client for risk behaviors: IV drug abuse, recurrent STDs.	Identifies clients at risk for infection.
Wash hands before and after caring for client. Teach client to wash frequently: before eating, before and after using the bathroom.	Friction and hot water remove many microorganisms from the hands and prevent their transmission.
Teach client to avoid contact with people with infections (large crowds, enclosed areas).	Protects client from infections spread by respiratory droplets.
Use and teach client's family to use clean gloves if handling body fluids; use masks, eye shields, and so forth as indicated. Do not recap needles; clean spills with bleach solution in the home.	Follows CDC guidelines to prevent transmission of blood-borne pathogens to caregiver or others in the family of client.
Monitor lab values as obtained for signs of infection risk (specify: cultures, CBC, ELISA, Western Blot, PCR, HIV culture, CD4, etc.).	Provides information about the microorganism causing the infectious process.
Use protective isolation techniques (gloves, mask, gowns for staff or visitors, etc.) for clients at high risk because of immune suppression.	Interventions protect immune-compromised client from contact with infection.
Administer drugs as ordered (specify: drug, dose, route, and times).	(Describe action of each drug related to the infectious agent.)
Administer prophylactic antibiotics prior to dental work, birth, and invasive procedures if ordered.	Prevents bacterial endocarditis in client at risk (e.g., hx of rheumatic fever, heart disease).
Monitor for side effects of medications (specify for each).	Provides information about client tolerance of the medication.
Provide emotional support and accurate information about the prognosis for the pregnancy (specify for each infectious agent the client has).	Provides information and support to help the client cope with a diagnosis that may endanger the fetus or herself.

INTERVENTIONS	RATIONALES
Refer client and family as indicated (specify: drug treatment programs, psychological counseling, and support groups, etc.).	Referrals provide additional information and assistance to client and family.

NIC: *Infection Protection*

Evaluation

(Date/time of evaluation of goal)

(Has goal been met? not met? partially met?)

(Does client deny s/s of infection? List s/s. Does client identify how to avoid infection? Use quotes)

(Revisions to care plan? D/C care plan? Continue care plan?)

HYPERTHERMIA

Related to: Physiologic response to infectious process.

Defining Characteristics: Increased body temperature (specify), warm, flushed skin, tachycardia.

Goal: Client will have a return to normal (specify range) body temperature by (specify date/time).

Outcome Criteria

✔ Client's temperature will be <102°F.

NOC: *Thermoregulation*

INTERVENTIONS	RATIONALES
Assess temperature (specify route), BP, pulse, and respiration every (specify time frame: e.g., q 2–4 hours).	Provides information about temperature changes, vital sign response: with ↑ temp, HR ↑, respiration ↑, BP may ↓ as a result of hypovolemia.
Assess client for dehydration: dry skin and mucous membranes, poor turgor, sunken eyes, output > intake, and so forth (specify how often).	Assessment provides information about hydration status. Hyperthermia causes fluid loss by metabolism, respirations, and diaphoresis.
Assess fetal heart tones (specify frequency or maintain on continuous EFM if condition warrants).	Maternal fever and dehydration cause fetal tachycardia. Hypovolemia may compromise placental flow and lead to fetal distress.

INTERVENTIONS	RATIONALES
Assess for contractions (specify to palpate or monitor with EFM for specified amount of time).	Maternal dehydration is implicated in uterine contractions which could lead to preterm labor and birth.
Provide ↑ fluids either by mouth or IV as ordered (specify: type of fluids, whether isotonic or hypotonic, amounts, routes, via pump, times, etc.).	Maintains hydration as fluid is lost from hyperthermia. (Isotonic fluids act as replacement only, hypotonic fluids cause fluid to move across membranes and back into the cells if severely dehydrated.)
Teach client to recognize dehydration (thirst, dry mouth, etc.) and to ↑ fluids early.	Prevents complication of preterm labor. Pregnant women have a ↑ need for fluids.
Monitor lab values as obtained (specify: cultures, etc.).	Lab tests may indicate which organism is responsible for fever.
Administer (or teach client to take) antipyretics only as ordered by health care provider (specify: drug, route, times, etc.).	(Specify action of drug in reducing temperature—aspirin is contraindicated during pregnancy because of its antiplatelet activity.)
Keep environmental temperature at 72° F, cover client with light blankets, add blankets if chilling occurs.	Promotes heat loss to the environment and promotes comfort, reduces chilling that may ↑ metabolic activity.
Encourage and provide for rest during illness.	Rest ↓ metabolic activity.

NIC: *Fever Treatment*

Evaluation

(Date/time of evaluation of goal)

(Has goal been met? not met? partially met?)

(What is client's temperature?)

(Revision to care plan? D/C care plan? Continue care plan?)

SOCIAL ISOLATION

Related to: Fear of rejection secondary to communicable disease.

Defining Characteristics: Client is diagnosed with (specify: HIV infection, AIDS, herpes, condyloma, etc.). Client reports feeling alone and being unable to make contact with others (specify with quotes).

Goal: Client will report ↑ social interaction by (date/time to evaluate).

Outcome Criteria

✔ Client will identify 2 strategies to ↑ social interactions.

✔ Client will verbalize correct information about her condition (specify others).

NOC: *Social Involvement*

INTERVENTIONS	RATIONALES
Establish a supportive relationship with client. Ensure privacy. Take time, use good eye contact and therapeutic communication techniques.	The client is vulnerable and benefits from the support of the nurse who shows respect and caring for the client as a worthy individual.
Teach client accurate information about the disease: agent, mode of transmission, and treatment options (specify for condyloma, herpes, HIV/AIDS, etc.).	Provides information with which to counter possible misconceptions about the condition.
Teach client how to avoid spread of the infection to others (specify: handwashing, condoms, abstinence during outbreaks, etc.). Verify understanding.	Empowers the client to care for herself and other people.
Explore misconceptions that the client and other people may have about the infection and how it is spread.	Identifies myths and misinformation about the infection.
Discuss ways to provide accurate information to others and when it would be important to do so (specify for each condition).	Helps to reduce fear of rejection by practicing how to tell others of the infection.
Ask client to describe her current social network: family, friends, co-workers, neighbors, and so forth.	Provides baseline information about client's social network.
Explore how client thinks her social network may change related to her diagnosis.	Validates the client's feelings, allows exploration of fears about how others will react to the diagnosis.
Provide a safe environment and encourage client to express her fears and feelings.	Empowers the client to work toward changing a situation she dislikes.
Assist client to plan two strategies to improve interaction with others during the next week.	Provides a beginning for improving social interaction within a specified time frame.

(continues)

(continued)

INTERVENTIONS	RATIONALES
Encourage client to initiate interaction with one other person she trusts in the next week.	Helps the client to be realistic and practice how to teach others factual information about the condition.
Provide simple written materials, videos, and so forth that client can use to teach others—help client to practice using the information.	Provides information and support from others who are coping with the same diagnosis.
Refer client to support groups as appropriate for this client (specify: HIV support groups, counseling, parenting groups, hobbies, etc.).	Gives client some options she may think of trying to meet new people who may be supportive.

NIC: *Socialization Enhancement*

Evaluation

(Date/time of evaluation of goal)

(Has goal been met? not met? partially met?)

(Describe strategies that client has chosen to improve social interaction.)

(Does client verbalize correct information about her diagnosis?)

(Revisions to care plan? D/C care plan? Continue care plan?)

INFECTION

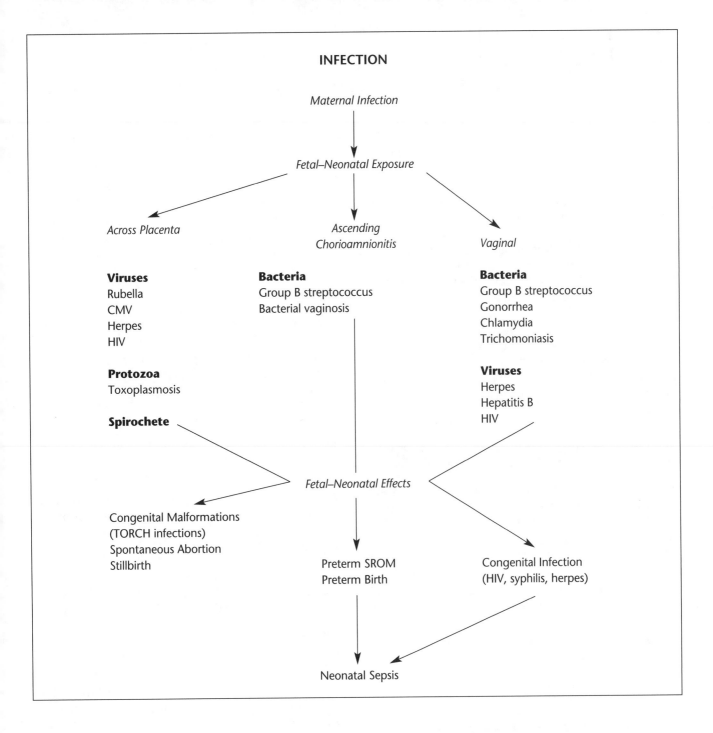

CHAPTER 1.7

SUBSTANCE ABUSE

The use of alcohol, tobacco, and illegal "street drugs" such as marijuana, cocaine (crack), heroin, PCP, and LSD can lead to an increase in perinatal mortality and morbidity. Miscarriage, malnutrition, infection, IUGR, placental abruption, stillbirth, preterm birth, congenital malformations, and mental retardation may result from maternal substance abuse during pregnancy.

All pregnant clients should be assessed for substance use in a caring and nonjudgmental manner. The client may delay seeking prenatal care for fear of reprisal. Clients frequently abuse several substances although they may only admit to one.

DEFINITIONS

- Psychological Dependence: The substance is used for pleasure or to avoid pain/problems. Results in intense craving and compulsive use.
- Physical Dependence: The body adapts to the chemical. Results in tolerance (dosage must be increased to produce the same effect) and withdrawal syndrome (uncomfortable physiological symptoms result from discontinuation of the chemical).
- Addiction: The substance-dependent person continues to use it in order to experience the pleasure *and* to avoid the discomfort of withdrawal.

MEDICAL CARE

- Urine toxicology screening: may be done at intervals during pregnancy
- Fetal well-being screening: ultrasounds, NST, BPP, and so forth—high risk pregnancy
- Referral to Alcoholics Anonymous, addiction counseling, or psychiatric consult if indicated.

- Heroin may not be discontinued abruptly as it will lead to decreased placental blood flow; methadone maintenance therapy may be used for women addicted to narcotics though it does cross the placenta

COMMON NURSING DIAGNOSES

  See BASIC CARE PLAN: PRENATAL HOME VISIT

See INEFFECTIVE HEALTH MAINTENANCE

Related to: Lack of understanding about effects of substance abuse during pregnancy. Lack of readiness to change behaviors detrimental to self and fetus.

Defining Characteristics: Client continues substance abuse during pregnancy. Client exhibits emotional fragility; behavior disorders; symptoms of abuse (specify).

 See DEFICIENT KNOWLEDGE: PRETERM LABOR PREVENTION

Related to: Inexperience or lack of understanding about the connection between substance abuse and preterm labor.

Defining Characteristics: Maternal substance abuse (specify) during pregnancy. Client expresses incorrect information about substance abuse or preterm labor (specify: e.g., "A seven-month baby does better than a nine-month baby.")

 See RISK FOR IMPAIRED GAS EXCHANGE: FETAL

Related to: Placental insufficiency secondary to substance abuse (specify).

ADDITIONAL NURSING DIAGNOSES

RISK FOR DELAYED GROWTH AND DEVELOPMENT: FETAL

Related to: Maternal substance abuse (specify) and ↓ nutrition.

Defining Characteristics: Inadequate maternal weight gain (specify). Evidence of SGA fetus or fetal IUGR (specify fetal size/gestational age); congenital defects (specify).

Goal: Fetus will experience appropriate growth and development during pregnancy.

Outcome Criteria

✔ Client's fundal height will be within 2 cm of value for gestational age between 18 and 30 weeks.

✔ Fetal growth and development appears appropriate on ultrasound—no fetal anomalies identified.

NOC: *Fetal Status: Antepartum*

INTERVENTIONS	RATIONALES
Assess fundal height (specify frequency: e.g., each visit, each week, etc.).	From approximately 18 to 30 weeks, fundal height in cms equals gestational age.
Assess maternal nutrition and weight gain (specify frequency). Reinforce nutrition teaching.	Substance abuse may lead to poor nutrition and inadequate weight gain.
Assess fetal heart tones by EFM (specify frequency).	Provides information on fetal well-being.
Teach mother to count and chart fetal movements and review (specify frequency).	The severely affected fetus may show a decrease in movement.
Perform tests for fetal well-being as ordered (specify: e.g., NST, CST, BPP, etc.) report non-reassuring results to caregiver.	Provides information about fetal well-being. Ensures health care provider is aware of testing results.
Monitor results of fetal testing (specify: Doppler flow studies; ultrasounds: fetal growth, physical anomalies, amniotic fluid volume (AFV). Amniocentesis: congenital anomalies, L-S ratio, phosphatidylglycerol levels, etc.).	Provides information about fetal warning signs: decreased cord blood flow, decreased AFV; cardiac or neurologic anomalies may accompany alcoholism; L-S ratio of 2:1 or more and/or PG presence indicate fetal maturity.
Explain all testing and results to client in terms she can understand.	Allows client to participate in care of her fetus.

INTERVENTIONS	RATIONALES
Teach client about the possible/ actual feral effects of her substance abuse (specify).	Client may be unaware of detrimental fetal effects of substance abuse.
Encourage client to abstain from substance abuse and praise efforts to do so.	Provides reinforcement for client attempts to abstain.
Refer client for substance abuse counseling or support groups (specify) if unable to stop on her own.	Provides additional encouragement and assistance to client trying to stop using substances.
Notify NICU, pediatrician, perinatologist, and/or neonatologist of fetal condition and plans for delivery.	Promotes multidisciplinary involvement in decisions regarding fetal care and delivery.

NIC: *Self-Responsibility Facilitation*

Evaluation

(Date/time of evaluation of goal)

(Has goal been met? not met? partially met?)

(What is fundal height/gestational age?)

(What are results of ultrasound? growth? development? anomalies?)

(Revisions to care plan? D/C care plan? Continue care plan?)

INEFFECTIVE COPING

Related to: Substance abuse behavior in response to stress.

Defining Characteristics: Client reports substance abuse (specify: alcohol, tobacco, cocaine, amounts, years of use, etc.). Client states she uses substance to cope with stress (specify, use quotes).

Goal: Client will cope effectively with stress without substance use by (date/time to evaluate).

Outcome Criteria

✔ Client will identify stresses that lead to addictive behaviors. Client will plan ways to avoid stress in personal life. Client will use effective coping strategies to deal with unavoidable stress.

NOC: *Coping*

INTERVENTIONS	RATIONALES
Establish rapport by conveying a nonjudgmental and caring attitude while presenting reality.	Clients who are substance abusers may have learned to be manipulative to avoid negative consequences.
Assist client to identify all substances she abuses, and approximate amounts used—allow time, suggest others if client hesitates.	Client may attempt to avoid admitting to all substances that are used or the amounts used.
Teach client about the effects of the substances she uses on herself and her fetus. Describe how each affects fetus and mother.	Provides information about the negative consequences of each substance.
Offer to assist client to develop more effective coping mechanisms.	Reassures client she is not alone and is worthy of the attention of the nurse.
Assist client to explore original reasons for substance abuse and any relapses if she has tried to stop.	Provides information about history and stimuli for substance abuse.
Assist client to identify current stress in her life, which accounts for continuing substance abuse.	Provides information about stresses in the client's current life.
For each stress identified, help client to plan a way to avoid the stress if possible.	Avoidance of "trigger" situations will make it easier to avoid using the substance.
Teach more effective coping techniques: relaxation, exercise, meditation, (specify).	Teaching provides information about possible effective coping strategies for handling stress.

INTERVENTIONS	RATIONALES
Encourage client to identify potential sources of emotional support (specify: family, significant other, support groups, etc.).	Social support influences the client's ability to effectively cope with stresses.
Praise client for attempts to stop substance abuse and encourage continued attempts if she has a relapse.	Provides positive reinforcement. Clients may have many relapses before finally being able to stop substance abuse.
Refer to appropriate professional support (specify: Alcoholics Anonymous, Narcotics Anonymous, psychiatric nurse counselors, or others as ordered: (e.g., psychiatrist, in-patient psychiatric unit, etc.).	The client may need more assistance than the nurse is prepared to offer. Support groups such as AA are often successful in helping clients to quit substance abuse.

NIC: *Coping Enhancement*

Evaluation

(Date/time of evaluation of goal)

(Has goal been met? not met? partially met?)

(List stresses client has identified)

(List ways client has decided to avoid specific stresses.)

(Describe coping strategies client has decided to use to cope with unavoidable stresses.)

(Revisions to care plan? D/C care plan? Continue care plan?)

SUBSTANCE ABUSE

Associated Factors
social attitudes/environment
stress, occupation (access)
low self-esteem, poor coping
skills, lack of knowledge,
familial substance abuse,
frequently uses combination
of substances, amounts used

Signs/Symptoms
delay in seeking care
hx of spontaneous abortion
stillbirth, LBW infants
malnutrition, dental decay
sinusitis, chronic URI's
cellulitis (track marks)
infections, poor personal hygiene

Maternal Substance Use
alcohol
tobacco
cocaine (crack)
heroin
PCP, LSD, others

Fetal–Neonatal Effects

spontaneous abortion
chromosome breakage
congenital heart defects
spinal anormalies
intestinal atresia
limb anomalies
brain anomalies
GU malformations
perinatal death
Fetal Alcohol Syndrome
developmental delays
mental retardation

Growth
LBW
IUGR
FTT

Maternal Effects

Cocaine: cardiac dysrhythmias
myocardial infarction, stroke, seizure
placental abruption, sudden death

CHAPTER 1.8

DOMESTIC VIOLENCE

One out of every three women may be physically or sexually abused during her lifetime. Acts of violence may escalate during pregnancy as the abuser views the pregnancy as threatening to an already low self-esteem. Physical violence is frequently aimed at the abdomen, breasts, or vagina of the pregnant woman. The cycle of violence includes periods of remorse when the abuser may be very loving and make promises to change. Many victims hold out hope that this phase can be attained on a permanent basis and therefore choose to stay in the relationship even though violence tends to increase over time.

Parents who were abused as children are more likely to abuse their own offspring. Dysfunctional parenting tends to perpetuate itself with increased abuse during times of crisis. Pregnancy may increase the stresses a family must cope with. When the pregnancy is complicated or results in a preterm birth, ill newborn, or neonate who is perceived as "difficult," the risk for child abuse increases.

UNIVERSAL SCREENING

All women should be screened for abuse during pregnancy. In addition to physical or psychosocial assessment findings that may indicate intentional injury, the nurse should ask each client the following questions:

1. Within the last year have you been hit, slapped, kicked, or otherwise physically hurt by someone? If yes, by whom? Total number of times?

2. Since you've been pregnant, have you been hit, slapped, kicked, or otherwise physically hurt by someone? If yes, by whom? Total number of times?

3. Within the last year, has anyone forced you to have sexual activities? If yes, by whom? Total number of times?

COMMON NURSING DIAGNOSES

 ### See BASIC CARE PLAN: HEALTHY PREGNANCY

 ### See BASIC CARE PLAN: PRENATAL HOME VISIT

 ### See ANXIETY

Related to: Threat of injury or death

Defining Characteristics: Client exhibits anxious behavior (specify e.g., poor eye contact, fidgeting, scanning for danger, etc.) Client verbalizes feelings of anxiety (specify: e.g., use quotes). Client appears frightened (specify: e.g., voice trembling, shaking, etc.).

 ### See SOCIAL ISOLATION

Related to: Inability to engage in satisfying social interactions

Defining Characteristics: Client reports lack of social support when asked (specify who the client identifies as support system). Client appears (specify: withdrawn, sad, shows poor eye contact). Client expresses loneliness imposed on her by others (specify: use quotes whenever possible).

ADDITIONAL NURSING DIAGNOSES

 ### RISK FOR INJURY

Related to: Continuation in a physically abusive relationship

Defining Characteristics: none, as this is a potential diagnosis

Goal: Client and fetus will not experience any injury by (specify date and time to evaluate).

Outcome Criteria:

✔ Client reports no physical abuse has taken place.

✔ Client has no observable injuries (specify what was observed, based on previous injuries).

✔ Fetus appears safe (specify indications of fetal well-being appropriate for gestational age).

NOC: *Knowledge: Personal Safety*

INTERVENTIONS	RATIONALES
Interview client alone in a private place. Ask partner to wait in another area during exam.	The client may be afraid to disclose information in front of an abusive partner.
Observe client for signs of physical abuse: bruising, grimacing, patches of hair loss, wearing extra clothing to conceal injuries	Observation provides the nurse with additional information to share with client.
Ask client if she has been hit, kicked, slapped, pushed, or otherwise physically abused since her last visit.	Assessment provides information about recent events.
Provide emotional support: let the client know that you are actively listening and recognize how difficult it must be for her to disclose this information.	The support and respect of the nurse helps the client to believe in herself.
Ask the client what she thinks about the safety of herself and her children at this time.	Encourages the client to explore safety issues.
Discuss signs of escalating danger that the client might become aware of: increased surveillance by the abusive partner, increasing jealousy and isolation, sexual abuse or rape, and increasing severity of threats including use of weapons or threats against pets, children, or other people.	Discussion may help the client to face the risks to herself and her children and acknowledge increasing danger.
Provide information about community resources available to help client and her children	Specify for client and community: include police, safe houses, etc.
Assist client to develop a safety plan for herself and her children to include: identification of a safe place to go to when she feels threatened, keeping an extra set of keys, important documents,	Helping the client to plan for her escape empowers the client to help protect herself.

INTERVENTIONS	RATIONALES
and some money with a trusted friend or in a safe deposit box that only she can get to.	
Praise client for disclosing the abuse and working on a safety plan for herself and her children.	Praise increases the client's self-esteem.
Document all findings including client statements, injuries, and care provided.	Documentation may become part of legal proceedings against the abuser.

NIC: *Security Enhancement*

Evaluation

(Date/time of evaluation of goal)

(Has goal been met? Not met? Partially met?)

(Did client report that no physical abuse took place since last visit? Use quotes.)

(Does client have any observable injuries?)

(Specify indications of fetal well-being appropriate for gestational age, e.g., fetal growth pattern, FHR, variability, accelerations.)

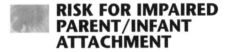

RISK FOR IMPAIRED PARENT/INFANT ATTACHMENT

Related to: (Specify: unplanned or unwanted pregnancy; unrealistic expectations of the infant; disappointment with the gender or appearance of the infant; sick or premature infant; parental immaturity, lack of a good role model, etc.)

Defining Characteristics: None, as this is a potential diagnosis.

Goal: Client will exhibit attachment behaviors toward the infant by (date/time to evaluate).

Outcome Criteria

✔ Client will (specify: e.g., hold and smile at baby; make eye contact and talk to infant appropriately; identify positive feelings about the baby; express a desire to learn to care for infant).

NOC: *Parent–Infant Attachment*

INTERVENTIONS	RATIONALES
Evaluate possible causes for impaired attachment: pain, difficult birth, unplanned pregnancy, infant doesn't meet expectations, lack of support from partner or family.	Provides information to guide nursing care.
Promote client comfort. Assist with hygiene, provide nourishment, and ensure that room is comfortable for client. Evaluate for pain and medicate if needed (specify drug, dose, route, and frequency).	Maternal discomfort interferes with attention necessary for attachment. The mother must have her needs met before she is able to meet the needs of the infant.
Assist the client to talk about the birth experience and her thoughts about the infant. Allow time to sit down with client and listen actively.	Assists the client to integrate her birth experience and have any questions answered. Indicates that the nurse is willing to help.
Explore with the client her feelings about being a mother. Ask her if she wants to be like her own mother or if there is another positive role model she would like to emulate.	Parenting is a learned role. Children who are abused may grow up to repeat the abuse with their own children.
Provide ample opportunity for client to interact with her infant. Promote skin-to-skin contact (specify how if baby is in the NICU or has been transported to another facility).	Close contact during the first few days of life enhances bonding.
Observe the client interacting with the infant. Point out characteristics of the baby. Help the client to identify how the baby responds to her voice and touch. Point out cues the infant sends to the mother.	The identification process includes recognition of how the infant is like the parents and how he is unique. Interaction between infant and mother enhance attachment.

INTERVENTIONS	RATIONALES
Assist the client to provide physical care for her baby. Reassure client that the staff will be available to teach and assist her with infant care. Provide videos or written materials to reinforce teaching.	The client may fear hurting the baby or may be reluctant to form attachment if the infant is pre-term or ill. Education assists the client to gain parenting skills and confidence.
Support the parent's efforts and praise positive interactions.	Reinforces new skills and positive parenting.
Encourage client to identify positive support systems she can rely on for assistance after discharge.	Social support may help the new parent develop skill and self-confidence.
Make referrals as appropriate.	Specify for client e.g., NICU parent support group, social services, DCFS, etc.)

NIC: *Attachment Promotion*

Evaluation

(Date/time of evaluation of goal)

(Has goal been met? Not met? Partially met?)

(Did client hold and smile at baby?)

(Did client make eye contact and talk to infant appropriately? Specify using quotes.)

(Did client identify positive feelings about the baby? What did she say?)

(Did client express a desire to learn to care for infant? Use quotes.)

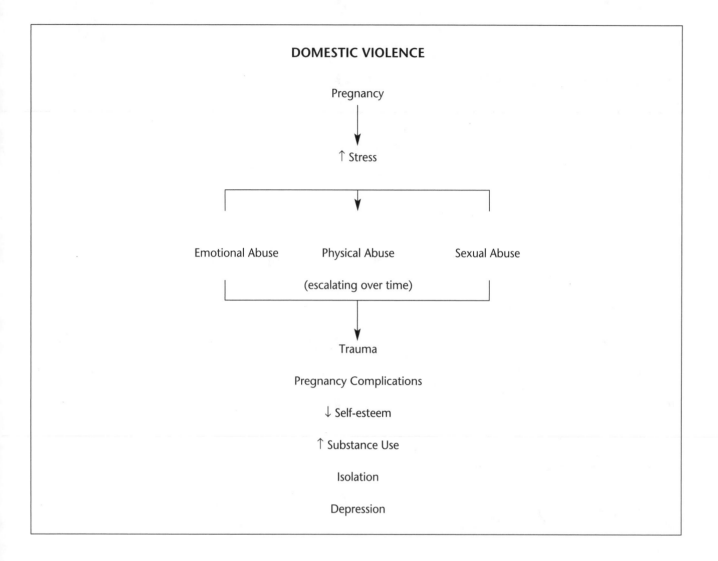

CHAPTER 1.9

DIABETES MELLITUS AND GESTATIONAL DIABETES

Diabetes mellitus is a metabolic disorder caused by inadequate insulin production or inability to adequately utilize insulin. Insulin is a hormone that moves glucose from the blood into the cells for energy use or storage. Diabetes mellitus may be broadly classified as Type I (insulin dependent, IDDM) or Type II (non-insulin dependent, NIDDM), depending on the severity of the deficit.

Gestational diabetes mellitus (GDM) results from the inability to meet the need for increased insulin production during pregnancy. The mother's body stores more glucose during the first half of pregnancy and later, the placental hormone hPL (hCS) works to resist maternal insulin, allowing more glucose to be available for the fetus. GDM may be controlled by diet alone or may require insulin injections.

RISK FACTORS

- Native American, Hispanic, or African-American heritage
- Family hx of diabetes
- Previous GDM
- Previous unexplained stillbirth
- Previous infant >9.5 pounds
- Maternal obesity
- Maternal age >30

PERINATAL COMPLICATIONS

- Pregnancy-induced hypertension (PIH)
- Bacterial infections
- Macrosomic infant
- Hydraminos
- Preterm birth

- Stillbirth (IDDM only)
- Congenital anomalies: heart defects, neural tube defects (IDDM only)
- Neonatal RDS, polycythemia, hyperbilirubinemia

MEDICAL CARE

- Dietary control: 30–35 kcal/kg of ideal body weight/day ADA diet with no concentrated sweets
- Blood glucose monitoring
- Medication: insulin (human)—oral hypoglycemic medications are contraindicated (teratogenic)
- Urine testing for glucose and ketones
- MSAFP at 16–18 weeks
- Fetal movement counts
- NST weekly from 28–32 weeks
- Ultrasound for anomalies, AFV, and fetal growth patterns
- Possible: CST, BPP, amniocentesis for lung maturity
- Possible induction at 38–39 weeks and/or cesarean delivery

COMMON NURSING DIAGNOSES

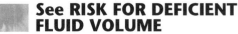 **See RISK FOR DEFICIENT FLUID VOLUME**

Related to: Osmotic dehydration secondary to hyperglycemia.

 See ANXIETY

Related to: Threat to biologic integrity secondary to complicated pregnancy. Threat to well-being of fetus secondary to maternal illness.

Defining Characteristics: Client expresses apprehension about self and fetal well-being (specify). Client exhibits physical tension (heart rate, BP, etc.).

See RISK FOR IMPAIRED GAS EXCHANGE: FETAL

Related to: Placental vascular changes secondary to poor glycemic control.

ADDITIONAL NURSING DIAGNOSES

RISK FOR INJURY: MATERNAL/FETAL

Related to: Fluctuations in internal environment: hyperglycemia or hypoglycemia.

Defining Characteristics: None, as this is a potential diagnosis.

Goal: Mother and fetus will not experience any injury from hyper-, hypoglycemia by (date/time to evaluate).

Outcome Criteria

✔ Client maintains fasting blood glucose between 80–105 mg/dL, and urine is negative for ketones.

✔ Fetal growth is appropriate for gestational age.

✔ Fetus moves at least 10 times in 2-hour count.

NOC: *Symptom Control*

INTERVENTIONS	RATIONALES
Assess client's blood glucose and HbA$_{1-c}$ as ordered (specify method and timing: e.g., FSBG, GTT, postprandial, q.i.d., q.d., weekly, etc.). Review client's home testing records at each visit.	Provides information about glycemic control during pregnancy: blood glucose >105 mg/dL fasting or 120 mg/dL 2 hour postprandial may require insulin administration. If HbA$_{1-c}$ is >8.5, fetus is at ↑ risk for congenital anomalies.
Assess urine for glucose and ketones (specify timing). Review client's home testing record at each prenatal visit.	Excess blood glucose spills into urine. Inability to use glucose leads to ↑ fat and protein metabolism resulting is ketoacidosis.
Monitor client's compliance with diet (specify: e.g., 2500 kcal ADA w/o concentrated sugar divided into 3 meals and 3 snacks daily).	GDM may be controlled by diet alone if client complies. This diet provides steady blood glucose levels throughout the day.

INTERVENTIONS	RATIONALES
Monitor client's self-administration of human insulin SC as ordered (specify: type, timing, and dosage).	Appropriate insulin administration maintains normal blood glucose levels w/o causing hypoglycemia: may be administered by insulin pump or injection.
Teach client to record daily "kick counts" after 28 weeks: After a meal, when baby is active, sit comfortably and count fetal movement until 10 "kicks" have been recorded. Call health provider if ↓ fetal movement, fewer than normal kicks, or <10 in 2 hours.	Fetal movement counts are an inexpensive way to provide daily information about fetal well-being without being invasive. A decrease in fetal movement may indicate distress. Allows client to be a participant in her care.
Explain purpose of MSAFP test at 16–18 weeks to r/o fetal neural tube defects.	Fetuses of mothers with IDDM and poor glycemic control are at ↑ risk for NTD.
Monitor fetal testing as ordered (specify: BPP, ultrasound, fetal echocardiogram, amniocentesis).	Provides information about fetal growth, complications, and lung maturity.
Assess client for signs of PIH at each prenatal visit (BP, wt gain, proteinuria, edema, and reflexes).	Client with diabetes is at higher risk for PIH.
Perform weekly NSTs as ordered from 28–32 weeks (or more frequently—specify), CST or OCT as ordered.	Reactive NST is reassuring sign of fetal well-being. Nonreactive NST needs further assessment such as CST or OCT.
Measure fundal height at each visit, compare to previous value, and correlate to estimated gestational age.	Macrosomic fetus is at risk for birth trauma, shoulder dystocia and may need cesarean delivery.
Coordinate referrals as ordered (specify: perinatologist, endocrinologist, diabetic nurse educator, dietitian, etc.).	Coordination of referrals insures continuity of care and communication between multiple health care providers.

NIC: *Hyperglycemia Management*
Hypoglycemia Management

Evaluation

(Date/time of evaluation of goal)

(Has goal been met? not met? partially met?)

(What is client's fasting blood glucose? What is fetal growth pattern relative to gestational age? How often is fetal movement felt in 2 hours?)

(Revisions to care plan? D/C care plan? Continue care plan?)

DEFICIENT KNOWLEDGE: DIABETES IN PREGNANCY

Related to: Lack of information about diabetes mellitus during pregnancy.

Defining Characteristics: (Specify: new diagnosis of GDM). Client (and significant other) verbalize lack of knowledge about diabetes during pregnancy—request information about pathophysiology, treatment, prognosis, self-care options (specify, use quotes).

Goal: Client (and significant other) will verbalize knowledge about gestational diabetes by (date/time to evaluate).

Outcome Criteria

✔ Client (and significant other) will verbalize an understanding of glycemic control during her pregnancy: diet, exercise, BG, and urine testing (insulin administration).

✔ Client (and significant other) demonstrate skills needed for control of diabetes during pregnancy (specify: e.g., blood glucose monitoring, urine dipsticks, SC insulin administration, etc.)

NOC: *Knowledge: Diabetes Management*

INTERVENTIONS	RATIONALES
Provide a comfortable environment for learning, invite client to include significant other, allow adequate time for questions.	Facilitates learning of complex content; significant other may provide support and reinforce learning at home.
Assess client and significant other's knowledge of diabetes mellitus and ability to learn needed skills.	Provides baseline data for planning education about diabetes and self-care—individualizes content to client learning level.
Describe maternal and fetal pathophysiology of GDM in simple terms: use visual aids and written materials; verify understanding.	Basic information the client needs to understand the condition and assess her physiologic responses.
Teach client and significant other about the physiologic rationale for the diet plan prescribed (specify: e.g., 2400 cal ADA, divided into 3 meals and 3 snacks, etc.).	Understanding the physiology will enhance compliance and allow the client to modify her diet based on activity levels and BG testing.

INTERVENTIONS	RATIONALES
Instruct client and significant other in proper use of blood glucose monitoring equipment. Demonstrate and have client perform a return demonstration.	Ensures client understands procedure and can perform skills correctly.
Teach client to perform urine testing for glucose and ketones: observe client's ability to read results accurately.	Ensures client is capable of testing urine and understands how to read results.
(If insulin is prescribed: Instruct client and significant other in insulin administration: include storage, drawing up accurate dosage, rolling vial to mix, draw up clear (Regular) insulin before cloudy (NPH) if mixing types, SC technique, rotation of sites—allow client to demonstrate skill at next dosage.)	Teaching promotes safe and accurate insulin administration technique—enhances self-esteem to master this skill.
Teach client to engage in regular nonstrenuous exercise such as walking or swimming and to adjust diet according to activity level.	Exercise promotes utilization of dietary CHO and may ↓ insulin need. May need to ↑ CHO intake before vigorous activity or ↓ insulin if ill.
Teach client and significant other the s/s of hypoglycemia (BG <70 mg/dL) and how to treat it: Immediately eat some simple carbohydrate—glass of fruit juice, honey, and so forth. Follow this with 15 gm of a complex carbohydrate such as a slice of toast or crackers and peanut butter, wait 15 minutes and retest BG.	Promotes recognition of condition and allows fast treatment to avoid complications. Empowers the client and significant other to recognize and handle situation. Simple CHO ↑ BG levels quickly but is metabolized quickly so needs to be followed with longer-lasting CHO to maintain blood levels.
Teach client and significant other the s/s of hyperglycemia, the dangers of diabetic ketoacidosis, and to check BG and notify health care provider (administer insulin).	Promotes recognition and fast treatment to avoid DKA.
Instruct client to report any signs of illness or infection to caregiver as diet or insulin needs may change quickly.	Clients with GDM are at greater risk of infection, which may result in DKA.
Instruct client to keep a record of all BG and urine testing, insulin administration, diet, and activity levels. Review record with client at prenatal visits.	Written record provides information about client's individual responses. Allows client to modify self-care as needed.

INTERVENTIONS	RATIONALES
Provide written reinforcement of all teaching topics, reassure client that you will return to review content (specify when). Suggest writing down questions.	Provides alternative source of information, reinforces content and ensures client's questions will be answered.
Refer client to other resources as needed (specify: Registered dietician, American Diabetic Association, support groups, etc.).	Resources provide additional information and support.

NIC: *Teaching, Disease Process*

Evaluation

(Date/time of evaluation of goal)

(Has goal been met? not met? partially met?)

(Do client and significant other verbalize understanding of: diet, exercise, BG, and urine testing [insulin administration]?)

(Did client and significant other demonstrate blood glucose monitoring, urine dipsticks, SC insulin administration, etc.?)

(Revisions to care plan? D/C care plan? Continue care plan?)

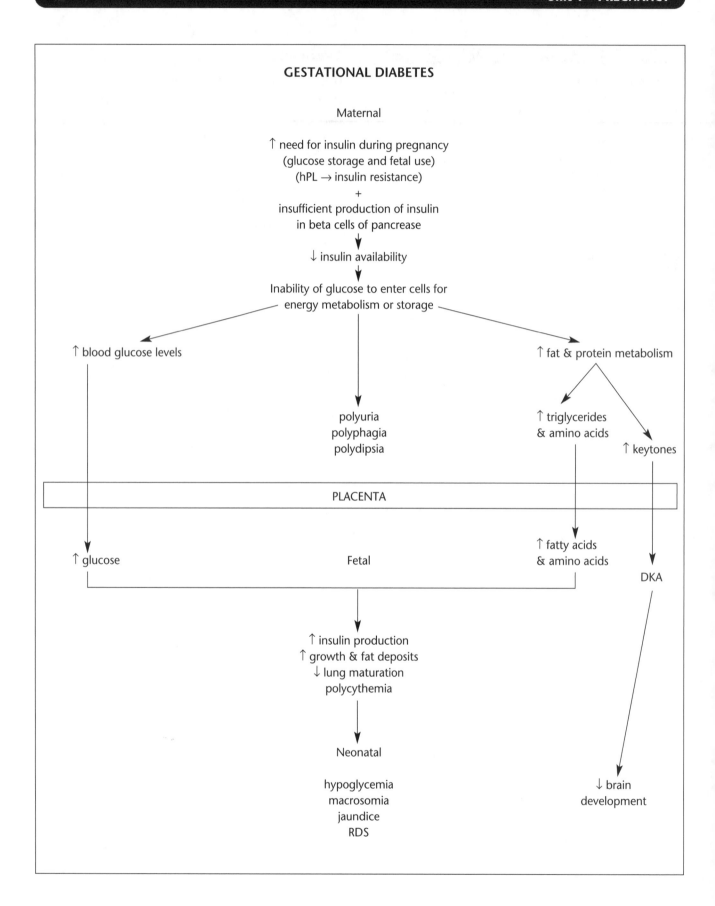

GESTATIONAL DIABETES

Maternal

↑ need for insulin during pregnancy
(glucose storage and fetal use)
(hPL → insulin resistance)
+
insufficient production of insulin
in beta cells of pancrease

↓ insulin availability

Inability of glucose to enter cells for
energy metabolism or storage

↑ blood glucose levels

polyuria
polyphagia
polydipsia

↑ fat & protein metabolism

↑ triglycerides
& amino acids

↑ keytones

PLACENTA

↑ glucose

Fetal

↑ fatty acids
& amino acids

DKA

↑ insulin production
↑ growth & fat deposits
↓ lung maturation
polycythemia

Neonatal

hypoglycemia
macrosomia
jaundice
RDS

↓ brain
development

CHAPTER 1.10

HEART DISEASE

Heart disease is the fourth leading cause of maternal mortality after hypertension, hemorrhage, and infection (Olds, London, Ladewig, 2000). Rheumatic fever is declining as a cause of heart disease but advances in treatment of congenital defects means that more of these women are now likely to become pregnant.

Pregnancy increases the workload of the heart. Cardiac output is increased from 15–25% by 8 weeks of gestation and peaks at 30–50% by midpregnancy. The left ventricle has an increased workload, pulse rates increase, and there is a decrease in peripheral and pulmonary vascular resistance. The diseased heart has a decreased cardiac reserve and may have difficulty adapting to these changes.

CLASSIFICATION OF HEART DISEASE (NYHA)

Clients with Class I and II heart disease have a potential for good pregnancy outcome. Those with Class III or IV are at risk for serious complications and may be advised to avoid pregnancy.

- Class I—Uncompromised: Physical activity is not limited by angina or symptoms of cardiac insufficiency
- Class II—Slightly Compromised: Comfortable at rest but normal activity causes fatigue, palpitations, dyspnea, or angina.
- Class III—Markedly Compromised: Comfortable at rest but less than ordinary activity causes excessive fatigue, palpitation, dyspnea, or angina
- Class IV—Severely Compromised: Unable to perform any activity without discomfort; may experience angina or signs of cardiac insufficiency while at rest

MEDICAL CARE

- Diagnostics: echocardiogram, chest X-ray, electrocardiogram, auscultation for murmurs, possible cardiac catheterization
- Medications: vitamins and iron, flu vaccine, Heparin (coumadin is teratogenic), thiazide diuretics, furosemide, cardiac glycosides (digitalis), prophylactic antibiotics for dental or surgical invasive procedures and for delivery
- Close monitoring to avoid excessive weight gain (24-lb. goal), anemia, fluid retention, PIH, and infection
- Plan for low forceps vaginal delivery with epidural anesthesia
- Hospitalization for Class III or IV prior to delivery with possible invasive hemodynamic monitoring

COMMON NURSING DIAGNOSES

See ANXIETY

Related to: Actual or perceived threat to biologic integrity secondary to effects of pregnancy on pre-existing heart disease.

Defining Characteristics: (Specify: client states feeling nervous; anxious, anticipates misfortune. Client exhibits physiologic signs of anxiety: trembling, palpitations, pallor, etc. Client reports cognitive signs of anxiety: unable to concentrate, confusion, etc.).

See RISK FOR INFECTION

Related to: Underlying heart disease and decreased cardiac reserve.

See ACTIVITY INTOLERANCE

Related to: Fatigue, insufficient oxygenation for normal activity.

Defining Characteristics: (Specify: client reports weakness and fatigue. Client exhibits shortness of breath, dyspnea, tachypnea with activity [specify level]. Specify changes in pulse and BP with activity.)

ADDITIONAL NURSING DIAGNOSES

DECREASED CARDIAC OUTPUT

Related to: Inability of the heart to adapt to hemodynamic changes of pregnancy secondary to mechanical, electrical, or structural alterations.

Defining Characteristics: Client reports (specify: fatigue, syncope, angina at rest, with normal activity, with exertion. Specify: ↓ BP, ECG changes, ↑ pulse, ↓ peripheral pulses, ↓ urine output, ↓ CVP, etc.).

Goal: Client will maintain adequate cardiac output during pregnancy (date/time to evaluate).

Outcome Criteria

✔ Client will maintain stable BP (Specify: e.g., systolic >100 mm Hg), pulses regular rhythm, rate <100, urine output >30 cc/hr.

NOC: *Vital Sign Status*

INTERVENTIONS	RATIONALES
Assess BP (specify sites) and apical pulse for 1 minute noting rate and rhythm, assess peripheral pulses (specify frequency).	Systolic BP <100 mm Hg, pulse >100 or irregular with ↓ peripheral pulses, may indicate ↓ C.O.
(Assess CVP or Swan Ganz readings if applicable [specify timing]—monitor for complications: trauma, infection, emboli, dysrhythmias, pneumothorax, etc.)	Central venous pressure provides information about circulating blood volume; Swan Ganz catheter provides information about pulmonary pressures.
Assess for changes in pulse and respirations associated with activity change (specify frequency). Compare to previous findings.	↓ C.O. results in tachycardia and tachypnea (respirations >24) with ↑ activity. Worsening condition indicates cardiac decompensation.
Assess for ECG changes (if applicable [specify timing]).	Dysrhythmias may cause ↓ C.O. or be symptomatic of ↓ cardiac function.

INTERVENTIONS	RATIONALES
Assess urine output (specify frequency: e.g., qh, q shift). Teach client to report if output estimated at <30 cc/hr.	Provides information about adequacy of C.O. relative to renal blood flow and the effect on renal function.
Assess fetal well-being (specify frequency: e.g., continuous, q shift, weekly etc.) FHR, reactivity, fetal movement counts, fundal height, and so forth.	Assessment provides information about adequacy of cardiac output and utero-placental blood flow, fetal oxygenation, and nutrition/growth.
Monitor lab values and test results: potassium, calcium, ECG, echocardiogram, amniocentesis, and so forth.	Assessment provides information about electrolytes critical for cardiac function; cardiac pathology; fetal maturity.
Administer drugs such as digitalis, ß-blockers, and calcium channel blockers, as ordered (specify: drug, dose, route, and times). For digoxin, assess apical pulse for 1 min and hold dose if HR <60—notify M.D. Monitor serum K⁺ levels.	Digitalis (cardiac glycoside) increases the strength of the myocardial contraction while decreasing the rate and workload of the heart (specify action of each drug relative to cardiac output) ↓ K⁺ increases risk of digitalis toxicity.
Assess for therapeutic and adverse effects of each drug (specify: e.g., s/s digitalis toxicity: anorexia, nausea, vomiting, bradycardia, and dysrhythmias).	Assessment provides information about the desired effect and early recognition of complications of drug therapy.
Assess social support and include family and/or significant other in teaching about conditions and care.	Client will need good social support for lifestyle changes needed during ↑ risk pregnancy.
Teach client med. administration (specify: e.g., for digitalis need to teach to take apical pulse) and adverse effects to report (signs of digitalis toxicity).	Teaching provides information to ensure safe administration of cardiac drugs.
Teach client to rest in bed for 10 hours at night and for 30 minutes after meals. Teach client to lie in left lateral position and to sit with feet elevated.	Resting decreases workload on the heart. These positions facilitate venous return and renal and uteroplacental perfusion.
Teach client use of antiembolism stockings if prescribed: teach to roll on, check pulses, color of toes, and sensation.	Antiembolism stockings prevent venous stasis and provide mechanical stimulation for venous return.
Teach client and family of need to limit activity to no more than light housework, not to climb stairs, and to avoid emotional stress (bed rest if ordered).	Limiting activity decreases cardiac workload—extent of limitations depends on degree of cardiac disease: Class III or IV may need complete bed rest.

INTERVENTIONS	RATIONALES
Teach client and significant other warning signs of cardiac decompensation to report immediately: progressive severe dyspnea, ↑ fatigue, tachycardia, palpitations, or syncope, chest pain on exertion.	Teaching allows for prompt treatment to prevent further complications such as CHF or dysrhythmias.
Refer to support groups if available, social service agencies, and so forth (specify).	Referrals may provide social or financial support.

NIC: *Cardiac Care*

Evaluation

(Date/time of evaluation of goal)

(Has goal been met? not met? partially met?)

(What is client's BP? Is systolic >100 mm Hg? What is client's pulse rate and rhythm? Is rate <100? What is client's urine output? Is output >30 cc/hr?)

(Revisions to care plan? D/C care plan? Continue care plan?)

EXCESS FLUID VOLUME

Related to: Compromised regulatory systems secondary to heart disease and ↑ circulating volume of pregnancy.

Defining Characteristics: Client reports dyspnea, shortness of breath, edema (specify where, how much: e.g., dependent, periorbital, +2, +3 . . . pitting). Intake > output (specify), ↑ wt. gain greater than expected for gestation (specify).

Goal: Client will not exhibit excess fluid retention by (date/time to evaluate).

Outcome Criteria

✔ Client will report ↓ dyspnea.

✔ Client will have ↓ edema (specify: e.g., < +2 dependent).

✔ Urine output will approximately equal intake.

✔ Weight gain will be no more than (specify based on gestation).

NOC: *Fluid Balance*

INTERVENTIONS	RATIONALES
Weigh client (at each prenatal visit) and compare to expected gain for gestation.	Unexplained weight gain is an early sign of fluid retention.
Assess for edema (at each visit): dependent, sacral (if lying), fingers (check rings), facial, and periorbital. Rate extent (+1, +2, etc.). Compare to previous findings.	Increased fluid volume of pregnancy and gravity may account for dependent edema (physiologic edema of pregnancy).
Assess skin turgor and striae gravidarum (stretch marks) development (at each visit).	Increased fluid retention in the extravascular spaces causes taut skin. Striae may develop rapidly as skin stretches.
Assess for other signs of PIH (at each visit): BP, hyperreflexia, epigastric pain, and visual disturbances. Assess urine for protein.	Clients with heart disease are at higher risk of developing PIH.
Assess for cough, respirations noting rate and ease. Auscultate lungs noting any rales (crackles), rhonchi, or wheezes (at each visit).	Cough, dyspnea, and tachypnea (>24) are signs of ↓ oxygenation possibly caused by pleural effusions resulting from FVE.
Assess for jugular (neck) vein distention (at each visit).	Jugular distention is an indication of systemic venous congestion.
Assess intake and output and urine specific gravity (specify time frame). Teach client to assess intake and output at home and to report urine output <30 cc/hr.	Oliguria indicates ↓ renal perfusion, which activates the renin-angiotensin–aldosterone system causing NA+, K+, and H$_2$O retention and ↑ specific gravity of of urine.
Administer diuretics as ordered early in the day (specify: drug, dose, route, times) and assess results (teach client to self-administer diuretics if indicated).	(Describe how specific drug works to cause diuresis.) Teaching client about medications enables her to participate in her care and assess for therapeutic or adverse effects.
Monitor lab results as obtained. Note serum albumin, sodium and potassium levels.	Monitoring labs provides information on fluid and electrolyte balance.
Assist client to plan a diet ↑ in iron and protein and essential nutrients with no added salt. Explain rationale for diet changes.	Low protein, ↑ sodium contributes to fluid retention. Iron is needed for hemoglobin. Understanding the rationale helps the client to comply.
Teach client to position herself with head and shoulders raised and a wedge under right hip to tilt uterus to the left.	Upright position facilitates breathing, and left uterine displacement increases renal and uteroplacental blood flow and fetal perfusion.
Instruct client and significant other to notify physician if client experiences ↑ dyspnea, tachypnea, a "smothering" feeling, cough, or hemoptysis.	Instruction allows for prompt treatment to avoid complications from congestive heart failure.

NIC: *Fluid Management*

Evaluation

(Date/time of evaluation of goal)

(Has goal been met? not met? partially met?)

(Does client report ↓ dyspnea?)

(Describe edema, does urine output approximately equal intake? What was client's wt gain?)

(Revisions to care plan? D/C care plan? Continue care plan?)

ALTERED TISSUE PERFUSION: PLACENTAL, CARDIOPULMONARY

Related to: Changes in circulating blood volume, secondary to heart disease.

Defining Characteristics: Specify: (pallor, cyanosis, ↓ BP [specify normal and present BP], ↑ capillary refill time [specify how many seconds], ↓ SaO$_2$ levels [specify], anemia [specify Hgb & Hct], fetal IUGR, and/or late decelerations on EFM).

Goal: Client will experience adequate cardiopulmonary and placental tissue perfusion by (date/time to evaluate).

Outcome Criteria

✔ Client's BP will be > (specify: e.g., 100/60 mm Hg). SaO$_2$ will be ≥ 95%.

✔ Fetal growth will be appropriate for gestational age.

✔ FHR will be 110–160 with average variability and no late decelerations.

NOC: *Circulation Status*

INTERVENTIONS	RATIONALES
Assess BP and pulses, skin color and temperature, mucous membrane color, capillary refill time, SaO$_2$ (if available), clubbing of fingers/toes, and level of consciousness (LOC) (state how often).	Assessment provides information about circulation: CO, oxygenation at the capillary level, chronicity of hypoxemia, oxygenation of the CNS.
Assess fetal growth compared to expected rate, and monitor FHT for rate (110–160), variability, and accelerations or	Assessment provides information on placental function. Changes in baseline FHR with loss of variability or late decelerations

INTERVENTIONS	RATIONALES
decelerations. Perform NST or OCT as ordered (state when to assess fetal well-being).	indicate ↓ oxygenation or placental perfusion.
Assess client for anemia: monitor labwork as obtained (e.g., Hgb & Hct).	Tissue oxygenation is dependent on adequate hemoglobin levels.
Provide oxygen via face mask or nasal cannula at (specify rate) as ordered.	Provides supplemental oxygen to tissues.
Administer cardiac glycoside medications (or others) as ordered (specify: drug, dose, route, time). Monitor for therapeutic and adverse effects.	Cardiac glycosides promote CO by slowing and strengthening contraction of the myocardium (specify action of other drugs). Prevents complications of drug therapy.
Teach client to rest in left lateral position or semi-Fowler's with a wedge under right hip and to change position at least q 2h.	Rest and positioning facilitate placental perfusion. Position change prevents skin breakdown from continuous pressure on one area.
Provide egg-crate mattress and extra pillows for client on bed rest. Provide ROM exercises as needed (specify timing). Assess skin condition during bath noting any reddened areas.	Interventions prevent development of pressure sores from ↓ tissue perfusion over bony prominences.
Teach client to avoid tight or restrictive clothing.	Tight clothing may further ↓ circulation.
Teach client to do daily "kick counts" of fetal movement.	Provides information on fetal oxygenation.
Reinforce measures to ensure optimal oxygenation: diet, iron and vitamins, and no smoking.	Reinforcement supports the client in making lifestyle changes to improve tissue perfusion.

NIC: *Circulatory Care*

Evaluation

(Date/time of evaluation of goal)

(Has goal been met? not met? partially met?)

(Specify client's BP. What is SaO$_2$ level? Is fetal growth appropriate for gestational age? What is baseline FHR? Are there any accelerations or decelerations?)

(Revisions to care plan? D/C care plan? Continue care plan?)

HEART DISEASE

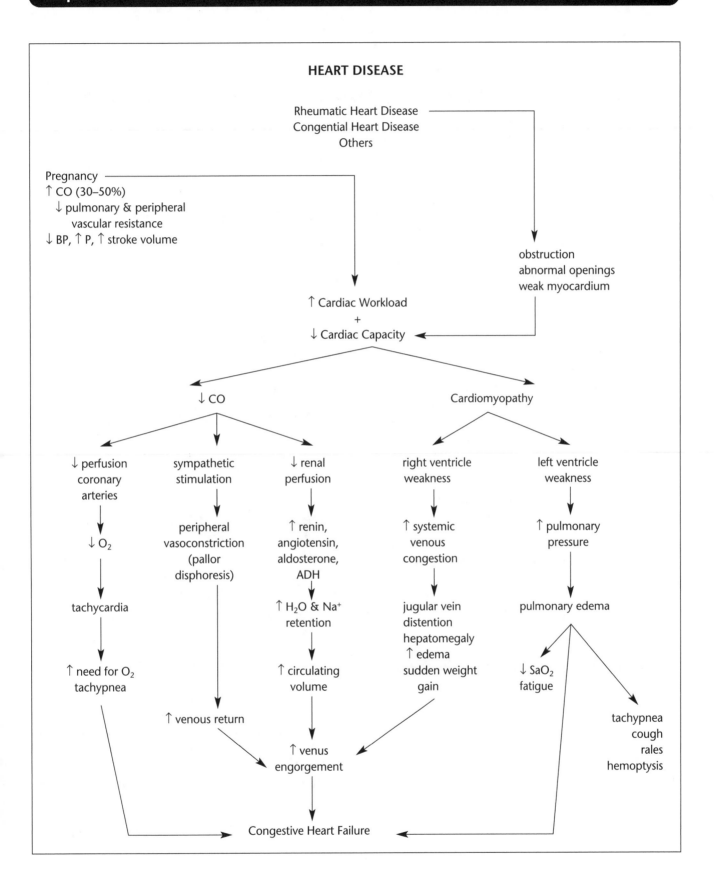

Rheumatic Heart Disease
Congential Heart Disease
Others

Pregnancy
↑ CO (30–50%)
 ↓ pulmonary & peripheral
  vascular resistance
↓ BP, ↑ P, ↑ stroke volume

obstruction
abnormal openings
weak myocardium

↑ Cardiac Workload
+
↓ Cardiac Capacity

↓ CO   Cardiomyopathy

↓ perfusion   sympathetic   ↓ renal   right ventricle   left ventricle
coronary   stimulation   perfusion   weakness   weakness
arteries

↓ O_2 ↑ renin,   ↑ systemic   ↑ pulmonary
                    peripheral   angiotensin,   venous   pressure
                    vasoconstriction   aldosterone,   congestion
                    (pallor   ADH
tachycardia   disphoresis)
                                        ↑ H_2O & Na^+ jugular vein   pulmonary edema
                                        retention   distention
                                                         hepatomegaly
↑ need for O_2 ↑ circulating   ↑ edema   ↓ SaO_2
tachypnea   volume   sudden weight   fatigue
                                                         gain
                    ↑ venous return
                                                                                              tachypnea
                                        ↑ venus   cough
                                        engorgement   rales
                                                                                              hemoptysis

                                        Congestive Heart Failure

CHAPTER 1.11

PREGNANCY-INDUCED HYPERTENSION

Pregnancy-induced hypertension (PIH) is defined as persistent BP readings of 140/90 mm Hg or higher (or an elevation of more than 30 mm Hg systolic or more than 15 mm Hg diastolic over baseline BP) which develops during pregnancy.

Pre-eclampsia is diagnosed when hypertension is combined with proteinuria (of 300 mg/L or more in a 24 hour specimen) and or pathologic edema. The edema is generalized, not dependent, and can be assessed in the hands and face. Pre-eclampsia is further divided into mild and severe. Severe pre-eclampsia is diagnosed when the diastolic BP is >110 mm Hg or the client experiences persistent 2+ or more proteinuria (or >4 g/L in 24 hours). Ominous signs of severe pre-eclampsia are severe headache, visual disturbances, and epigastric pain. These signs may indicate impending eclampsia.

Eclampsia is PIH that progresses to maternal convulsions. High maternal and fetal mortality and morbidity is associated with eclampsia.

PIH usually develops in the third trimester. An exception to this is found in molar pregnancies when severe PIH can develop during the first 20 weeks. The cause of PIH is unknown with theories including immunologic factors and abnormal prostaglandin synthesis. The only known cure is delivery.

RISK FACTORS

- Primigravida
- Primipaternity
- Maternal age <18 or >35
- Family hx of PIH
- Large uterine mass: multiple gestation, fetal hydrops (Rh sensitization), diabetes mellitus
- African-American heritage, hx chronic renal or vascular disease
- Molar pregnancy

COMPLICATIONS

- Complications are the result of vasospasm and vascular damage
- Congestive heart failure
- Cerebral: edema, ischemia, seizures, hemorrhage/ stroke → coma, death
- Pulmonary edema
- Portal hypertension → hepatic hematomas and rupture
- Retinal detachment
- Coagulopathy: HELLP, DIC
- Fetal hypoxia and malnutrition: IUGR, fetal distress
- Placental abruption

MEDICAL CARE

- Mild pre-eclampsia (BP <150/100, no evidence of IUGR): bed rest, evaluation twice a week
- BP sustained >150/100: hospitalization, bed rest
- Severe pre-eclampsia (BP ≥160/110, proteinuria, edema, ominous s/s: severe headache, visual disturbances, epigastric pain, oliguria): hospitalization, stabilization, and delivery (induction or cesarean)
- Medications—MgSO$_4$ IV or IM (prevents convulsions) and hydralazine (Apresoline) po, or IV (lower BP). Cervical ripening if indicated, pitocin induction, possibly betamethasone IM (induce fetal lung maturity)
- Laboratory tests: Hgb & Hct, platelets, serum creatinine, BUN, liver enzymes, coagulation studies, 24 hour urine for protein and creatinine clearance.
- Fetal testing: u/s, fetal size, NST, OCT, BPP, AFV, amniocentesis for lung maturity

COMMON NURSING DIAGNOSES

 ### See ANXIETY

Related to: Actual or perceived threat to biologic integrity of mother and fetus secondary to complication of pregnancy.

Defining Characteristics: Client expresses feelings of apprehension or nervousness (specify). Client exhibits physical signs of tension or anxiety (specify: e.g., trembling, diaphoresis, insomnia, etc.).

 ### See ACTIVITY INTOLERANCE

Related to: Prescribed bed rest secondary to hypertensive complication of pregnancy.

Defining Characteristics: Client exhibits increased BP >15 mm Hg with activity. Client reports weakness, fatigue (specify) after activity.

 ### See RISK FOR IMPAIRED GAS EXCHANGE: FETAL

Related to: Placental separation secondary to vascular damage and hypertension.

ADDITIONAL NURSING DIAGNOSES

RISK FOR INJURY: MATERNAL AND FETAL

Related to: Tonic–clonic convulsions.

Defining Characteristics: None, as this is a potential diagnosis.

Goal: Client and fetus will not experience injury from convulsions by (date/time to evaluate).

Outcome Criteria

✔ Client does not exhibit tonic–clonic convulsions, FHR remains between 110–160 without late decelerations.

NOC: *Symptom Control*

INTERVENTIONS	RATIONALES
Assess maternal BP, P, R (specify frequency: e.g., q 5–15 min, q h).	Assessment provides information about escalation of hypertension, that may precede convulsions.
Assess DTRs (specify frequency) and compare to baseline prenatal DTRs: 0 = no reflexes +1 = hyporeflexia +2 = normal DTR +3 = brisk DTR +4 = very brisk, with clonus	Hyperreflexia, especially with clonus, indicates cerebral irritation, which may precede convulsions. MgSO$_4$ toxicity may first be suspected with absent DTRs.
Assess for signs of worsening condition (specify timing): headache, N&V, visual disturbances, or epigastric pain.	Assessment provides information on increased CNS irritability and portal hypertension—ominous signs indicating imminent convulsions.
Provide decreased sensory stimulation: dim lights, provide a quiet atmosphere, limit visitors to significant other.	Interventions decrease cerebral stimulation. Significant other may provide reassurance and comfort.
Initiate and monitor MgSO$_4$ administration IV via pump or IM (Z-track) as ordered (specify dose & time). Report respiration <12 and d/c MgSO$_4$—support respirations and give calcium gluconate.	MgSO$_4$ is a CNS depressant that ↓ acetylcholine release at motor neurons that prevent convulsions. May cause resp. depression/arrest.
Inform client of expected side effects of IV administration: feeling of warmth.	Teaching prepares client for expected sensations to avoid anxiety.
Maintain strict bed rest. Keep side rails up (x4) and padded (with bath blankets), keep oral airway at bedside.	Interventions prevent injury from tonic–clonic movements. Airway is available to maintain airway during seizure.
Monitor magnesium levels as obtained: 6–8 mg/100 ml—therapeutic range 8–10 mg/100 ml—patellar DTR disappears 12+ mg/100 ml—respiratory depression	Monitoring levels provides information on therapeutic range and helps avoid magnesium toxicity or respiratory arrest.
Monitor hourly urine output and inform physician if <30 cc/hr.	The kidneys excrete MgSO$_4$—intervention prevents toxic accumulation.
Keep calcium gluconate at the bedside for emergency use.	Calcium reverses respiratory depression caused by magnesium toxicity.

(continues)

(continued)

INTERVENTIONS	RATIONALES
Administer antihypertensive medications as ordered (specify: e.g., hydralazine) and per protocol (e.g., give IVP slowly over 1 minute, assess BP q 2–3 minutes etc.).	Describe action of specific medications (e.g., hydralazine ↓ BP by direct action on arterial smooth muscle.
Implement continuous EFM and assess for changes in fetal well-being (specify frequency of documentation).	Fetal monitoring provides information about baseline rate or late decelerations. Convulsions may interrupt placental perfusion or lead to placental abruption.
Inform client and significant other about all procedures and medications provided.	Information decreases anxiety about unfamiliar therapies.
If client has a convulsion: insert the airway if possible, protect client from injury, note duration and activity during seizure, assess airway and fetal well-being after seizure, perform vaginal exam. Stay with client and have someone else notify the physician.	Interventions protect the client from injury; provide information about CNS activity during convulsion and fetal response; cervix may become completely dilated during a seizure.
Keep other caregivers (specify: e.g., perinatologist, neonatologist) informed of client and fetus condition.	Informing the caregivers ensures continuity of care and allows a team approach to ensure maternal/fetal well-being.

NIC: *Seizure Precautions*

Evaluation

(Date/time of evaluation of goal)

(Has goal been met? not met? partially met?)

(Has client had a convulsion? What is FHR baseline? Any late decelerations?)

(Revisions to care plan? D/C care plan? Continue care plan?)

DEFICIENT FLUID VOLUME

Related to: Fluid shift to the extravascular space secondary to ↓ plasma protein and colloid osmotic pressure.

Defining Characteristics: Edema (describe e.g., 3+ pitting, periorbital, etc.), abnormal weight gain (specify), ↓ urine output (described), ↑ hematocrit (specify) s/s pulmonary edema (specify: cough, rales, etc.).

Goal: Client will maintain intravascular fluid volume by (date/time to evaluate).

Outcome Criteria

✔ Client will exhibit decreased edema (specify: e.g., 2+ or less), increased urine output (specify hourly amount), hematocrit will return to normal for pregnancy (specify: e.g., <40%).

NOC: *Fluid Balance*

INTERVENTIONS	RATIONALES
Assess for edema (specify frequency): +1 = slight pedal and pretibial edema +2 = marked dependent edema +3 = edema of hands, face, periorbital area, sacrum +4 = anasarca with ascites	Assessment provides information on the extent of the fluid shift from intravascular to extravascular spaces. Provides information about improvement of condition.
Position client on her left side, maintain strict bed rest as ordered. Suggest client remove jewelry and give to significant other.	Left lateral positioning facilitates renal and placental perfusion. Jewelry may become constrictive with edema.
Insert Foley catheter (as ordered) and measure strict hourly intake and output, check urine specific gravity, and assess urine for protein.	Retention catheter provides information about urine output and fluid balance. Output <30 ml/hr or sp. gravity >1.040 indicates severe hypovolemia.
Maintain IV fluids via pump as ordered (specify fluid type and rate: e.g., LR at 60 cc/hr). Assess site (specify frequency) for redness, edema, or tenderness.	IV provides venous access and careful fluid replacement. Pump protects against accidental fluid overload. Assessment provides information about IV infiltration or infection.
(Assess & monitor hemodynamics via CVP line or Swan Ganz catheter if inserted. Norms: CVP—R atrium: 5–15 mm Hg; pulmonary artery wedge pressure—8–12 mm Hg.)	Assessment provides accurate measurement of intravascular fluid volume. Complications include trauma, infection, emboli, and cardiac dysrhythmias.
Auscultate lungs (specify frequency). Note any changes: for example, development of a cough or rales that don't clear after 2–3 deep breaths. Notify caregiver.	Assessment provides information about the development of pulmonary edema.

INTERVENTIONS	RATIONALES
Explain all procedures and rationales to client and significant other.	Explanation decreases anxiety about unfamiliar events.

NIC: *Fluid Monitoring*

Evaluation

(Date/time of evaluation of goal)

(Has goal been met? not met? partially met?)

(Describe edema, hourly urine output, and latest hematocrit level)

(Revisions to care plan? D/C care plan? Continue care plan?)

INEFFECTIVE TISSUE PERFUSION: CEREBRAL, HEPATIC, RENAL, PLACENTAL, PERIPHERAL

Related to: Vasospasm, coagulopathies secondary to vascular endothelial damage.

Defining Characteristics: Client reports (specify: severe headache, blurred vision or "seeing spots," nausea, epigastric pain, ↓ fetal movement). (Specify: hyper-reflexia [specify], oliguria [specify], proteinuria, IUGR, fetal distress, fetal demise, ↓ platelets, ↑ AST and ALT, bleeding gums, petichiae, etc.).

Goal: Client and fetus will experience adequate tissue perfusion by (date/time to evaluate).

Outcome Criteria

✔ Client will deny any headache, visual disturbances, or epigastric pain.

✔ Client will have platelet count >100,000/mm³, liver enzymes (AST & ALT) WNL (specify for lab), fetal heart rate will remain between 110–160 without late decelerations.

NOC: *Tissue Perfusion*

INTERVENTIONS	RATIONALES
Assess temp (q 2 h), BP, P, R (q 15–30 minutes or specify).	Assessment provides ongoing information about physiologic changes.
Assess LOC, monitor for severe headaches and hyperreflexia (specify frequency).	Assessment provides information about neurologic perfusion and irritation.

INTERVENTIONS	RATIONALES
Assess for nausea and vomiting, epigastric pain, or jaundice. Monitor lab work for liver enzymes (AST [SGOT] and ALT [SGPT]).	Assessment and monitoring provide information about hepatic perfusion, distention, portal hypertension, and liver damage.
Assess intake and urine output via Foley catheter, monitor urine sp. gravity and proteinuria. Monitor lab work as obtained: BUN, serum creatinine, and uric acid.	Assessment provides information about renal perfusion, GFR, and damage to glomerular endothelium.
Monitor fetal growth pattern using fundal height, serial ultrasound measurements (if provided).	Assessment provides information about placental perfusion and transfer of nutrients to the fetus.
Provide continuous EFM (if indicated). Monitor FHR for ↑ or ↓ baseline, wandering baseline, ↓ variability, or late decelerations. Notify caregiver.	Continuous EFM provides information about ↓ placental perfusion and impaired gas exchange to the fetus.
Assess client's skin condition, color, temperature, turgor, and edema (specify frequency).	Assessment provides information about client's peripheral perfusion.
Monitor client for HELLP syndrome: hemolysis, ↑ liver enzymes, and ↓ platelets.	HELLP syndrome may be associated with severe preeclampsia.
Monitor client for the development of disseminating intravascular coagulation (DIC): easy bruising, epistaxis, bleeding gums, hematuria, petechiae, or conjunctival hemorrhages.	Clients with PIH may develop DIC, which may result in spontaneous hemorrhage. Infection or fever reduces platelets further.
Administer acetaminophen as ordered for elevated temperature. Monitor for signs of infection.	Aspirin is thrombocytopenic. Acetaminophen does not affect platelets.
Keep client's caregiver informed of client's status and new information as obtained.	Client's condition may deteriorate quickly. Delivery is indicated with HELLP regardless of EGA.
Transfuse blood products and coagulation factors as ordered per agency protocol.	Intervention provides replacement of necessary blood and clotting components.
Provide emotional support to client and family. Explain all equipment and procedures. Arrange for health care providers to meet with client and family to discuss plans. Arrange for significant other (family) to tour NICU if indicated.	Illness and the potential for a poor outcome may frighten client and family. Knowledge decreases anxiety related to unfamiliar events and equipment.

NIC: *Circulatory Care*

Evaluation

(Date/time of evaluation of goal)

(Has goal been met? not met? partially met?)

(Does client deny any headache, visual disturbances, or epigastric pain? What is the platelet count? Are liver enzymes [AST and ALT] WNL [specify for lab]? What is FHR? Are there any late decelerations?)

(Revisions to care plan? D/C care plan? Continue care plan?)

DEFICIENT DIVERSIONAL ACTIVITY

Related to: Isolation and inability to engage in usual activity secondary to prolonged bed rest/hospitalization.

Defining Characteristics: Client reports boredom, depression (specify with quotes), flat affect, complaining, or appears disinterested.

Goal: Client will engage in diversionary activities as condition permits by (date/time to evaluate).

Outcome Criteria

✔ Client will plan and participate in three appropriate activities within limitations imposed by illness.

NOC: *Leisure Participation*

INTERVENTIONS	RATIONALES
Assess desired activities and limitations imposed by physician's order, or client condition.	Assessment provides information about client's desires and their congruency with the medical regimen.
Plan to spend quality time with client (specify: e.g., 1 hour each day).	Validates client's concerns and worth as a person.
Explain rationales for limitations to client and significant other.	Understanding rationale for limits improves compliance.
Assist client and significant other to develop a list of diversionary activities allowed in the plan of care.	Intervention involves client and significant other in plan of care.

INTERVENTIONS	RATIONALES
Suggest additional activities client may not think of: e.g., books on tape, music therapy, computer activities (Internet if available) and games, needlework, scrapbooks, and so forth.	Suggestions provide options for diversionary activities—stimulates thinking about additional ideas.
Suggest that client and family may like to decorate the hospital room with pictures, cards, window painting, and so forth.	Suggestions promote personalization of the environment and provide diversionary activity for the client.
Allow client to make decisions regarding timing of routine care whenever possible (e.g., bathe in the evening rather than morning).	Decision making promotes a sense of control over daily activities.
Encourage visitors (including children) if client's condition allows. Suggest scheduling visits throughout the day and evening—allow flexible hours.	Visitors provide social support. Scheduling avoids having all visitors come at once.
For clients with a small social support network, suggest having pastoral care or a volunteer come visit client.	Suggestion promotes social diversion for clients who have few visitors.
Consider allowing a favorite pet to visit in client's room.	Pet visits may help meet client's emotional needs and provide diversion.
Suggest an outing on a stretcher if condition allows and physician agrees.	A change of scenery may provide stimulation and diversion for client.
Suggest an occupational therapy referral for client (or play therapist if available, for an adolescent).	Referrals promote age-appropriate diversionary activity.

NIC: *Recreation Therapy*

Evaluation

(Date/time of evaluation of goal)

(Has goal been met? not met? partially met?)

(Has client planned and participated in at least three diversionary activities? Specify.)

(Revisions to care plan? D/C care plan? Continue care plan?)

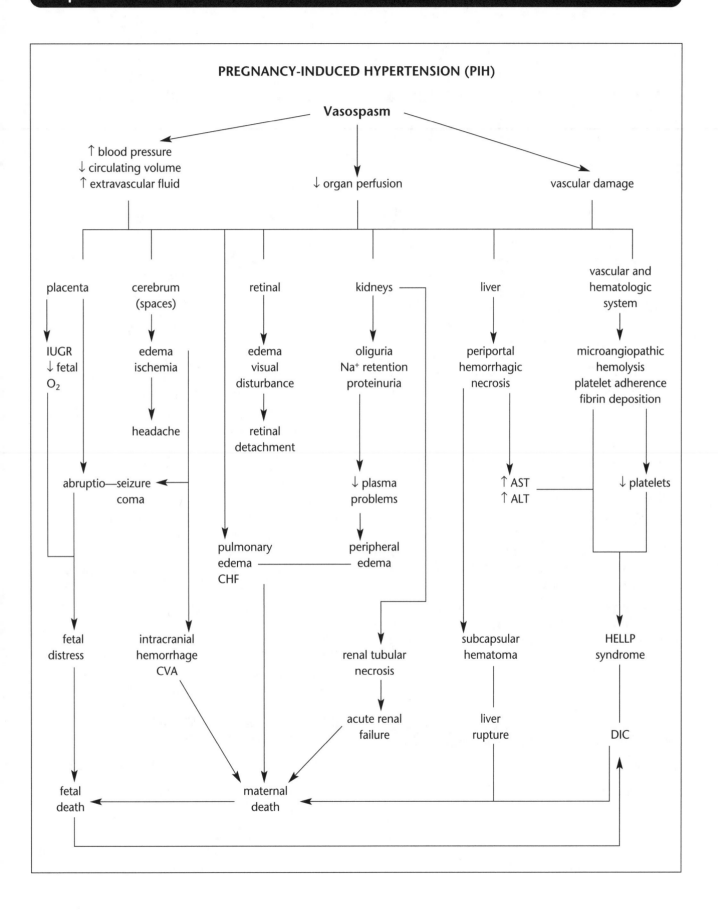

PREGNANCY-INDUCED HYPERTENSION (PIH)

Vasospasm

↑ blood pressure
↓ circulating volume
↑ extravascular fluid

↓ organ perfusion

vascular damage

placenta

cerebrum (spaces)

retinal

kidneys

liver

vascular and hematologic system

IUGR
↓ fetal O$_2$

edema ischemia

edema visual disturbance

oliguria
Na$^+$ retention
proteinuria

periportal hemorrhagic necrosis

microangiopathic hemolysis
platelet adherence
fibrin deposition

headache

retinal detachment

↓ plasma problems

abruptio—seizure coma

↑ AST
↑ ALT

↓ platelets

pulmonary edema
CHF

peripheral edema

fetal distress

intracranial hemorrhage
CVA

renal tubular necrosis

subcapsular hematoma

HELLP syndrome

acute renal failure

liver rupture

DIC

fetal death

maternal death

CHAPTER 1.12

PLACENTA PREVIA

Placenta previa is an abnormally low implantation of the placenta in proximity to the internal cervical os. As the cervix softens, late in the second trimester and then dilates, the placenta is pulled away, opening the blood-filled intervillous spaces and possibly rupturing placental vessels. The result is bleeding which may be mild or torrential. Often the first episode of bleeding is mild and resolves spontaneously. As pregnancy progresses however, the cervical changes increase, and bleeding episodes become more profuse. The classic sign of placenta previa is painless, bright red vaginal bleeding.

Placenta previa is classified as:

- Total previa—the placenta completely covers the internal cervical os
- Partial previa—the placenta covers a part of the internal cervical os
- Marginal previa—the edge of the placenta lies at the margin of the internal cervical os and may be exposed during dilatation
- Low-lying placenta—the placenta is implanted in the lower uterine segment but does not reach to the internal os of the cervix.

Low-lying placentas or previas diagnosed by ultrasound early in pregnancy often resolve as the uterus and placenta both grow. This is called placental migration. Previas noted after 30 weeks gestation are less likely to migrate and more likely to cause significant hemorrhage.

RISK FACTORS

- Advanced maternal age
- Multiparity
- Previous uterine surgery
- Large placenta (multiple gestation, erythroblastosis)
- Maternal smoking

MEDICAL CARE

- Ultrasound exams to determine migration of an early-diagnosed previa or classification of the previa as total, partial, marginal, or low-lying
- With a small first bleed, client may be sent home on bed rest if she can return to a hospital quickly.
- If bleeding is more profuse, client is hospitalized on bed rest with BRP, IV access; labs: Hgb & Hct, urinalysis, blood group and type and cross-match for 2 units of blood on hold, possible transfusions; goal is to maintain the pregnancy until fetal maturity.
- No vaginal exams are performed except under special conditions requiring a double set-up for immediate cesarean birth should hemorrhage result.
- Low-lying or marginal previas may be allowed to deliver vaginally if the fetal head acts as a tamponade to prevent hemorrhage.
- Cesarean birth, often with a vertical uterine incision, is used for total placenta previa.

COMMON NURSING DIAGNOSES

 See ACTIVITY INTOLERANCE

Related to: Enforced bed rest during pregnancy secondary to potential for hemorrhage.

Defining Characteristics: Specify: (e.g., client exhibits weakness, palpitations, dyspnea, confusion, etc.).

 See RISK FOR IMPAIRED GAS EXCHANGE: FETAL

Related to: Disruption of placental implantation.

See DEFICIENT DIVERSIONAL ACTIVITY

Related to: Inability to engage in usual activities secondary to enforced bed rest and inactivity during pregnancy.

Defining Characteristics: Specify: (e.g., client states she is bored or depressed about bed rest. Client exhibits flat affect, appears inattentive, yawning, is restless, etc.).

ADDITIONAL NURSING DIAGNOSES

 ### DEFICIENT FLUID VOLUME: MATERNAL

Related to: Active blood loss secondary to disrupted placental implantation.

Defining Characteristics: Describe bleeding episode (amount, duration, painless/painful, abdomen soft/hard), ↓ BP, ↑ P & R ↓ urine output (specify values), pale, cool skin, ↑ capillary refill (specify).

Goal: Client will exhibit improved fluid balance by (date/time to evaluate).

Outcome Criteria

✔ Client will experience no further vaginal bleeding; pulse <100; BP > (specify for individual client); capillary refill <3 seconds.

NOC: *Fluid Balance*

INTERVENTIONS	RATIONALES
Assess color, odor, consistency, and amount of vaginal bleeding: weigh pads (1 g = 1 cc).	Provides information about active bleeding versus old blood, tissue loss, and degree of blood loss.
Assess hourly intake and output.	Provides information about maternal and fetal physiologic compensation for blood loss.
Assess BP and P (specify frequency) and note changes. Monitor FHR.	Assessment provides information about possible infection, placenta previa, or abruption. Increasing abdominal girth suggests active abruption.
Assess abdomen for tenderness or rigidity—if present, measure abdomen at umbilicus (specify frequency). Assess temperature (specify: e.g., q 2–4h).	Assessment provides information about development of infection. Warm, moist, bloody environment is ideal for growth of microorganisms.
Assess SaO₂, skin color, temperature, moisture, turgor, and capillary refill (specify frequency).	Assessment provides information about blood volume, O_2 saturation, and peripheral perfusion.

INTERVENTIONS	RATIONALES
Assess for changes in LOC; note complaints of thirst or apprehension.	Assessment provides information about cerebral perfusion.
Provide supplemental humidified oxygen as ordered via face mask or nasal cannula at 10–12 L/min.	Intervention increases available oxygen to saturate decreased hemoglobin.
Initiate IV fluids as ordered (specify the fluid type and rate).	IV replacement of lost vascular volume.
Position client supine with hips elevated if ordered or left lateral position if stable (specify).	Position decreases pressure on placenta and cervical os. Left lateral position improves placental perfusion.
Monitor lab work as obtained: Hgb & Hct, Rh and type, cross-match for 2 units RBCs, urinalysis, etc. Arrange portable ultrasound as ordered.	Lab work provides information about degree of blood loss; prepares for possible transfusion. Ultrasound provides information about the cause of bleeding.
Determine if client has any objections to blood transfusions—inform physician.	Client may have religious beliefs related to accepting blood products.
Administer blood transfusions as ordered with client consent per agency procedure (specify).	Provides replacement of blood components and volume.
Monitor closely for transfusion reaction following agency policy and procedures (specify).	Potentially life-threatening allergic reaction may result from incompatible blood.
Provide emotional support; keep client and family informed of findings and continuing plan of care.	Support and information decrease anxiety and help client and family to anticipate what might happen next.
Administer prenatal vitamins and iron as ordered; provide a diet high in iron: lean meats, dark green leafy vegetables, eggs, whole grains.	Diet and vitamins replace nutrient losses from active bleeding to prevent anemia—iron is a necessary component of hemoglobin.
(Prepare client for cesarean birth if ordered: e.g., severe hemorrhage, abruption, complete previa at term, etc.)	Cesarean birth may be necessary to resolve the hemorrhage or prevent fetal or maternal injury.

NIC: *Hypovolemia Management*

Evaluation

(Date/time of evaluation of goal)

(Has goal been met? not met? partially met?)

(When was last bleeding noted? What is client's BP, P, capillary refill time?)

(Revisions to care plan? D/C care plan? Continue care plan?)

FEAR

Related to: Threat to maternal and/or fetal survival secondary to excessive blood loss.

Defining Characteristics: Specify (Client states she is frightened [quotes]; client is crying, trembling, eyes are dilated. Client complains of muscle tension, dry mouth, palpitations, inability to concentrate, etc.).

Goal: Client will exhibit decreased fear by (date/time to evaluate).

Outcome Criteria

✔ Client will identify her fears and methods to cope with each.

✔ Client will report a decrease in fearfulness.

NOC: *Fear Control*

INTERVENTIONS	RATIONALES
Provide adequate time for discussion and a calm environment.	Calm environment and unhurried discussion promote a decrease in anxiety.
Validate the perception that the client, family are feeling fearful.	Validation provides information about client's behavior.
Assist client and family to identify specific fears.	Assistance allows identification of frightening thoughts.
Listen actively to client and family's perception of threat.	Active listening promotes understanding of client and family's perceptions.

INTERVENTIONS	RATIONALES
Provide accurate and honest information about client's condition and expected plan of care.	Fears may be based on unrealistic imaginings or misunderstanding.
Assist client and family to identify ways to cope with fears (e.g., preparation for getting to the hospital quickly should bleeding begin).	Planning a response to cope with situation may alleviate feelings of helplessness.
Suggest and teach relaxation techniques, creative visualization, etc.	Interventions promote relaxation and a sense of control.
Assess degree of fearfulness after discussion. Validate client's feelings and plan for further discussion as needed.	Evaluates effectiveness of teaching and discussion. Provides continual support.
Arrange for other health providers to talk with client as appropriate (specify: e.g., pastoral care, NICU staff, etc.).	Increased information may help client and family to feel calmer about possible outcomes.

NIC: *Coping Enhancement*

Evaluation

(Date/time of evaluation of goal)

(Has goal been met? not met? partially met?)

(List fears client verbalized. Does client report a decrease in fearfulness?)

(Revisions to care plan? D/C care plan? Continue care plan?)

PLACENTA PREVIA

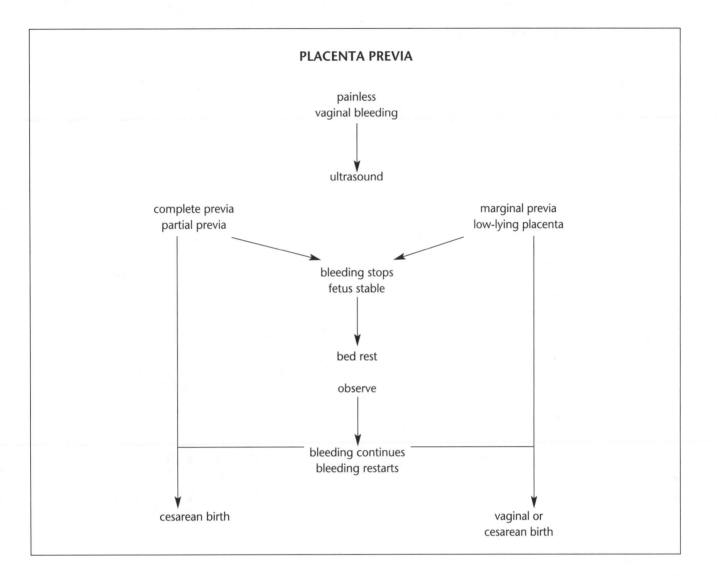

painless
vaginal bleeding

↓

ultrasound

complete previa   marginal previa
partial previa   low-lying placenta

bleeding stops
fetus stable

↓

bed rest

observe

↓

bleeding continues
bleeding restarts

cesarean birth   vaginal or
                                                   cesarean birth

CHAPTER 1.13

MULTIPLE GESTATION

The incidence of multi-fetal pregnancies is increasing because of use of drugs that induce ovulation and other infertility technologies such as in vitro fertilization (IVF).

The fetuses may either be monozygotic (identical) resulting from one ovum that divides, or dizygotic (fraternal) where more than one ovum is released and fertilized. This can be determined by examination of the placenta(s) and membranes or DNA studies after birth. Monozygotic twins are at greater risk for discordancy (twin-to-twin transfusion) and cord entanglement.

PHYSIOLOGIC RISKS

- Spontaneous abortion, malformations
- Preterm birth, LBW
- Abnormal growth: discordancy, IUGR
- Increased incidence of PIH
- Maternal anemia, PP hemorrhage
- Placenta and cord accidents
- Abnormal fetal presentation

MEDICAL CARE

- Close observation: prenatal visits q 2 weeks until 26 weeks, then weekly.
- Serial (monthly) ultrasounds to assess growth of each fetus and try to determine if monozygotic or dizygotic fetuses.
- Increased iron (60–100 mg) and folic acid (1 mg) is usually prescribed.
- Maternal hemoglobin may be checked each trimester.
- Tests for fetal well-being beginning at 30 weeks—NST, BPP, possibly Doppler flow studies and amniocentesis to determine L/S ratios.

- More frequent vaginal exams to rule out preterm effacement and dilatation of cervix.
- Bed rest may be prescribed from 28–30 weeks (earlier if cervical changes are noted) until birth.
- Cesarean birth is planned for about 50% of twin pregnancies, and for almost all with greater numbers of babies because of abnormal presentations.

COMMON NURSING DIAGNOSES

 See BASIC CARE PLAN: HEALTHY PREGNANCY

Increase calorie intake by 300 kcal per fetus per day. (Twin pregnancy should gain 40–45 pounds.)

 See BASIC CARE PLAN: PRENATAL HOME VISIT

 See DEFICIENT KNOWLEDGE: PRETERM LABOR PREVENTION

Related to: Inexperience with multiple gestation pregnancy.

Defining Characteristics: Client has not experienced preterm labor before, is unaware of sensations of PTL. Client is at increased risk for preterm birth: multiple gestation (specify: twins, triplets, etc.).

 See RISK FOR IMPAIRED GAS EXCHANGE: FETAL

Related to: Decreased oxygen supply secondary to complications of multiple gestation (specify: monozygotic multiple pregnancy, cord entanglement, placental insufficiency, twin-to-twin transfusion, etc.).

ADDITIONAL NURSING DIAGNOSES

 ANXIETY

Related to: Fears for well-being of mother and fetus secondary to complicated pregnancy.

Defining Characteristics: Client verbalizes anxiety about pregnancy outcome (specify: feels physically threatened, afraid babies will die, can't sleep, etc.). Client rates anxiety as a (specify) on a scale of 1 to 10 with 1 being no anxiety and 10 being the most.

Goal: Client will demonstrate a ↓ in anxiety by (date and time to evaluate).

Outcome Criteria

✔ Client will rate anxiety as a (specify) or less on a scale of 1 to 10 with 1 being least, 10 most.

✔ Client will appear calm (specify: not crying, no tremors, HR <100, etc.).

NOC: *Anxiety Control*

INTERVENTIONS	RATIONALES
Assess for physical signs of anxiety: tremors, palpitations, tachycardia, dry mouth, nausea, or diaphoresis.	Anxiety may cause the "fight or flight" sympathetic response. Some cultures prohibit verbal expression of anxiety.
Assess for mental and emotional signs of anxiety at each visit: nervousness, crying, difficulty with concentration or memory, and so forth.	Anxiety may interfere with normal mental and emotional functioning.
Ask client to rate anxiety on a scale of 1 to 10 with 1 being calm and 10 very anxious.	Rating allows measurement of anxiety level and changes.
Provide reassurance and support: acknowledge anxiety, allow time for discussion, and use touch (if culturally appropriate).	Severe anxiety may interfere with the client's ability to take in information. These measures may help ↓ anxiety levels.
Ask client how she usually copes with anxiety and discuss if this would be helpful now.	Allows identification of adaptive coping mechanisms versus maladaptive (e.g., smoking, alcohol, etc.).
Encourage client to involve significant other(s) in attempts to identify and cope with anxiety.	Significant others are also under stress during complicated pregnancy.
When client is calmer, validate concerns and provide client with factual information about complications of pregnancy and what will be done to lessen the risks (specify: NST, BPP, bed rest, perinatologist, etc.).	Client may be overly fearful. Understanding empowers the client to participate in her own care by understanding the risks and treatment options that may be offered.
Assist client to plan coping strategies for anxiety during	Developing a plan to address anxiety promotes a sense of

INTERVENTIONS	RATIONALES
pregnancy. Suggest the following possibilities: breathing and relaxation, creative imagery, music, biofeedback, talking to self, and so forth (suggest others).	control, which enhances coping ability.
Arrange a tour of the NICU if appropriate. Prepare client and significant other for what they will see and hear in the unit.	Familiarity decreases fear of the unknown. Preparation decreases anxiety.
Provide information about counseling or support groups as appropriate (specify: groups for parents of multiple gestation, congenital anomalies, etc.).	Severe anxiety may require individual counseling. Support groups provide reassurance and coping strategies.

NIC: *Anxiety Reduction*

Evaluation

(Date/time of evaluation of goal)

(Has goal been met? not met? partially met?)

(How does client rate her anxiety now? Does client appear calm? Specify: not crying, smiling, pulse 72, etc.)

(Revisions to care plan? D/C care plan? Continue care plan?)

ACTIVITY INTOLERANCE

Related to: Prescribed bed rest during pregnancy.

Defining Characteristics: Client reports (specify: weakness, fatigue, difficulty concentrating, etc.). Client is physically de-conditioned (specify: has lost weight, short of breath, weak pulse, etc.). Client reports psychological symptoms (specify: boredom, depression, etc.).

Goal: Client will experience minimal negative effects from enforced bed rest during pregnancy by (date/time to evaluate).

Outcome Criteria

✔ Client will participate in exercises for bed rest as approved by her care provider.

✔ Client will identify three activities to combat boredom and depression during bed rest.

NOC: *Activity Tolerance*

INTERVENTIONS	RATIONALES
Plan time to spend with client (specify: e.g., 15 minutes q shift if hospitalized), sit down, listen actively to client's concerns.	Clients report that caring and empathy from nurses is most helpful.
Assess client's perception of the need for bed rest; correct any misunderstandings. Reinforce positive outlook.	Intervention assists client to comply with bed rest. Thinking about helping the baby helps the client to tolerate enforced bed rest.
Assess BP, pulse, breath sounds, and muscle strength (specify time frame). Ask client how she feels physically (e.g., weak, tired, nauseated, s.o.b., etc.).	Bed rest results in ↓ cardiac output, ↓ aerobic capacity, muscle atrophy, ↓ GI motility, and fluid and electrolyte changes.
Assess client's perception of the main stresses of bed rest (e.g., boredom, role strain, sleep disturbance, etc.).	Isolation and confinement may lead to emotional and family conflict. Sleep disturbances are common as client naps during the day.
Assist client to plan three activities she can do in bed to cope with the stresses (specify: reading, writing lists, phone calls, music, TV, needlework, etc.).	Planning empowers the client to take control of her situation and plan individualized activities to cope with the stresses of bed rest.
Teach client to eat 6 small meals a day, rather than 3 large ones. Include 8 glasses of water a day, increase intake of fiber and fresh fruits and vegetables.	Decreased appetite, wt. loss, indigestion, heartburn, and constipation are common with prolonged bed rest.
Teach client to avoid lying flat on her back: side-lying or high Fowler's (if permitted) are preferred.	Supine position may cause uterine compression of the inferior vena cava, which can lead to hypotension and fetal distress.

INTERVENTIONS	RATIONALES
Collaborate with client's health provider to have a physio-therapist (PT) teach client exercises that can be done on bed rest.	Intervention provides safe exercise to ↓ the ill effects of bed rest. Exercises need to be chosen that don't stimulate contractions.
Review and reinforce exercises (specify when: e.g., at each visit).	Review and reinforcement provide feedback to client about performing exercises correctly.
Share with caregiver recent research indicating that bed rest is not necessarily beneficial during complicated pregnancy.	Discussion promotes research-based practice. The nurse acts as a client advocate.

NIC: *Energy Management*

Evaluation

(Date/time of evaluation of goal)

(Has goal been met? not met? partially met?)

(Does client exercise as prescribed? Describe routine, times, etc.)

(Which three activities has client identified to combat the boredom and depression of bed rest?)

(Revisions to care plan? D/C care plan? Continue care plan?)

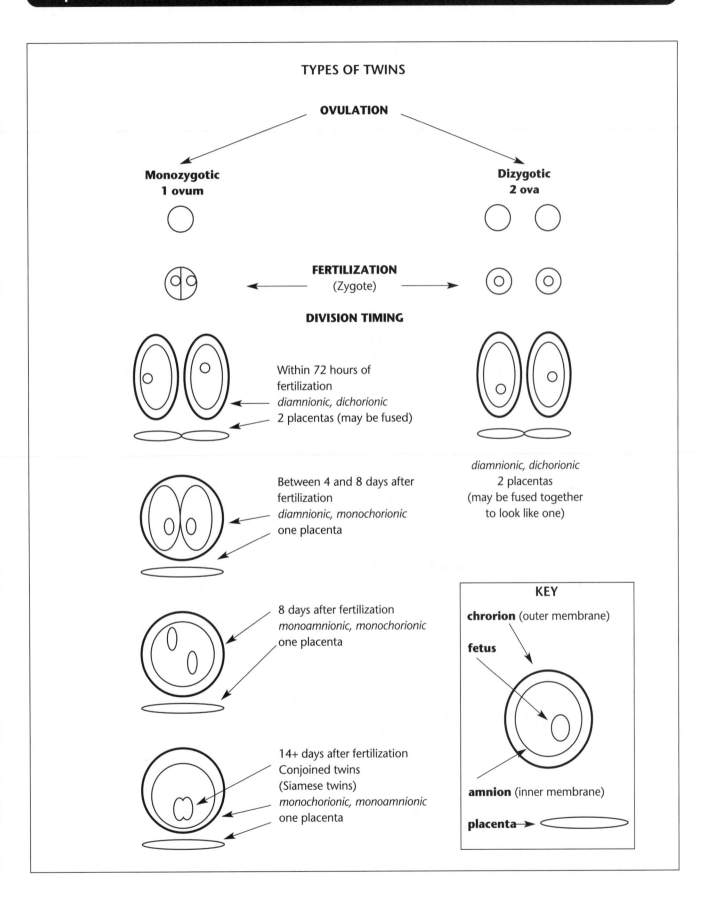

TYPES OF TWINS

OVULATION

Monozygotic
1 ovum

Dizygotic
2 ova

FERTILIZATION
(Zygote)

DIVISION TIMING

Within 72 hours of
fertilization
diamnionic, dichorionic
2 placentas (may be fused)

diamnionic, dichorionic
2 placentas
(may be fused together
to look like one)

Between 4 and 8 days after
fertilization
diamnionic, monochorionic
one placenta

8 days after fertilization
monoamnionic, monochorionic
one placenta

14+ days after fertilization
Conjoined twins
(Siamese twins)
monochorionic, monoamnionic
one placenta

KEY

chrorion (outer membrane)

fetus

amnion (inner membrane)

placenta

CHAPTER 1.14

PRETERM LABOR

A term pregnancy lasts from 38 to 42 weeks after the LNMP. Preterm labor refers to progressive uterine contractions, after 20 weeks and before 38 weeks gestation, that result in cervical change (effacement and dilatation). Preterm is a description of fetal age, not maturity or size.

Preterm birth is the number one cause of neonatal morbidity and mortality. Preterm birth may result from preterm labor, spontaneous preterm rupture of membranes, or the baby may be delivered early because of severe maternal or fetal illness. Infants born between 24 and 34 weeks have the highest incidence of complications. Complications may result in permanent physical and mental disabilities. Advances in neonatal intensive care have resulted in improved outcomes for infants born after 24 weeks of gestation.

The exact cause of preterm labor is unknown as is the exact mechanism that begins term labor. All pregnant women should be assessed for risk factors and monitored carefully during pregnancy.

RISK FACTORS

- Previous preterm labor or birth
- Infection: maternal or fetal
- Chronic maternal illnesses: heart disease, kidney disease, diabetes mellitus
- Uterine or cervical anomalies or scarring, DES exposure, trauma, abdominal surgery
- Pregnancy factors: multiple gestation, ↑ amniotic fluid (hydramnios), PIH, placenta previa or abruption, SROM
- Low socioeconomic status

MEDICAL CARE

- Frequent prenatal visits and assessments for clients at risk

- Home uterine monitoring, decreased activity, bed rest, po tocolytics, subcutaneous terbutaline pump
- Hospitalization, hydration, antibiotics as indicated
- Tocolytics: $MgSO_4$, ß-adrenergic receptor agonists (ritodrine, terbutaline), others: prostaglandin inhibitors, calcium channel blockers
- Testing: urinalysis, GBS, fetal fibronectin, u/s amniocentesis: L/S ratio, phosphatidylglycerol
- Corticosteroids to ↑ fetal lung maturity
- Cervical cerclage for incompetent cervix

COMMON NURSING DIAGNOSES

See ANXIETY

Related to: Threat to fetal well-being secondary to preterm labor/SROM.

Defining Characteristics: Specify: (e.g., client is trembling, eyes dilated, shaking, crying, etc. Client verbalizes anxiety about fetal well-being).

See ACTIVITY INTOLERANCE

Related to: Prescribed bed rest or decreased activity secondary to threat of preterm labor.

Defining Characteristics: Specify: (e.g., client reports feelings of weakness, fatigue, shortness of breath, etc.).

See DEFICIENT DIVERSIONAL ACTIVITY

Related to: Inability to engage in usual activities secondary to attempts to avoid preterm labor and birth.

Defining Characteristics: Specify: (e.g., client reports feelings of boredom or depression related to bed rest or lack of activity).

ADDITIONAL NURSING DIAGNOSES

 ### RISK FOR INJURY: MATERNAL/FETAL

Related to: Risk for preterm birth. Adverse effects of drugs used to prevent preterm birth.

Defining Characteristics: None, as this is a potential diagnosis.

Goal: Client and fetus will not experience preterm birth or injury from drugs used to stop preterm labor by (date/time to evaluate).

Outcome Criteria

✔ Contractions will stop. FHR will remain 110–160 with accelerations. No cervical change.

✔ Client's BP will remain >100/70 (or specify for client), pulse <120 (or specify), respirations >14, DTRs 2+ (or specify for client).

NOC: *Symptom Control*

INTERVENTIONS	RATIONALES
Position client on left side as much as tolerated. Change to right side if client becomes uncomfortable—avoid supine position.	Positioning facilitates uteroplacental perfusion. Supine position causes compression of the inferior vena cava by the heavy uterus, ↓ blood flow to the heart and ↓ BP and placental perfusion.
Explain all procedures and equipment to client and significant other. Provide accurate information while providing emotional support.	Client and significant other may be experiencing high anxiety and need repeated explanations.
Place external fetal monitor on client; also assess uterine contractions by palpation to determine frequency, intensity, and duration (specify frequency).	External tocodynamometer does not provide information on contraction intensity, may not show preterm labor contractions.
Assess FHR for baseline rate, variability, accelerations, or decelerations (specify frequency).	Assessment provides information about fetal well-being.
Perform sterile vaginal exam if indicated (as ordered)—limit exams.	Vaginal exam provides information about fetal presentation and labor progress—excessive exams may introduce infection or stimulate labor.

INTERVENTIONS	RATIONALES
Place client on cardiac monitor if ordered. Obtain baseline vital signs. Monitor for tachycardia or dysrhythmias.	Beta-adrenergic agonists (ritodrine, terbutaline) may cause hypotension from relaxation of smooth muscle resulting in tachycardia and additional stress on the heart.
Start an IV with designated fluids (specify) at ordered rate (specify) via IV pump. Provide bolus if ordered then reduce rate as ordered (specify).	Provides venous access, hydration, and a port for piggyback medications.
Prepare piggyback IV tocolytic medication as ordered or per policy (specify: e.g., drug strength, dose, IV solution). Piggyback tocolytic to mainline IV and begin infusion via pump at designated rate (specify loading dose and titration).	Careful preparation of tocolytic drugs ensures the proper dose will be given. Piggyback allows the drug to be discontinued while maintaining venous access. Pump ensures the client receives the right dose.
Teach client about side effects of the drugs; (specify: MgSO$_4$ causes feelings of warmth, flushing, terbutaline or ritodrine may cause ↓ BP, tachycardia (mom and baby), feeling "jittery," possible N&V).	Teaching prepares client for unfamiliar sensations, ↓ anxiety for client.
Monitor maternal vital signs, breath sounds, and DTRs as ordered or per protocol for drug (specify).	Monitoring provides information about response to drug.
Monitor hourly I&O—notify physician if output <30 cc/hr. Assess skin turgot, mucous membranes (specify frequency).	Monitoring provides information about fluid balance. Adequate renal function is necessary for excretion of the drugs.
Apply TED hose if ordered.	Compression stockings facilitate venous return from extremities.
Discontinue tocolytic and notify physician if signs of complications develop (specify: for ß-adrenergics, chest pain, >6 PVCs/hr, s.o.b., maternal HR >140, FHR >200, etc.; for MgSO$_4$, respirations <12, absent DTRs, etc.).	Discontinuing the drug prevents serious complications from tocolytic medications: cardiac dysrhythmias, pulmonary edema, and respiratory depression.
Monitor labs as obtained noting potassium and glucose levels if ß-adrenergics are used, magnesium level if MgSO$_4$ is used (specify).	Monitoring labs provides information about complications of drug therapy: hyperglycemia, hypokalemia, and magnesium toxicity.

(continues)

(continued)

INTERVENTIONS	RATIONALES
Keep antidotes to medications at bedside (specify: calcium gluconate for MgSO$_4$, beta-blockers may be used for ß-adrenergic tocolytics).	Antidotes reverse the action of drugs (specify for drug used).
Administer p.o. tocolytics as ordered (specify: when, drug, dose, and time).	(Describe action of p.o. tocolytic.) Allows client to be maintained without IV meds.
Provide and monitor results of fetal testing as ordered: amniocentesis for L/S ratio, PGs, NST, etc.	Fetal testing provides information on fetal maturity and well-being.
Administer glucocorticoids IM as ordered (specify: dose, timing). Explain rationale to parents.	Glucocorticoids may be given between 28–34 weeks and delivery delayed for 24–48 hours in an attempt to hasten fetal lung maturity.
Arrange for a NICU nurse to talk with client and family about preterm infants and the NICU environment.	Consultation provides anticipatory information to client at risk for preterm birth.
Ensure that all involved health care providers are kept informed of client's status.	An informed health care team ensures readiness and continuity.

NIC: *Medication Management*

Evaluation

(Date/time of evaluation of goal)

(Has goal been met? not met? partially met?)

(Have contractions stopped? Is FHR between 110–160 with accelerations? What are client's v/s: BP, P, R, and DTRs?)

(Revisions to care plan? D/C care plan? Continue care plan?)

 ## DEFICIENT KNOWLEDGE: PRETERM LABOR PREVENTION

Related to: Unfamiliarity with preterm labor (signs/symptoms, and prevention).

Defining Characteristics: Client reports that she doesn't know the s/s of preterm labor (specify with quote). Client is at risk for preterm labor (specify: substance abuse, multiple gestation, IDDM, etc.).

Goal: Client will verbalize ↑ knowledge about preterm labor by (date/time to evaluate).

Outcome Criteria

✔ Client will describe s/s of preterm labor (specify: regular contractions, lower back pain, pelvic pressure, cramps, etc.).

✔ Client will describe steps to take to avoid preterm labor (specify: drink 2–3 quarts/day, void q 2h, stop smoking, report early s/s UTI, etc.).

NOC: *Knowledge: Labor and Delivery*

INTERVENTIONS	RATIONALES
Assess client's risk factors for preterm labor, education level, and ability to understand teaching (provide interpreter if needed).	Assessment provides information to guide planning an individualized teaching program to ensure client understanding.
Provide a comfortable quiet setting for teaching—invite family to participate in session(s).	Interventions decrease distractions and promote learning; family may reinforce teaching and help client comply.
Assess client's understanding of the risks of preterm labor and birth for her baby.	Some clients may believe that preterm infants have few problems or that 7 month babies do better than 8 month gestations (old wives' tale).
Correct any misconceptions and provide information on fetal lung development.	Accurate information encourages compliance.
Help client to identify Braxton–Hicks contractions she may be experiencing: if she says she doesn't have any, ask her if the baby ever "balls up" (or other terms to help understanding) and explain that this is a contraction.	Assistance empowers the client to recognize mild uterine contractions. Many women are unaware that Braxton–Hicks are contractions even if they are not painful.
Teach client to palpate Braxton–Hicks contractions at the fundus, moving fingertips around. Teach to time frequency of contractions from the start of one contraction to the beginning of the next. Praise efforts.	Teaching promotes self-care and assessment skills. The fundus is the thickest part of the uterus where contractions are most easily felt.
Teach client to lie down on her left side 2 or 3 times a day and palpate for contractions noting fetal movements ("kick counts") and to keep a journal of findings.	Teaching promotes awareness of sensations of contractions and fetal movement. Journal provides a written record of activity.
Teach client other s/s of preterm labor to report: dull low back	Teaching empowers client to recognize subtle signs of preterm

INTERVENTIONS	RATIONALES
pain, pelvic pressure, abdominal cramping with or without diarrhea, or an increase in vaginal discharge (especially if watery or bloody); other s/s of infection.	labor. Client may not experience contractions as such.
Teach client s/s of urinary tract infections to report: frequency, urgency or burning on urination. Teach to wash hands and wipe from front to back after using the bathroom.	Urinary tract infections may precede preterm labor. Hand washing and wiping front to back prevents fecal contamination of urethra or vagina.
Instruct client to drink a glass of water or juice every hour, or 2–3 quarts/day and to void at least every 2h while awake.	Dehydration or a distended bladder may increase uterine irritability/activity.
Teach client to avoid overexertion, heavy lifting, or staying in one position for long periods (sitting or standing). Have employer contact physician if this is a problem.	Teaching helps client avoid ligament and muscle strain, changing position facilitates circulation, uteroplacental perfusion, and venous return.
Instruct client to avoid nipple stimulation and possibly avoid sexual intercourse or to use condoms as advised by caregiver.	Instruction avoids activity that may cause the release of oxytocin from posterior pituitary gland. Semen contains prostaglandins that may affect uterine activity.
Teach proper administration of p.o. tocolytics if ordered (specify: drug, dose, route, times, etc.). Teach side effects to call physician for (specify).	(Describe action of specific drug as it relates to uterine activity. Specify why these side effects are dangerous.)
Arrange for additional teaching if terbutaline pump and/or home uterine monitoring is to be used.	Additional instruction provides information the client needs if these modalities are ordered.

INTERVENTIONS	RATIONALES
Encourage client to stop smoking if indicated—refer to support group or smoking cessation program.	Smoking has been implicated in preterm labor.
Instruct client that if she feels an unusual increase in contractions to drink a large glass of water and lie down on her left side. If pattern continues for 20–30 minutes or becomes more intense to call the physician or go to the hospital for evaluation.	Instruction allows client to have some control over evaluation of preterm labor.
Praise client and family for ability to comply with instructions and reinforce that each day labor is held off is another day for her baby's lungs to mature.	Provides encouragement and incentive for compliance.
Provide pamphlets, books, videos, and refer client and family to support groups if available.	Reinforces teaching, may provide additional coping ideas.

NIC: *Teaching, Individual*

Evaluation

(Date/time of evaluation of goal)

(Has goal been met? not met? partially met?)

(What signs of preterm labor can client identify? What steps to avoid preterm labor does client verbalize?)

(Revisions to care plan? D/C care plan? Continue care plan?)

PRETERM LABOR

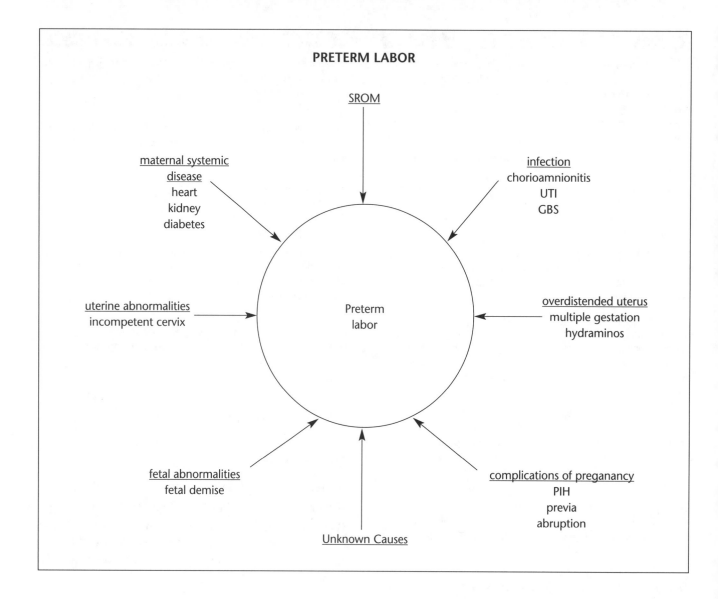

SROM

maternal systemic
disease
heart
kidney
diabetes

infection
chorioamnionitis
UTI
GBS

uterine abnormalities
incompetent cervix

Preterm
labor

overdistended uterus
multiple gestation
hydraminos

fetal abnormalities
fetal demise

complications of preganancy
PIH
previa
abruption

Unknown Causes

CHAPTER 1.15

PRETERM RUPTURE OF MEMBRANES

Preterm rupture of the fetal membranes describes ruptured membranes before 38 weeks of gestation. The term refers to the gestational age of the fetus at the time of rupture. Premature rupture of membranes (PROM) describes membrane rupture before the onset of labor. PROM may occur with either term or preterm gestations. The terminology for ruptured membranes with no labor before 38 weeks gestation would be preterm premature rupture of membranes or PPROM.

Like preterm labor, the exact cause of preterm rupture of membranes is unknown. Infection, which may not be clinically apparent, is often implicated and is also one of the most serious complications.

COMPLICATIONS

- Gross rupture early in pregnancy: amputation deformities from adhesion of amnion (amniotic bands) to fetal parts; musculoskeletal deformities from fetal compression; pulmonary hypoplasia
- Infection: chorioamnionitis; maternal postpartum endometritis; neonatal sepsis
- Abnormal presentation (breech, transverse lie)
- Prolapsed cord
- Possible abruption
- Severe decelerations during labor from cord compression

RISK FACTORS

- Maternal/fetal infection: UTI; cervicitis
- Overdistended uterus: multiple gestation, polyhydraminos
- Preterm labor and factors that cause preterm labor
- Incompetent cervix
- Maternal trauma

MEDICAL CARE

- Confirmation of rupture of membranes: nitrazine test; sterile speculum exam to visualize fluid and cervix; ferning test of fluid
- Determination of gestational age of fetus: LNMP, ultrasound measurements, and possible amniocentesis to determine L/S ratio and presence of PG
- Expectant management: monitor for infection and contractions—may discharge to home on bed rest with BRP after stabilization
- Urinalysis and daily CBC
- Vaginal cultures for gonorrhea, group B streptococcus; possible antibiotic therapy if positive; if infection is evident, the fetus is delivered by induction or cesarean
- Serial fetal testing: daily NST, biophysical profiles (BPP), ultrasound estimation of amniotic fluid index (AFI), possible weekly amniocentesis for lung maturity
- May give corticosteroids (betamethasone) to enhance fetal lung maturation—may use tocolytics to prevent birth for 24 to 48 hours after administration
- If fetus is mature, may carefully induce labor after waiting 12 hours for labor to ensue naturally

COMMON NURSING DIAGNOSES

See ANXIETY

Related to: Threat to maternal or fetal well-being secondary to risk for infection or preterm birth.

Defining Characteristics: Specify: (Client reports increased worry and anxiety. Client exhibits difficulty remembering information, crying, etc.).

See ACTIVITY INTOLERANCE

Related to: Enforced bed rest during complicated pregnancy.

Defining Characteristics: Specify: (Client reports feeling weak or tired; decreased muscle tone, constipation, etc.).

 ## See DEFICIENT DIVERSIONAL ACTIVITY

Related to: Inability to engage in usual activity due to enforced bed rest.

Defining Characteristics: Client reports boredom, depression (specify). Client exhibits withdrawal, sleeps more than usual, etc. (specify).

 ## See RISK FOR INJURY: MATERNAL/FETAL

Related to: Tocolytic drugs used to delay birth for administration of glucocorticoids.

ADDITIONAL NURSING DIAGNOSES

 ## RISK FOR INFECTION: MATERNAL/FETAL

Related to: Site for organism invasion secondary to preterm rupture of fetal membranes.

Defining Characteristics: None, as this is a potential diagnosis.

Goal: Client and fetus will not experience infection related to preterm rupture of membranes by (date/time to evaluate).

Outcome Criteria

✔ Client's temperature will be <99.5° F, amniotic fluid will remain clear with no offensive odor.

NOC: *Risk Control*

INTERVENTIONS	RATIONALES
Confirm rupture by testing external fluid (no vaginal exams) with nitrazine paper. Note date and time of rupture.	Positive nitrazine test provides documentation of rupture date and time. Vaginal exam might introduce microorganisms.

INTERVENTIONS	RATIONALES
Apply external fetal monitor; assess fetal well-being and palpate for uterine contractions (specify frequency of monitoring).	Assessment provides information about fetal well-being and preterm labor.
Assist caregiver with sterile speculum exam, ferning test, and vaginal cultures—monitor the lab results.	Interventions provide information about membrane status and possible infection.
Obtain specimens for CBC and urinalysis as ordered (specify: e.g., daily CBC)—monitor the lab results.	Laboratory studies provide information about possible inflammation and infectious processes.
Administer antibiotics as ordered (specify drug, dose, route, time).	(Specify action of individual drug.)
Provide accurate information and emotional support to client and family. Allow time for questions.	Client and family may be anxious and confused about prognosis for their baby.
Assess client's temperature q 2–4 hours (specify). Notify caregiver if >99.5° F.	Assessment provides information about the development of infection.
Monitor color, amount, and odor of vaginal discharge. Notify caregiver if increased amount, color changes, or foul odor is noted.	Thick foul-smelling fluid may indicate chorioamnionitis; increased fluid loss may put the fetus at risk for cord prolapse.
Maintain client on bed rest with BRP (shower) if ordered.	Bed rest may decrease the amount of active fluid loss.
Assist/instruct client in good hygiene practices: hand washing technique, perineal care. If client wants to wear a peri pad for leakage, instruct her to change it at least every 2 hours.	Teaching helps prevent the spread of microorganisms from the environment to the genital area. Moist, warm peri pad provides a favorable environment for organism growth.
Monitor fetal well-being: perform daily NSTs as ordered, note presence of variable decelerations; arrange other testing as ordered (specify: e.g., BPP, amniocentesis for L/S ratio and PG, ultrasound for AFI).	Monitoring provides information about fetal stress, which may result from sepsis; cord compression, maturity, and amount of amniotic fluid.
If client is to be discharged to home, teach her to read a thermometer accurately, to take her temperature every 4 hours, remain on bed rest with BRP, avoid sexual intercourse, and	Teaching promotes safety and self-care. Some clients have difficulty reading a regular thermometer, signs of infection may necessitate delivery.

INTERVENTIONS	RATIONALES

notify her physician for: temp
>99.5° F, uterine tenderness/
contractions, ↑ leakage, or
foul-smelling discharge.

NIC: *Infection Protection*

Evaluation

(Date/time of evaluation of goal)

(Has goal been met? not met? partially met?)

(What is client's temperature? Is fluid clear with no foul odor?)

(Revisions to care plan? D/C care plan? Continue care plan?)

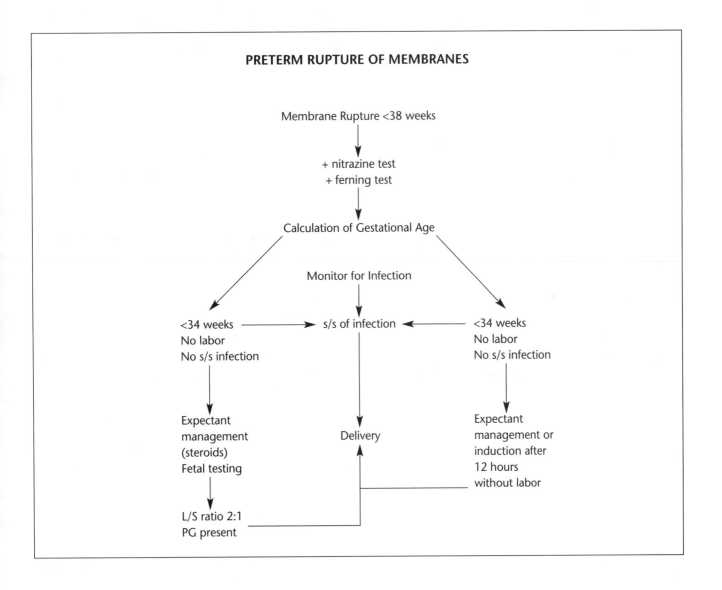

PRETERM RUPTURE OF MEMBRANES

Membrane Rupture <38 weeks

\+ nitrazine test
\+ ferning test

Calculation of Gestational Age

Monitor for Infection

<34 weeks
No labor
No s/s infection → s/s of infection ← <34 weeks
No labor
No s/s infection

Expectant
management
(steroids)
Fetal testing

Delivery

Expectant
management or
induction after
12 hours
without labor

L/S ratio 2:1
PG present

CHAPTER 1.16

AT-RISK FETUS

Most serious maternal illnesses of complications of pregnancy create risks for the fetus too. Teratogens may seriously disrupt development of the embryo. Maternal anemia or poor nutrition may result in inadequate oxygen and nutrients for the developing fetus. Abnormal maternal blood components may also affect the fetus as in hyperglycemia or Rh isoimmunization. Anything that interferes with placental or cord perfusion decreases fetal gas and nutrient/waste exchange. Cord entanglement can lead to fetal death or distress during labor.

The fetus at risk should be closely monitored throughout pregnancy. Interventions are designed to provide an optimum intrauterine environment. Once viability has been reached, the risks of preterm birth are weighed against the risks of continuing in a hostile uterine environment.

RISK FACTORS

- Serious maternal disease: heart, kidney, hypertension, and others
- Maternal anemias
- Diabetes mellitus
- Infections (STD, bacterial, HIV)
- Multiple gestation
- Oligohydraminos or polyhydraminos
- Rh isoimmunization
- PIH, HELLP, DIC
- Placenta previa/abruption
- Preterm ruptured membranes or labor
- IUGR, fetal anomalies
- Postterm pregnancy (42+ weeks)
- Substance abuse

MEDICAL CARE

- Testing: CVS, NST, OCT, ultrasound, BPP, Doppler flow studies, amniocentesis, PUBS, fetal echocardiogram, MRI, and so forth.
- Medications given to the mother: iron supplements, oxygen, insulin, Rh immune globulin, antibiotics, antivirals, tocolytics, glucocorticoids
- Fetal blood transfusion, fetal surgery
- Induction or cesarean delivery if indicated

COMMON NURSING DIAGNOSES

See ANXIETY

Related to: Perceived threat to fetal well-being secondary to complications of pregnancy; maternal illness; identified fetal anomalies.

Defining Characteristics: Specify: (Client reports feeling anxious, upset about prognosis for her baby. Client is crying, angry, trembling, etc.).

See ANTICIPATORY GRIEVING

Related to: Potential for fetal death or injury.

Defining Characteristics: Specify: (Client and family express distress over fetal prognosis, exhibit indications of denial, anger, guilt, etc.).

ADDITIONAL NURSING DIAGNOSES

DEFICIENT KNOWLEDGE: FETAL TESTING

Related to: Lack of experience or information about fetal testing (specify tests).

Defining Characteristics: Client and family verbalize unfamiliarity with the prescribed test or misinformation about the tests (specify: use quotes).

Goal: Client and family will gain knowledge about the suggested fetal test(s) by (date/time to evaluate).

Outcome Criteria

✔ Client and family will describe the testing procedure and risks and benefits of the proposed fetal testing.

NOC: *Treatment Procedure*

INTERVENTIONS	RATIONALES
Assess client and family's previous understanding or perception of the proposed fetal testing (specify tests).	Assessment provides baseline information to plan needed teaching content.
Reinforce caregiver explanations of the test including preparation needed, actual procedure, duration, information to be gained (benefits) and when the results will be available. Identify any risks to fetus or mother (specify for each test). Use visual aids, videos, or written information as indicated.	Provides information the client and family need to make informed decisions about fetal testing. Primary caregiver is responsible for informing the client of risks/benefits. Explanation helps the client and family to evaluate the proposed testing. Visual aids and written information enhances understanding.
Allow time for questions about the testing or fetal condition that indicates a need for testing. Ask client about cultural or religious concerns if indicated.	An unhurried approach promotes understanding and comfort. Clients from some cultures may need to be encouraged to ask questions, some religions disallow blood transfusions.
Provide emotional support without encouraging false hopes. Encourage family and friends' support of client and significant other.	Honesty and support helps client and significant other to express and cope with fears.
Verify understanding of material presented. Correct misunderstandings.	Ensures that client and S/O correctly understand teaching content.
Refer client for further information to her physician, perinatologist or others (specify: e.g., genetic counselor).	Referrals provide client with additional sources of information.

NIC: *Teaching, Procedure/Treatment*

Evaluation

(Date/time of evaluation of goal)

(Has goal been met? not met? partially met?)

(Do client and family describe the test procedure, risks and benefits? Use quotes.)

(Revisions to care plan? D/C care plan? Continue care plan?)

RISK FOR IMPAIRED GAS EXCHANGE: FETAL

Related to: Specify: insufficient placental function, altered cord blood flow, ↓ oxygen-carrying capacity of maternal blood (anemia, substance abuse), fetal hemolysis, and so forth.

Defining Characteristics: None, as this is a potential diagnosis.

Goal: Fetus will demonstrate adequate gas exchange for intrauterine environment by (date/time to evaluate).

Outcome Criteria

✔ Fetal growth will be appropriate for gestational age (fundal height, ultrasound), FHR between 110–160 without late or severe variable decelerations.

NOC: *Respiratory Status: Gas Exchange (Fetal)*

INTERVENTIONS	RATIONALES
Assess fetal growth pattern compared to expected rate using serial fundal height or ultrasound reports.	Assessment provides information about adequacy of placental nutrient transfer to rule out IUGR.
Monitor maternal lab work for anemia or Rh sensitization (antibody titers, indirect Coombs test) as obtained.	Provides information about O_2-carrying capacity of blood; antibodies may cause hemolysis of fetal RBCs.
Teach client to take iron supplements as ordered and avoid substance abuse to enhance the amount of oxygen available for the fetus.	Teaching promotes compliance with medical regimen, helps client to participate in caring for her fetus.

(continues)

(continued)

INTERVENTIONS	RATIONALES
Assess any vaginal discharge: fluid, bleeding, and so forth (specify frequency if active loss).	Assessment provides information about cause of hypovolemia, anemia, potential for cord compression.
Assess FHR for baseline rate, variability, accelerations, and decelerations (specify frequency).	Assessment provides information about oxygenation, cord compression, placental perfusion.
Perform NST, OCT, etc. as ordered. Assist with other tests as appropriate (specify for each test ordered). Monitor results.	Testing provides information about fetal reserve; other tests may indicate cause of impaired gas exchange.
Explain all procedures and equipment to client and significant other. Provide reassurance and emotional support.	Decreases anxiety about unfamiliar procedures and anxiety about the condition of the fetus.
Position client on left side or semi-Fowlers with wedge under right hip.	Facilitates placental perfusion by avoiding compression of the vena cava.
Monitor intake and output, assess hydration: skin turgot, mucous membranes, and urine sp. gravity (specify frequency).	Monitoring provides information about maternal fluid balance and placental perfusion.
Assess maternal BP and pulse (specify frequency).	Maternal hypotension may lead to tachycardia and ↓ placental perfusion.
Ensure adequate hydration: oral or IV fluids as ordered (specify p.o. amounts/hr, IV fluid, & rate).	Dehydration may affect placental perfusion leading to inadequate gas exchange for the fetus.

INTERVENTIONS	RATIONALES
Provide humidified oxygen at 10–12 L/min via facemask or n/c as needed (specify: e.g., sickle cell crisis, late decelerations).	Interventions provide ↑ oxygen for the fetus.
Administer medications as ordered (specify drug, dose, route, time, e.g., Rh immune globulin [RhoGAM], SC terbutaline for a prolapsed cord, etc.).	(Describe action of specific drug related to factors that alter fetal gas exchange.)
Arrange for tour of NICU if indicated by fetal condition or prognosis. If client is unable to tour unit, have NICU nurse come talk to her.	Impaired gas exchange for the fetus may necessitate NICU stay because of preterm delivery or other perinatal problems.

NIC: *Airway Management (Fetal)*

Evaluation

(Date/time of evaluation of goal)

(Has goal been met? not met? partially met?)

(What is fetal growth compared to expected size for gestation?)

(What is FHR? Are there decelerations?)

(Revisions to care plan? D/C care plan? Continue care plan?)

AT-RISK FETUS

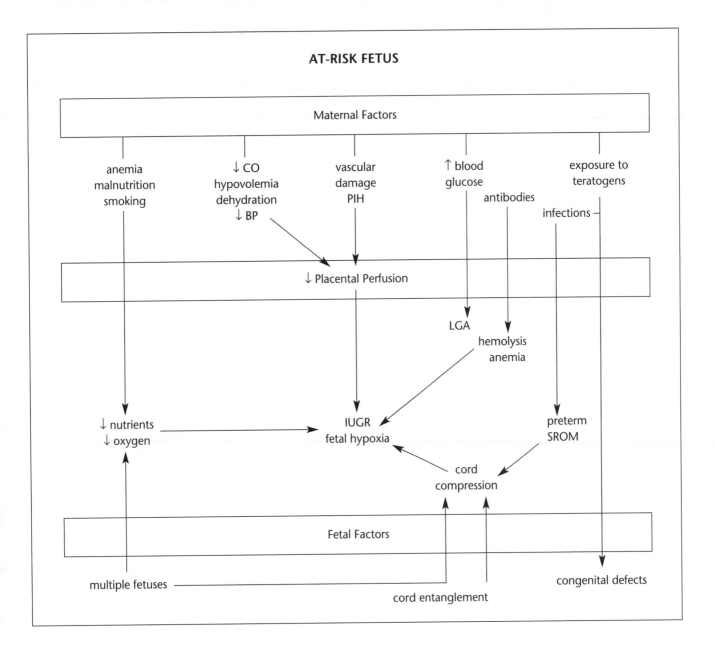

CHAPTER 1.17

INFERTILITY

Infertility is defined as the lack of conception after 12 months of unprotected intercourse. Primary infertility describes a woman who has never conceived and the term, secondary infertility, is used if a woman has conceived in the past but is unable to do so again. The incidence of infertility in the United States is estimated at approximately 8% of couples desiring to have children.

Infertility treatment begins with thorough history, assessment, and evaluation of both partners to identify the presumed cause. Infertility testing may be embarrassing and expensive. Nurses provide necessary emotional support and act as client advocates during this stressful time.

ESSENTIAL FERTILITY FACTORS

- Ovulation must occur
- Fallopian tubes must be patent
- Healthy sperm, in adequate numbers, must be ejaculated near the cervix
- Cervical mucus must be hospitable to sperm to allow passage into the uterus
- The endometrium must be hormonally prepared to receive the conceptus
- Adequate hormones must be produced to maintain the pregnancy

MEDICAL CARE

INFERTILITY TESTING

- Evaluation of lifestyle factors: stress, substance use, employment
- Assessment of ovulation: BBT, cervical mucus
- Hormone assessment: FSH, LH, TSH, progesterone, prolactin
- Semen analysis
- Postcoital test (Huhner test)

- Hysterosalpingography
- Laparoscopy

TREATMENT

- Pharmacologic: ovulation stimulants, hormones, danazol, bromocriptine, and so forth
- Surgical: lysis of adhesions, repair of varicocele, and so forth
- Artificial insemination (husband or donor)
- In vitro fertilization (IVF), GIFT, ZIFT
- Surrogate mother/gestational carrier
- Adoption

COMMON NURSING DIAGNOSES

See ANXIETY

Related to: Perceived threat of not being able to have children.

Defining Characteristics: Specify for couple (one or both clients report feelings of anxiety; one or both exhibit physiologic signs of anxiety: pallor, crying, tremors, etc.).

See DECISIONAL CONFLICT: INFERTILITY OPTIONS

Related to: Risks versus benefits of infertility treatment options

Defining Characteristics: (Specify for couple: e.g. couple verbalize uncertainty about choices; couple report having difficulty agreeing on treatment options, etc.).

ADDITIONAL NURSING DIAGNOSES

DEFICIENT KNOWLEDGE: INFERTILITY

Related to: Infertility testing and treatment options.

Defining Characteristics: (specify for couple: couple express a lack of understanding about infertility testing and treatment; couple ask for information—use quotes).

Goal: Couple will learn about infertility testing and treatment options.

Outcome Criteria

✔ Clients will identify the basic steps of infertility testing.

✔ Clients will express treatment options that may be available to them.

NOC: *Knowledge: Treatment Regimen*

INTERVENTIONS	RATIONALES
Assess the current understanding the clients have about infertility testing and treatment.	Provides information on current knowledge-level of clients.
Review reproductive anatomy physiology with couple. Include the menstrual cycle, spermatogenesis, ovulation, conception, and implantation. Use visual aids and models as needed (specify).	Review helps clients to understand the purpose of tests and treatment modalities.
Teach clients that interference with the reproductive anatomic or physiologic processes may lead to infertility. Point out physiologic barriers using models (e.g., blockage of fallopian tubes, varicoeles).	Teaching and use of visual aids help the clients to understand mechanical barriers to conception.
Briefly discuss hormonal imbalances that may interfere with fertility: FSH, LH, progesterone, prolactin, androgens.	Fertility requires appropriate release of reproductive hormones.
Inform clients about the usual infertility physical exams and lab work (specify, e.g., BBT, cervical biopsy, hormone assays, hysterosalpingography, Huhner test, etc.). Describe treatment options for infertility (specify for clients if cause is known): Ovulation stimulants (Clomid), hormones, hysterosalpingography performed to avoid disrupting a fertilized ovum, surgical or	Provides information for couple to consider.

INTERVENTIONS	RATIONALES
laparoscopic removal of adhesions and scarring, artificial insemination, in vitro fertilization GIFT, and surrogate gestational carriers.	
Allow time for questions and discussion. Encourage clients to express feelings about infertility and testing.	Infertility is complex both physiologically and emotionally.
Refer clients to support groups if indicated (specify).	Information from someone who has experienced the problem is often helpful.
Encourage couple to think about the information presented and make an appointment to begin testing if desired.	Allows time for thought about infertility, testing, and treatment.

NIC: *Teaching, Sexuality*

Evaluation

(Date/time of evaluation of goal)

(Was goal met? Not met? Partially met?)

(Did couple learn about infertility testing and treatment options?)

(Did clients identify the basic steps of infertility testing?)

(Did clients express treatment options that may be available to them?)

POWERLESSNESS

Related to: Inability to control fertility.

Defining Characteristics: Subjective or objective indications of anger, apathy, depression (specify for client). Client expresses feeling helpless (specify, e.g., client states thoughts about babies/children interfere with work, socialization, home life, etc.). Couple report difficulties in relationship (specify, e.g., client feels that the partner "doesn't care").

Goal: Client will express increased feelings of control by (date/time to evaluate).

Outcome Criteria

✔ Clients will identify fertility options (specify).

✔ Clients will report that they have agreed on a course of action.

NOC: *Health Beliefs: Perceived Control*

INTERVENTIONS	RATIONALES
Ask clients to identify difficult situations that they, as a couple, have experienced in the past and how they handled it as a couple.	Provides information about the ability of the couple to control events in their life.
Assess for knowledge about infertility and treatment options that have been suggested by the health care provider.	Provides information about the client's grasp of the physiologic basis for the problem.
Encourage effective communication between clients and their health care provider: Suggest that they write down questions and be sure they understand options thoroughly.	Clients may feel embarrassed or shy about asking reproductive questions. Incomplete information interferes with the ability to make decisions.
Provide information about self-help or support groups for couples with similar infertility diagnoses (specify).	Provides information and additional support from experienced couples to increase the client's feelings of control over their problem.
Assist couple to identify which fertility options they would consider and which are unacceptable to them. (Specify for clients: e.g., artificial insemination with husband sperm only or mixed with donor sperm, in vitro fertilization, surrogate carrier, adoption.)	Allows the couple a sense of control over multiple options.
Encourage couple to make a decision about the next step they want to pursue related to fertility even if it is to just put off any decisions for 6 months.	Actively engaging in decision-making increases the personal sense of control and self-esteem.

NIC: *Self-Esteem Enhancement*

Evaluation

(Date/time of evaluation of goal)

(Was goal met? Not met? Partially met?)

(Did clients identify fertility options ? State options.)

(Did clients agree on a course of action? Specify what they said here.)

 INEFFECTIVE SEXUALITY PATTERNS

Related to: Fear of continued failure to conceive.

Defining Characteristics: Couple report concerns about or a disturbance in their usual sexual behaviors and identity (Provide specific information obtained from couple e.g., "I don't feel like a real woman anymore," "I have trouble maintaining an erection when she is so tense.")

Goal: Couple will resume previous sexuality patterns by (date/time to evaluate).

Outcome Criteria

✔ Clients will identify stressors that affect their sexual relationship.

✔ Clients will report that sexual relationship is satisfying for both of them.

NOC: *Self-Esteem*

INTERVENTIONS	RATIONALES
Provide for privacy and a nonhurried discussion with couple. Express willingness to discuss feelings and concerns that the couple are willing to talk about.	Clients may feel that sexuality is very personal and private. Reassures clients that the nurse will not be intrusive when they object.
Ask clients to describe their sexual history together and how it has changed. Remain nonjudgmental and matter-of-fact.	Provides information about pattern of sexuality prior to infertility and allows the couple to identify alterations.
Describe the relationship between stress and sexual functioning. Ask clients to identify how the stress of infertility may be interfering with their sexuality.	Provides an external "reason" for the problem and encourages the couple to identify specific stressors.
Encourage the couple to have open discussions with each other about the need for closeness, touch, and expressions of love that don't always culminate in sexual intercourse.	Infertility clients may be so obsessed with conception that they forget other aspects of a loving relationship.
Promote a sense of humor if couple can tolerate it (specify) about the infertility treatment options such as planning intercourse to meet ovulation timing.	Humor releases tension, decreasing the negative effects of stress.
Suggest that clients plan specific ways to cope with the stressors of infertility and regain their previous sexual satisfaction.	Encourages clients to gain insight and control over stressors.

INTERVENTIONS   RATIONALES

Refer clients as needed (specify
e.g., sex therapist, physician,
etc.).

NIC: *Sexual Counseling*

Evaluation

(Date/time of evaluation of goal)

(Was goal met? Not met? Partially met?)

(Did clients identify stressors that impact their sexual
   relationship? Specify stressors using quotes if
   possible.)

(Did clients report satisfaction with their sexual relationship? Specify subjective data.)

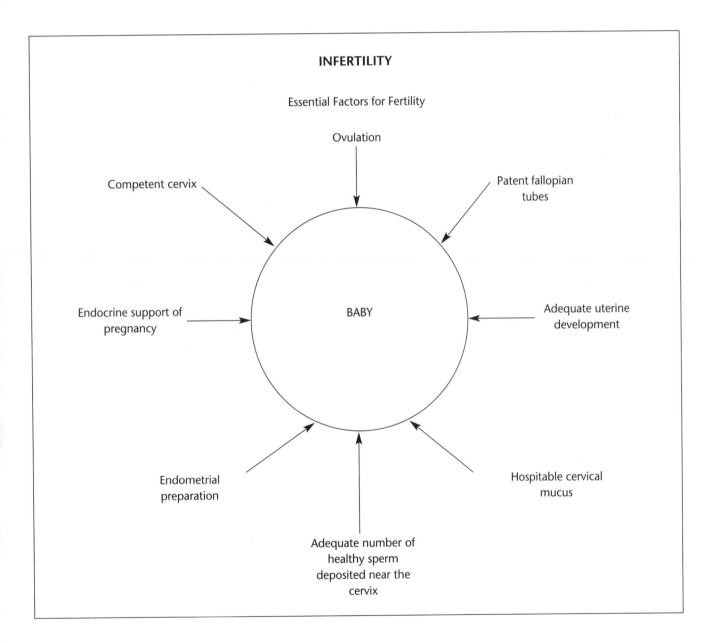

INFERTILITY

Essential Factors for Fertility

Ovulation

Competent cervix

Patent fallopian
tubes

BABY

Endocrine support of
pregnancy

Adequate uterine
development

Endometrial
preparation

Hospitable cervical
mucus

Adequate number of
healthy sperm
deposited near the
cervix

UNIT 2
INTRAPARTUM

CHAPTER 2.0

LABOR AND BIRTH

Vaginal birth is a normal physiologic process that begins with softening of the cervix (ripening) and increased uterine contractility. The contractions become stronger and more regular causing effacement (thinning) and dilatation of the cervix, and descent of the fetus. Once the cervix is completely dilated, second stage contractions are assisted by maternal pushing efforts and the infant is born. Following a brief respite, the placenta and membranes are expelled and the uterus contracts to prevent excessive bleeding.

Approximately one-fourth of pregnant women in the United States today will give birth by cesarean section for various reasons. Nurses have done much to make this surgical experience a time of family bonding and celebration.

The goal of nursing care is to facilitate the natural progression of labor and delivery, safeguard the surgical client, and encourage family participation. Cultural sensitivity and client advocacy are important attributes of the labor and delivery nurse. Risk assessment for both mother and fetus begins with a review of the prenatal record followed by an admission assessment and continual assessments throughout labor and birth.

STAGES OF LABOR

- 1st Stage: Begins with onset of regular uterine contractions and ends with complete dilatation of the cervix (10 cms); divided into: Latent Phase: 0 to 4 cms dilatation, Active Phase: 4 to 8 cms dilatation, and Transition Phase: 8 to 10 cms
- 2nd Stage: From complete dilatation of the cervix to birth of the baby
- 3rd Stage: From birth of the baby to delivery of the placenta
- 4th Stage: Immediate postbirth recovery lasting from 1 to 4 hours

PHYSIOLOGIC CHANGES

- Cardiovascular: during contractions: ↑ maternal CO, ↑ BP, ↓ P as uteroplacental blood is shunting back into maternal circulation ↑ WBCs during labor
- Respiratory: ↑ respiratory rate; may hyperventilate causing respiratory alkalosis
- Gastrointestinal: ↓ motility and digestion; may experience nausea and vomiting of undigested food

PSYCHOLOGICAL CHANGES

- Latent Phase: May be talkative and excited that labor has started
- Active Phase: Becomes more serious and focused on contractions; concerned about ability to cope with discomfort
- Transition Phase: Client becomes more irritable and may lose control during contractions; convinced that she can't do it; very introverted or sleeping between contractions
- 2nd Stage: Works hard at pushing and sleeps or appears exhausted between contractions
- 3rd Stage: Client is usually elated with birth of baby and pushes on request to deliver placenta
- 4th Stage: Client is alert and ready to bond or breast feed her baby; may be talkative and hungry

FETAL ADAPTATION

During the peak of a moderate contraction (at 50 mm Hg pressure) placental blood flow stops and the fetus must rely on oxygen reserves. Uterine resting tone between contractions is required to replenish oxygen supplies.

TABLE 2.1 Passageway, Passenger, and Powers

PASSAGEWAY	PASSENGER	POWERS
Maternal Pelvis & Soft Tissues	*Fetal Size Presentation, Position*	*Uterine Contractions*
Pelvic Types	**Lie**	**Frequency**
gynecoid (50%) ◯ android ♡ anthropoid ⬭ platypelloid ⬭	longitudinal transverse	Irregular Regular amount of time from the beginning of one contraction to the beginning of the next
Pelvic Planes	**Attitude**	
	flexed	**Duration**
Inlet: Diagonal Conjugate: ≥12.5–13 cm	**Presentation**	length of time from the beginning to the end of the average contraction
Midpelvis: Interspinous Diameter: ≥10.5 cm	cephalic breech	**Intensity**
Outlet: Transverse Diameter: ≥10 cm	**Position**	strength of the contraction as palpated mild, moderate, strong, or
Cervix	Left or Right Anterior or Posterior Occiput, Sacrum OA, OP, ROA, ROP, LOA, LOP, SA, SP, RSA, RSP, LSA, LSP	measured by an intrauterine pressure catheter (IUPC) in mm Hg
ripe soft & elastic w/o scarring anterior	**Fetal Head Size**	**Resting Tone**
Vagina & Perineum	overlapping of skull bones (molding)	allows uteroplacental perfusion between contractions
soft and elastic w/o extensive scarring	**Fetal Shoulder Size**	
	shoulder dystocia clavicular fracture	

Position
Maternal positioning
may shorten labor

Psyche
Maternal anxiety and
tension may lengthen labor

TABLE 2.2   Intrapartum Care Path

	ASSESSEMENTS	ACTIVITY	COMFORT TEACHING	NUTRITION	OTHER
Latent Phase	Admission assessment, VS, vaginal exam prn nitrazine/fern urine dip for protein, UA, CBC, contractions EFM X 20 min BP, P, R, and FHR assessment q lh (low risk) q 30" (high risk) Temp q 4 h until ROM then q 2 h	Ambulation if membranes intact or with SROM and head engaged	Explain all procedures & equipment, include S/O and family Review/teach breathing and relaxation techniques for labor	Clear liquids (light meals)	Social service consult as indicated
Active Phase	BP, P, R, ctx & FHR assessment q 30" (low risk) q 15" (high risk) Vag exam as needed	Ambulation if desired, rocking chair, bed on L side	Assist with breathing & relaxation, whirlpool, massage, music, birth ball, medications as desired	Clear liquids sips & chips IV fluids	Notify anesthesia for epidural (if desired)
Transition	Observe bloody show, signs of 2nd stage: grunting, pushing, hiccoughs, emesis	Bedrest or chair desired, hands & knees for OP	Support S/O back pressure for OP, effleurage as desired		Notify physician or CNM & prepare for delivery for multipara
2nd Stage	BP, P, R, ctx & Fetal response to pushing q 15" (low risk) q 5" (high risk)	Squatting or side lying to push; avoid breath-holding or supine position	Teach physiologic 2nd stage. Describe sensations Cool wash cloth, perineal massage		Notify physician CNM & prepare for delivery as indicated
Birth	Time of birth Apgar @ 1 & 5 min	As desired	Allow to hold infant if stable		As needed
3rd Stage	Time, maternal BP, P, R				Oxytocics after placenta
4th Stage	Temperature BP, P, R, fundus/lochia episiotomy & bladder checks q 15 min X 4, q 30 min X 2, q h X 2 then routine infant physical exam, gestational age assessment		Breast feeding, bonding with family Encourage voiding Peri care, ice pack if needed	Regular diet	Infant: eye prophylaxis, vitamin K wt., length Arm/leg bands, footprints, fingerprints

CHAPTER 2.1

BASIC CARE PLAN: LABOR AND VAGINAL BIRTH

The nursing care plan is based on a thorough review of the prenatal record, nursing admission assessment, and continual assessments during labor. Specific client-related data should be inserted wherever possible and within parentheses.

NURSING DIAGNOSES

 ### HEALTH SEEKING BEHAVIORS: LABOR

Related to: Desire for a safe labor and vaginal birth of a healthy newborn.

Defining Characteristics: Client seeks medical care for perceived signs of labor. Client states (specify: e.g., "I think I'm in labor; my water broke; is my baby okay?"). (List appropriate subjective/objective data.)

Goal: Client continues health seeking behaviors throughout pregnancy.

Outcome Criteria

✔ Client will verbalize agreement with the plan of care for labor (specify: EFM, IV, birth plan requests, etc.).
✔ Client participates in self-care during labor.

NOC: *Health Promoting Behavior*

INTERVENTIONS	RATIONALES
Interview client alone. Establish rapport, ensure privacy, listen attentively and observe nonverbal cues (provide an interpreter prn).	Privacy allows client to provide information and express concerns openly.
Assess client's chief complaint (reason for seeking care).	Assessments need to be adapted to client condition with prioritization of activities.

INTERVENTIONS	RATIONALES
If in active labor, quickly assess stage of labor and fetal well-being; notify caregiver of client's status. Assess client's knowledge of labor and birth (childbirth classes, other births she's experienced).	Assessment provides information about individual learning needs.
Ask client who she would like to have present during her labor and birth. Allow family to be present as client wishes.	The nurse acts as a client advocate in allowing desired support people and keeping others out of the client's room.
Teach client and significant others about equipment (specify: e.g., EFM) and procedures (specify: e.g., labs, IV) that have been ordered by her caregiver. Explain rationales for each. Allow time for questions.	Teaching empowers client and significant other to become participants in labor and birth.
Modify plan of care based on client's requests (e.g., female caregivers only) if safe to do so. Collaborate with caregiver for changes in routine orders (specify: e.g., no enema, no EFM).	Modifying routine care shows respect for the client as an individual with the right to participate in decisions regarding care.
Teach (review) stages and phases of labor with client. Inform client of her current status and how her baby is adapting to labor.	Information helps client to evaluate how she feels compared to her labor status, and provides reassurance that her baby is also being cared for.
Inform client of timing of routine vital signs and fetal assessments, and when vaginal exams might be done. Orient client to the setting (call lights, phone system, etc.) and show how she may adapt it for comfort (e.g., lighting switches, thermostat, extra blankets, etc.).	Information about expected interventions helps the client understand what is happening. Knowledge empowers the client to control aspects of her environment to ↑ comfort during labor.

(continues)

(continued)

INTERVENTIONS	RATIONALES
Encourage client to stay out of bed as long as possible to allow position to help advance her labor. Provide nonskid slippers and robe for ambulation, suggest rocking chair when she is tired of walking (birthing ball or whirlpool if available—specify use).	Encouragement promotes healthy behaviors to facilitate the progress of normal labor.
Provide emotional support and praise as needed to encourage client and significant other to cope with the demands of labor and birth.	Emotional support and praise reinforce client and significant other's sense of control during labor.

NIC: *Health Education*

Evaluation

(Date/time of evaluation of goal)

(Has goal been met? not met? partially met?)

(Does client verbalize agreement with the plan of care for labor? [Specify EFM, IV, birth plan requests, etc.])

(Does client participate in self-care during labor? Specify: e.g., walking, etc.)

(Revisions to care plan? D/C care plan? Continue care plan?)

 EFFECTIVE THERAPEUTIC REGIMEN MANAGEMENT

Related to: Physiologic and psychological challenges of labor.

Defining Characteristics: Client states (specify: e.g., "I can handle this now; I think I'll switch to the other breathing"). Client uses breathing/relaxation techniques (specify others) effectively during labor.

Goal: Client will continue to be able to effectively manage her labor by (date/time to evaluate).

Outcome Criteria

✔ Client adapts breathing techniques as labor progresses (specify).

✔ Client is able to relax during and between contractions (other specifics as appropriate).

NOC: *Symptom Control*

INTERVENTIONS	RATIONALES
Praise client's efforts to cope with labor contractions and significant other's coaching ability throughout labor and birth.	Praise reinforces client's belief in her ability to manage labor and birth, and significant other's coaching ability.
Inform client and significant other of labor progress and what changes to expect before they occur. Provide approximate time frames (e.g., transition will probably last < an hour for a multipara).	Information and anticipatory guidance help client and significant other to feel some control over events. Transition is the most difficult part of labor.
Suggest alternative coping techniques if client is having difficulty (specify: e.g., changes in position, breathing pattern, focus point/keep eyes open, pressure over sacrum, music, massage, cool wash cloth, birthing ball, whirlpool, etc.).	Client and significant other may benefit from alternative methods of coping with the discomfort of labor.
Remind client to relax during and between contractions. Assist significant other to evaluate degree of client's relaxation.	Relaxation saves energy and decreases the fear–tension–pain cycle by decreasing tension.
Role model coaching and support during contractions if needed, then encourage significant other to take over role.	Role modeling shows significant other how to help the client. Significant other may feel overwhelmed by the competence of staff and need encouragement to participate.
Reassure client that if she feels she needs pain medication that she can still participate actively in the birth of her baby.	Reassures the client that she is not a failure if she needs pharmacologic help to cope with the discomfort of labor.
Inform client when she is close to second stage. Provide constant support to client and significant other during the contractions of transition and second stage.	Information allows client to evaluate what is happening. Client and significant other may need extra support to handle the intensity of transition and second stage.
Encourage client to begin bearing-down efforts when she feels the urge to push.	Maternal efforts are more effective when the fetus has descended far enough to initiate Ferguson's reflex.
Instruct client to bear down at the peak of the contraction for no more than 6 seconds at a time and to exhale or make noise if she wishes.	Physiologic management of second stage causes less stress to the fetus than sustained maternal breath holding.

INTERVENTIONS	RATIONALES
Encourage client to change positions frequently during second stage (e.g., sitting in chair, on birthing ball, squatting, walking, hands and knees, etc.).	Position changes facilitate descent of the fetus and empower the client to be in control of her birthing.
Show significant other the fetal head as it comes into view. Allow client to touch the baby's head as desired.	Seeing or touching the baby's head reinforces maternal efforts to give birth.
Offer praise to client and significant other for their good work after the birth.	Praise reinforces family's bonding and positive memories of their birth experience.

NIC: *Anticipatory Guidance*

Evaluation

(Date/time of evaluation of goal)

(Has goal been met? not met? partially met?)

(Did client adapt breathing techniques as labor progressed? Specify.)

(Was client able to relax during and between contractions?)

(Revisions to care plan? D/C care plan? Continue care plan?)

 ## RISK FOR INJURY: MATERNAL AND FETAL

Related to: Dystocia, cephalopelvic disproportion, fetal malposition or presentation, precipitous birth, and so forth.

Defining Characteristics: None, as this is a potential diagnosis.

Goal: Client and her infant will not experience any injury during labor and birth (evaluate after birth).

Outcome Criteria

✔ Client's labor progress will be within the normal pattern on a labor curve.

✔ The fetus will descend at ≥ 1 cm/hr during second stage.

NOC: *Safety Status: Physical Injury*

INTERVENTIONS	RATIONALES
Review prenatal record for pelvic measurement, length of previous labors, and size of infant.	Review provides information about the passageway and pelvic adequacy; identifies clients at risk for precipitous births or dystocia.
Assess fetal lie, presentation, and attitude using Leopold's maneuvers. Inform caregiver of abnormalities.	Assessment provides information about the fetus as passenger.
Perform baseline vaginal exam; repeat only as needed to determine progress. Assess presentation, position, station, membrane status and effacement and dilatation of the cervix during vaginal exams. Document progress (on a labor curve).	Assessment provides information about progress of labor, fetal position, and descent. Use of a labor curve allows comparison with the normal patterns for primiparas or multiparas.
Assess contraction frequency, duration, intensity, and uterine resting tone q 30" during active labor (q 15" if high risk), and q 15" during second stage (q 5" if high risk). Palpate contractions if external EFM is being used. If IUPC is used, document intensity in mm Hg.	Assessment provides information about contraction and adequacy of uterine resting tone. External EFM does not provide information on intensity. Contraction intensity with IUPC is measured in mm Hg: 30–40 = mild, 50–60 = moderate, 70–80 = strong.
Assess fetal well-being on same schedule as contractions by auscultation or EFM. Assess and document baseline FHR, variability and periodic and nonperiodic changes (according to agency protocol, specify).	Assessment provides information about fetal oxygenation and adequacy of oxygen reserves during contractions.
Encourage client to change position frequently during labor: walk, sit on birthing ball, in rocking chair, and so forth.	Position changes may facilitate dilatation fetal descent through the pelvis.
Notify caregiver of nonreassuring FHR and institute independent nursing measures as appropriate: decrease or discontinue oxytocin if infusing, initiate maternal position changes, give oxygen at 8–12 L/min via face mask, IV fluids, perform vaginal exam, and so forth.	Independent nursing measures are designed to improve fetal oxygenation by decreasing uterine contractions, relieving cord compression, providing supplemental oxygen, increasing perfusion, and identifying factors that may be causing the distress.
Notify caregiver if client is not making expected labor progress (e.g., dilatation of ≥ 1cm/hr in active labor, descent of ≥ 1cm/hr in 2nd stage.	Timely notification alerts caregiver to possible dystocia, need for augmentation with oxytocin, or a reevaluation of pelvic adequacy.

(continues)

(continued)

INTERVENTIONS	RATIONALES
Keep client and significant other informed of labor progress and fetal well-being.	Information allows client and significant other to anticipate what will happen and to participate in decisions.
If infant experiences shoulder dystocia at birth, assist caregiver in applying McRoberts maneuver: flex mother's thighs onto abdomen, apply suprapubic pressure to rotate shoulder under symphysis.	Shoulder dystocia occurs after the head delivers, when the anterior fetal shoulder becomes lodged behind the symphysis pubis. McRobert's maneuver widens the angle of the pelvic outlet.

NIC: *Electronic Fetal Monitoring: Intrapartum*

Evaluation

(Date/time of evaluation of goal)

(Has goal been met? not met? partially met?)

(Was client's labor progress within the normal labor curve?)

(Did the fetus descend at >1 cm/hr during second stage?)

(Revisions to care plan? D/C care plan? Continue care plan?)

RISK FOR INFECTION: MATERNAL/FETAL

Related to: Invasive procedures and ruptured membranes during labor and birth.

Defining Characteristics: None, as this is a potential diagnosis.

Goal: Client and fetus will not experience infection from invasive procedures used during labor and birth by (date/time to evaluate).

Outcome Criteria

✔ Client's temperature will remain <100° F; newborn's temp will be <98.9° F.

NOC: *Risk Control*

INTERVENTIONS	RATIONALES
Review prenatal record for GBS status and provide intrapartum antimicrobial prophylaxis as ordered.	Group B streptococcus colonized in the reproductive tract may cause an overwhelming neonatal sepsis.

INTERVENTIONS	RATIONALES
Assess maternal temperature q 4h until membranes rupture, then q 2h until birth.	Assessment provides information about inflammatory processes.
Assess maternal pulse and FHR baseline according to protocol for stage of labor.	Maternal and fetal tachycardia may indicate infection.
Assess amniotic fluid for color and odor during each vaginal exam. Limit vaginal exams.	Foul-smelling or thick, cloudy amniotic fluid may indicate chorioamnionitis. Bacteria may be introduced during vaginal exams.
Assess any invasive devices (e.g., catheter, IV, continuous epidural) for s/s of infection: redness, edema, discomfort, warmth, etc. q 4h or as indicated.	Systematic assessment provides information about inflammation and infectious processes allowing early treatment.
Maintain medical asepsis by frequent hand washing; use clean gloves when in contact with body fluids.	Frequent hand washing prevents the spread of pathogens; clean gloves protect the caregiver from pathogens.
Use sterile technique per agency protocol for invasive procedures (e.g., IV therapy, vaginal exams, placement of a spiral electrode, AROM, catheterization, etc.).	Sterile technique prevents the introduction of microorganisms into sterile areas of the body.
Change under-buttocks pads frequently (at least q 2h) to keep client dry. Keep epidural dressing dry. Provide perineal care as needed, cleaning from front to back.	Interventions promote cleanliness and avoid a moist dark environment where bacteria may multiply. Front-to-back cleansing prevents fecal contamination of vagina/urethra.
Maintain a clean environment: ensure that housekeeping has cleaned the room (OR), equipment, and bathroom (whirlpool); empty trash as needed.	Cleaning prevents the spread of nosocomial infections within the hospital.
Avoid sharing equipment with other clients or other units in the hospital.	Equipment should be designated for obstetrics only to prevent cross-contamination.
Encourage client to void q 2h during labor. Provide privacy, run water, and so forth to stimulate urination. Teach s/s of UTI to report: frequency, urgency, burning.	Urinary stasis during pregnancy provides an optimum environment for bacterial growth. Voiding frequently avoids the need for catheterization. Teaching allows early identification of a UTI.

INTERVENTIONS	RATIONALES
Wash perineum prior to vaginal birth (per hospital protocol) using sterile technique. Wash from front to back using a new sponge for each wipe—clean labia first and wash over the vagina last.	Cleaning the perineum ↓ the number of microorganisms that may invade the vagina or lacerations during birth.
For cesarean birth, perform abdominal scrub and shave–prep (per agency protocol), remove scalp electrode, assist with maintenance of sterile technique during the surgery.	Interventions ↓ the number of microorganisms that may be introduced into the abdominal cavity and uterus during surgery.
After the placenta has delivered and any suturing is completed, apply a perineal pad (ice pack if indicated) front to back without touching the inner surface. Teach client how to apply peri pads.	Peri pad discourages the introduction of microorganisms to the vagina, episiotomy, or lacerations. Ice, ↓ edema. Application avoids fecal contamination.
(For cesarean birth, observe and maintain the sterile abdominal dressing.)	A wet dressing provides a medium for microorganism growth.
Wear clean gloves to provide immediate care to the newborn and until after the first bath.	Clean gloves protect the caregiver from blood-borne pathogens.
Delay newborn vitamin K injection or other invasive procedures until after the first bath.	Removal of maternal body fluids ↓ possibility of injecting pathogens into the fetus.
Assess infant's temperature, pulse, and respirations at birth. Note how long membranes have been ruptured.	Assessment provides information about possible sepsis (tachycardia, tachypnea). Prolonged rupture of membranes prior to birth increases the risk for infection.
Administer newborn eye prophylaxis as ordered (specify medication & dose). Cleanse eyes first.	Eye prophylaxis prevents neonatal opthalmic infections (specify action of drug that is used).
If removing epidural catheter per anesthesia order, note that entire catheter is withdrawn, assess puncture site for redness, edema, and drainage. Apply a Band-Aid.	Interventions rule out any retained fragments of catheter; local signs of inflammation or infection, a Band-Aid protects puncture site.
Monitor lab results for signs of infection. Notify caregiver if s/s of infection develop in client or infant.	Monitoring lab work allows early identification and treatment of infections.

NIC: *Infection Protection*

Evaluation

(Date/time of evaluation of goal)

(Has goal been met? not met? partially met?)

(What is client's temperature? What is newborn's temperature?)

(Revisions to care plan? D/C care plan? Continue care plan?)

RISK FOR DEFICIENT FLUID VOLUME

Related to: ↓ p.o. intake, ↑ losses.

Defining Characteristics: None, as this is a potential diagnosis.

Goal: Client will not experience a fluid volume deficit by (date/time to evaluate).

Outcome Criteria

✔ Client will maintain urine output of 30 cc/hr or greater, mucous membranes will remain moist, BP ≥ (specify for client).

NOC: *Fluid Balance*

INTERVENTIONS	RATIONALES
Review client hx for risk factors for hemorrhage (specify: e.g., overdistended uterus, clotting problems, etc.).	Provides information about client's propensity for perinatal hemorrhage.
Monitor client's BP, P, and R (specify frequency).	Hypovolemia results in ↓ BP; the body compensates by vasoconstriction and ↑ P. ↓ volume leads to hypoxia and ↑ R.
Assess intake and output every hour during labor and recovery.	Assessment provides information about fluid balance.
Assess skin color, temp, turgor, and moisture of lips/mucous membranes (specify frequency).	Pale, cool skin, poor skin turgor, and dry lips or membranes may indicate fluid loss/dehydration.
Encourage p.o. fluid intake (specify: type & amounts) during labor if allowed.	Oral fluid intake promotes fluid replacement for insensible losses during labor.
Initiate and maintain IV fluids and/or blood products as ordered (specify fluids and rate).	Provides replacement of fluid and/or blood losses.

(continues)

(continued)

INTERVENTIONS	RATIONALES
Monitor lab results as obtained (specify: e.g., Hgb, Hct, urine sp. gravity, clotting studies, etc.).	Changes in Hgb and Hct indicate the extent of blood loss. ↑ sp. gravity may indicate fluid loss. Clotting studies indicate the client at ↑ risk for hemorrhage.
Monitor vaginal losses: bloody show and amniotic fluid. Notify caregiver of excessive bloody show or if fetus develops severe variable decelerations.	Monitoring provides information about abnormal blood loss: possible placental abruption, or need for amnioinfusion to prevent fetal cord compression.
Note any unusual bleeding (e.g., from injection sites, gums, epistaxis, petichiae) and inform caregiver.	Abnormal bleeding may indicate a clotting abnormality.
After delivery of the placenta, assess uterine position, tone and color and amount of lochia; observe for hematomas and note integrity of incisions (specify frequency).	Assessments provide information about uterine displacement and tone; vaginal blood loss, hidden bleeding, and wound dehiscence.
Encourage frequent emptying of the bladder after birth (catheterize as needed). Massage the uterus if boggy, guarding over the symphysis. Administer oxytocics as ordered (specify: drug, dose, route, time).	Bladder distension may inhibit uterine contraction leading to excessive bleeding. Massage stimulates uterine tone (over-stimulation may cause relaxation), (specify action of drug ordered).

INTERVENTIONS	RATIONALES
Estimate blood loss by counting or weighing peri pads. Soaked pad in 15 min is excessive. (1 gm = 1 cc if weighing pads).	The degree of blood loss may not be apparent from appearance of vaginal discharge. Estimation helps determine replacement requirements.
Notify caregiver if bleeding continues after nursing interventions.	Continued blood loss may indicate retained placental fragments or a cervical laceration.

NIC: *Fluid Monitoring*

Evaluation

(Date/time of evaluation of goal)

(Has goal been met? not met? partially met?)

(What is client's urine output? Is it 30 cc/hr or greater? Are mucous membranes moist? What is client's BP? Is it ≥ (specify for client)?)

(Revisions to care plan? D/C care plan? Continue care plan?)

CHAPTER 2.2

BASIC CARE PLAN: CESAREAN BIRTH

Clients may be scheduled for a cesarean birth for several reasons including pelvic contracture, abnormal fetal presentation (e.g., transverse lie, breech), complete placenta previa, active genital herpes, or a previous cesarean with a classical uterine incision.

Complications that arise during labor that may lead to cesarean birth include prolapsed cord, fetal distress, failure to progress, and cephalopelvic disproportion (CPD).

COMMON NURSING DIAGNOSES

 See RISK FOR INFECTION: MATERNAL/FETAL

Related to: Site for organism invasion secondary to surgery.

 See RISK FOR DEFICIENT FLUID VOLUME

Related to: Excessive losses secondary to wound drainage.

ADDITIONAL NURSING DIAGNOSES

 ANXIETY

Related to: Threat to biologic integrity secondary to invasive procedure and concern for fetal well-being.

Defining Characteristics: Client states (specify using quotes: e.g., "I'm nervous; frightened; tense" etc.). Client is trembling, crying; has ↑ pulse, ↑ BP (specify other physiologic signs of anxiety).

Goal: Client will cope effectively with anxiety by (date/time to evaluate).

Outcome Criteria

✔ Client reports ↓ anxiety; pulse and BP are within normal limits (specify for client).

✔ Client appears calmer: is no longer crying, not trembling.

NOC: *Anxiety Control*

INTERVENTIONS	RATIONALES
Assess client for physical and emotional signs of anxiety: trembling, crying, tachycardia, hypertension, dry mouth, or nausea.	Assessment provides information about emotional and sympathetic nervous system response to perceived threat.
Acknowledge client's anxiety. Provide information about fetal status, realistic reassurance and support: stay with client, speak slowly and calmly, use touch as indicated (note cultural variance in use of touch).	Acknowledgment validates client's feelings. Reassurance and support help the client to regain control. Personal space requirements and tolerance for touch varies with individuals and cultures.
Explain all procedures and equipment on a level client can understand. Provide information about expected neonatal care. Repeat information as needed.	High anxiety may interfere with concentration and ability to process information. Understanding decreases anxiety about unfamiliar experiences.
Include significant other in teaching and support. Encourage a support person to participate in cesarean birth if appropriate.	Significant other may also be anxious about surgical interventions. Presence of a support person decreases client's anxiety.
Teach coping mechanisms (specify: e.g., relaxation and breathing techniques, visualization, etc.) to client and significant other.	Effective coping helps the client and significant other to increase feelings of self-control during stressful experience.
If client is to have cesarean, teach about what will happen during and after the birth, frequent v/s, need to turn, cough, deep breathe, incision pain and relief methods available (specify: e.g., epidural morphine, PCA pump, IM narcotics, splinting incision with pillow, etc.).	Preoperative teaching provides anticipatory guidance about the postoperative interventions and how client can help herself. Knowledge of pain relief measures helps ↓ anxiety about pain.

(continues)

(continued)

INTERVENTIONS	RATIONALES
Introduce client and significant other to members of the surgical (and neonatal team if appropriate) and explain their roles in the birth.	Introductions validate the client's individuality and worth.
If client is to have general anesthesia, describe sensations she may feel, remain by her side and hold her hand until she is asleep.	Anticipatory guidance enhances the client's ability to cope when new sensations are felt. Touch may be especially reassuring at this time.
Describe sensations the client may feel if having epidural anesthesia: pressure, pulling and tugging, etc.	Anticipatory guidance enhances the client's ability to cope when new sensations are felt.
Describe what is happening during surgery and/or neonatal resuscitation.	Information decreases anxiety about unfamiliar scenes and sensations.
Ensure that client can see and touch infant before transfer.	Intervention promotes attachment and ↓ anxiety about newborn.
Arrange to visit the client on the 1st or 2nd postpartum day to review the birth and answer any questions.	Review and discussion assist the client to form an accurate impression of her birth experience.
Praise client and significant other for their effective coping skills after the birth.	Praise may reinforce positive coping skills in the future.

NIC: *Anxiety Reduction*

Evaluation

(Date/time of evaluation of goal)

(Has goal been met? not met? partially met?)

(Does client report ↓ anxiety? What is pulse and BP? Does client appear calmer? e.g., no longer crying, not trembling?)

(Revisions to care plan? D/C care plan? Continue care plan?)

ACUTE PAIN

Related to: Tissue trauma secondary to abdominal surgery, postdelivery uterine contractions.

Defining Characteristics: Client reports pain (specify degree using a scale of 1 to 10 with one being least, 10 being most), facial grimace, crying, guarding of incision, and so forth (specify).

Goal: Client will experience a decrease in pain by (date/time to evaluate).

Outcome Criteria

✔ Client reports decreased pain (specify depending on what was reported first: e.g., <5 on a scale of 1 to 10).

✔ Client is relaxed, not grimacing or crying, appropriate guarding of incision.

NOC: *Pain Control*

INTERVENTIONS	RATIONALES
Assess location and character of pain when the client reports discomfort. Assess for cultural variations in pain response if indicated (e.g., Asian client may smile and deny any pain even with abdominal surgery).	Assessment provides information about the cause of pain: may be incisional, uterine, or may indicate a complication such as hematoma. Different cultures have varied accepted responses to pain, which may differ from the nurse's.
Assess client's perception of pain intensity using a scale of 1 to 10 with 1 being the least and 10 being the most pain.	Assessment provides quantitative information about client's perception of pain and guides the choice of medications. Level of pain is what the client says it is.
Administer appropriate pain medication as ordered (specify drug, dose, route, times. Instruct pt in PCA pump use if indicated).	(Specify rationale for choosing the drug: e.g., is drug contraindicated if breast feeding? Describe action of specific drug.)
Assess client for pain relief (specify timing for particular drug given). Observe for adverse effects (specify for drug: e.g., itching, urinary retention with epidural morphine).	Assessment provides information about client's response to medication.
Keep narcotic antagonist (naloxone) available if client has received narcotic analgesia.	Naloxone reverses the effects of narcotics in cases of overdose.
Assist client to change positions, encourage ambulation as soon as possible. Provide a comfortable environment (temperature, lighting, etc.).	Position changes decrease muscle tension, ambulation decreases flatus, comfortable environment enhances relaxation.
Teach client to ask for pain medication before pain becomes severe or before planned activity.	Pain medication is more effective and less is needed if given before pain is severe. Premedication affords pain relief for activity.

INTERVENTIONS	RATIONALES
Teach client nonpharmacological interventions: (specify: e.g., splinting incision with pillow, rolling to side before rising from bed, etc.).	(Specify rationale: e.g., splinting and rolling to the side prevents traction on the incision site.)
Offer nonpharmacological pain interventions if desired: e.g., therapeutic touch, back rub, music, etc.	Nonpharmacological interventions may use distraction or the gate-control theory to ↓ pain perception.
Teach client about the physiology of after-pains (relate to breast-feeding as indicated).	Understanding the physiology may ↓ anxiety and pain perception associated with after-pains.
Notify caregiver if pain is not controlled or if complications are suspected.	Caregiver may order a different analgesic or decide to re-evaluate the client.

NIC: *Pain Management*

Evaluation

(Date/time of evaluation of goal)

(Has goal been met? not met? partially met?)

(What degree of pain does client report? Is client calm? relaxed? not grimacing, etc.? Describe client's activity.)

(Revisions to care plan? D/C care plan? Continue care plan?)

RISK FOR PERIOPERATIVE-POSITIONING INJURY

Related to: Positioning and loss of normal sensory protective responses secondary to anesthesia.

Defining Characteristics: None, as this is a potential diagnosis.

Goal: Client will not experience any positioning injury for duration of anesthesia.

Outcome Criteria

✔ Client's BP remains ≥ (specify for client).

✔ Client denies any leg or back pain after anesthesia wears off.

NOC: *Safety Status: Physical Injury*

INTERVENTIONS	RATIONALES
Assess client for any previous back or leg injuries or conditions that may be affected by surgical position.	Assessment provides information about pre-existing risk factors for perioperative injury.
Assist with positioning for epidural anesthesia as needed.	Proper positioning facilitates introduction of the epidural catheter and avoids client injury.
If client has epidural anesthesia, protect her legs from possible falls or torsion injury/side rails ↑ × 2, guard legs if knees are raised to insert Foley, and so forth.	Interventions protect the client's legs from falling and hyperextending the hip joint.
Position client supine on the operating table with a wedge under her right hip and a pillow under her head. Apply safety straps. Align spine and neck at all times. Tilt the table to the left as ordered.	Safety strap prevents client falls. Alignment presents nerve injury. Tilting the uterus to the left facilitates maternal venous return and uteroplacental perfusion.
Evaluate fetal heart rate prior to abdominal scrub and draping.	Assessment provides information about placental perfusion.
Ensure that client's legs are in a natural, aligned position without crossed ankles before draping (inform client not to cross ankles if preparing for general anesthesia). Assist anesthesia provider with natural positioning of client's arms at side or on arm board.	Natural positioning prevents torsion and prolonged mechanical pressure on nerves and circulatory system during surgery.
Use padding for bony prominences (e.g., pad arm boards, heels, etc.).	Padding decreases pressure over bony areas, which can interfere with circulation.
After surgery is completed, move client to a stretcher using a roller and draw sheet and enough staff to maintain client's body alignment during move.	Maintaining alignment prevents torsion or twisting of the client's body. Providing adequate staff prevents staff injuries.
Assess client's skin condition as she is being cleaned up after surgery. Note any reddened or blanched areas.	Assessment provides information about possible tissue injury.
Assess return of motor and sensory function in legs as epidural wears off. Maintain safety precautions (side rails up, etc.) until client has full use of extremities.	Assessment provides information about when client may safely use her legs again.
Notify caregiver and anesthesia provider of any unusual findings or complaints.	Notification allows caregiver to investigate possible injury.

NIC: *Positioning: Intraoperative*

Evaluation

(Date/time of evaluation of goal)

(Has goal been met? not met? partially met?)

(Did client's BP remain ≥ (what was specified for client)? Does client deny any leg or back pain after anesthesia has worn off?)

(Revisions to care plan? D/C care plan? Continue care plan?)

RISK FOR IMPAIRED PARENT/INFANT ATTACHMENT

Related to: Barriers to or interruption of attachment process secondary to surgical routine or illness of mother/infant.

Defining Characteristics: None, as this is a potential diagnosis.

Goal: Client will demonstrate appropriate attachment behaviors by (date/time to evaluate).

Outcome Criteria

✔ Parents will hold infant following birth.
✔ Parents and infant will make eye contact.
✔ Parents will verbalize positive feelings towards infant.

NOC: *Parent–Infant Attachment*

INTERVENTIONS	RATIONALES
Assess maternal feelings towards the fetus prior to birth (e.g., "Do you have a name chosen?" Note nonverbal cues).	Assessment provides information about prenatal attachment to the fetus.
Inform parents of fetal responses as assessed by FHR prior to birth.	Information helps the parents view fetus as a real baby.
Assess cultural expectations of the parents and their families related to mother–baby care after birth. Solicit information about dietary needs, and who is expected to care for the infant. Share information with all staff.	Assessment provides information about cultural variations (e.g., in some cultures the mother is expected to rest while others care for the infant). Cold foods may be prohibited during the puerperium.
Provide parents with an opportunity to see and touch the baby immediately after birth. If infant needs resuscitation, allow parents to see and touch infant prior to transfer to nursery.	Mothers and infants are ready to form attachment in the first few minutes after birth. If the infant is ill, seeing and touching the baby reduces parental anxiety and fosters attachment.

INTERVENTIONS	RATIONALES
Delay eye prophylaxis and any unnecessary procedures until parents have had an opportunity to hold infant for 30 minutes to 2 hours (per protocol).	Eye prophylaxis may interfere with the infant's ability to see his parents' faces. The first period of sensitivity lasts 30–90 minutes.
For cesarean births with general anesthesia, allow the father (or significant other) to be present after induction to bond with the infant.	Allowing father to be present fosters parent–infant attachment even if mother is asleep.
For cesarean births, take infant to recovery room with mother and encourage her to hold and breast feed infant if desired.	Postoperative clients, who are not too sedated, are able to interact with their baby just as vaginal birth mothers do.
For vaginal births, keep the infant with the parents. Teach parents about assessments and interventions as they are performed.	Attachment requires proximity. Involvement in assessments and interventions facilitates the beginning of parenting skills.
Administer pain medications to the mother as needed (specify).	Pain may distract the client from attachment and bonding with her infant.
(Encourage and facilitate breast-feeding immediately after birth if indicated.)	Early breast-feeding provides lactose for the infant after the stress of labor; nipple stimulation causes a release of oxytocin for the mother: ↑ uterine contraction and ↓ vaginal bleeding.
Encourage parents to hold their baby skin-to-skin (kangaroo care).	Skin-to-skin positioning provides warmth for the infant and facilitates attachment.
Promote bonding by pointing out attractive features of the infant and his response to the parents.	Intervention helps parents adjust their idealized thoughts about the baby with the real baby.
Praise parental caregiving skills as indicated.	Parenting is a learned process. Praise promotes self-esteem.
Assess attachment behaviors of parents: eye contact, touch, and verbalization about the baby. Share observations with caregiver and postpartum staff.	Failure to make eye contact, avoidance of touch, or negative expressions may indicate attachment problems, which need to be evaluated further.
If infant is ill and taken to nursery, take parents to see infant as soon as client is stable. Encourage parents to participate in caring for infant in the nursery as possible.	Interventions foster attachment and reduce parental anxiety. If infant is very ill, parents may be afraid to touch or care for their baby.

INTERVENTIONS	RATIONALES
If infant is transferred to another facility, provide parents with photos and mementos of the infant before transport and the phone number of the facility.	Interventions promote attachment and information until the client is reunited with her infant.
If mother is too ill to care for infant, or if cultural prescriptions interfere with infant care, encourage father or other family member to stay in room.	Family-centered care promotes attachment with all family members.
Refer parents as needed (specify: e.g., social services, congenital anomaly support groups, grief support, etc.).	Intervention provides additional assistance for parents having difficulty with attachment or supports cultural beliefs.

NIC: *Attachment Promotion*

Evaluation

(Date/time of evaluation of goal)

(Has goal been met? not met? partially met?)

(Did parents hold infant following birth? Did parents and infant make eye contact? Did parents verbalize positive feelings towards infant? Specify using quotes.)

(Revisions to care plan? D/C care plan? Continue care plan?)

CHAPTER 2.3

FAILURE TO PROGRESS

Failure to progress refers to labor dystocia with a lack of progressive cervical dilatation and/or fetal descent. Systematic assessment of the "P's" of labor may help define the cause. Evaluation of the powers may show that the contractions are too weak or uncoordinated. A discrepancy between fetal size or position (passenger) and the pelvis (passageway) may inhibit fetal descent. High maternal anxiety (psyche) and maternal positioning may also interfere with labor progress.

MEDICAL CARE

- Evaluation of fetal size, presentation, position, and pelvic adequacy
- AROM or oxytocin augmentation may be initiated if uterine hypotonus is diagnosed and CPD ruled out
- Forceps or vacuum extraction may be tried if the problem develops in the second stage
- Cesarean delivery for CPD

COMMON NURSING DIAGNOSES

 ### See RISK FOR INJURY: MATERNAL AND FETAL

Related to: Cephalopelvic disproportion, dystocia, prolonged labor, etc.

 ### See ANXIETY

Related to: Perceived threat to self or fetus secondary to prolonged labor with lack of progress.

Defining Characteristics: Client expresses feelings of helplessness and tension, expresses worry about fetal well-being (specify, using quotes). Client exhibits signs of anxiety (specify: e.g., crying, withdrawn, or angry and critical, etc.).

ADDITIONAL NURSING DIAGNOSES

 ### FATIGUE

Related to: Increased energy expenditure and discouragement secondary to prolonged labor without progress.

Defining Characteristics: (Specify length and progression of client's labor.) Client states (specify: e.g., "I'm so tired, I can't do this anymore"). Client is (specify: uncooperative, crying, lethargic, listless, irritable, etc.).

Goal: Client will experience a decrease in physical and mental fatigue by (date/time to evaluate).

Outcome Criteria

- ✔ Client verbalizes understanding of plan of care.
- ✔ Client rests between contractions.
- ✔ Client is cooperative and not crying (specify other objective measurements).

NOC: *Energy Conservation*

INTERVENTIONS	RATIONALES
Allow client to express feelings of frustration and fatigue. Validate concerns.	Interventions validate client's perceptions of the experience.
Provide physical and emotional support to client and significant others.	Client may expend more energy being distressed. Family may also be tired.
Inform client and significant others about expected labor progress and realistic evaluation of client's labor pattern.	Client and family may have unrealistic expectations about labor progress.
Assess for the causes of failure to progress: powers, passenger, passageway, position, and psyche.	Assessment provides information about possible causes and infers solutions to the problems of failure to progress.

INTERVENTIONS	RATIONALES
Notify caregiver of lack of progress, client's fatigue and assessment findings.	Information assists caregiver in determining a plan of care for client.
Explain medical plan of care to client and significant other (specify: e.g., sedation, augmentation).	Explanation helps dispel feelings of helplessness and hopelessness.
Ensure hydration by providing fluids as ordered. Suggest fruit juices (if cesarean is unlikely) or IV solutions with added dextrose. Provide refreshments for significant other if desired.	Dehydration and starvation contribute to fatigue during labor. Significant other may neglect personal needs when focusing on client.
Provide a calm environment; dim lights, ↓ volume on monitor, ask extra visitors to leave. Assist client to conserve energy by resting between contractions, and accepting sedation if indicated.	Decreased environmental stimulation promotes rest. Client may feel that she is failure if she accepts medication.
Instruct client in relaxation techniques and mental imagery. Offer soothing music, a back rub, or massage as indicated.	Interventions promote conservation of energy and positive thoughts facilitating mental and physical relaxation.
Encourage significant other to rest also. Provide pillows and blankets if needed.	Support person may also be fatigued and anxious, adding to client's distress.
Keep client and significant other informed of labor progress, fetal status, and changes in plan of care.	Information promotes a sense of trust and relaxation.

NIC: *Energy Management*

Evaluation

(Date/time of evaluation of goal)

(Has goal been met? not met? partially met?)

(Does client verbalize understanding of plan of care? Is client resting between contractions? Is client cooperative and not crying? Specify other objective criteria.)

(Revisions to care plan? D/C care plan? Continue care plan?)

DISTURBED ENERGY FIELD

Related to: Slowing or blocking of energy flow secondary to labor.

Defining Characteristics: Disruption of the client's energy field as perceived by nurse experienced in therapeutic touch (specify: e.g., temperature, color, disruption, or movements of the visual field).

Goal: Client will regain harmony and energy field balance by (date/time to evaluate).

Outcome Criteria

✔ Client reports feelings of relief after therapeutic touch.

✔ Labor progress resumes.

NOC: *Well-being*

INTERVENTIONS	RATIONALES
Assess possible causes of failure to progress. If physiologic causes are not apparent, note if client exhibits psychological distress.	Assessment provides information about the possible causes of failure to progress. Psychological factors may hinder labor progress.
Explain therapeutic touch to client and assess client's desire for the intervention.	Client may not know about therapeutic touch as an intervention. Permission needs to be obtained and client safety assured before any intervention.
Reassure client that she may stop the procedure if she feels uncomfortable.	Reassurance may encourage client to try this intervention.
Notify a nurse qualified to perform therapeutic touch of client's request for the intervention.	Practitioners of therapeutic touch have had specialized instruction and supervised practice.
Provide privacy and avoid interruption of the process (e.g., time labor assessments to promote uninterrupted time for therapeutic touch).	Therapeutic touch is a very personal experience. The practitioner needs to focus on the client's energy field in order to facilitate the flow of healing energy.
Encourage and facilitate rest after therapeutic touch is completed.	Rest promotes harmony and balance of energy flow.
Evaluate client's verbal and nonverbal response to intervention. Monitor labor progress.	Evaluation provides information about effectiveness of intervention.

NIC: *Therapeutic Touch*

Evaluation

(Date/time of evaluation of goal)

(Has goal been met? not met? partially met?)

(Does client report feelings of relief? Specify using quotes. Has labor progressed? Specify changes in dilatation or descent.)

(Revisions to care plan? D/C care plan? Continue care plan?)

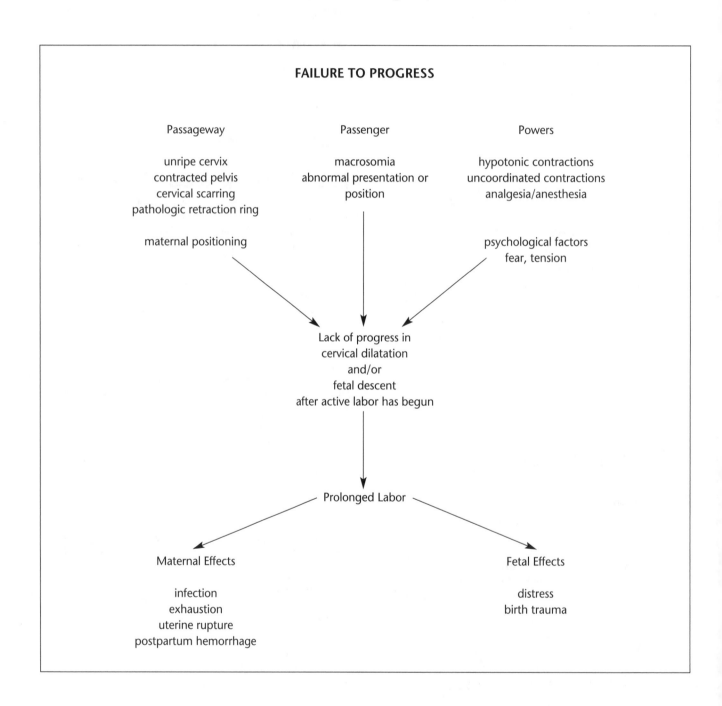

FAILURE TO PROGRESS

Passageway

unripe cervix
contracted pelvis
cervical scarring
pathologic retraction ring

maternal positioning

Passenger

macrosomia
abnormal presentation or
position

Powers

hypotonic contractions
uncoordinated contractions
analgesia/anesthesia

psychological factors
fear, tension

Lack of progress in
cervical dilatation
and/or
fetal descent
after active labor has begun

Prolonged Labor

Maternal Effects

infection
exhaustion
uterine rupture
postpartum hemorrhage

Fetal Effects

distress
birth trauma

CHAPTER 2.4

INDUCTION AND AUGMENTATION

Induction refers to artificial stimulation of labor before it has spontaneously started. Augmentation is artificial stimulation to enhance labor after it has begun naturally.

Reasons for induction include maternal and fetal conditions that prohibit continuing the pregnancy. These may include: severe PIH, fetal demise, IUGR, prolonged ruptured membranes, chorioamnionitis, diabetes mellitus or other severe maternal illnesses, and verified postterm pregnancy. Induction may be accomplished by use of cervical ripening agents if the cervix is unfavorable, followed by amniotomy, and oxytocin infusion. Augmentation usually consists of amniotomy and/or oxytocin infusion to increase the intensity and frequency of hypotonic uterine contractions.

Contraindications to induction or augmentation are contraindications to labor contractions and vaginal birth. These include fetal distress, complete placenta previa, active genital herpes, CPD, previous classical uterine incision, and fetal mal presentation. Care should be taken to verify fetal gestational age prior to inducing labor.

MEDICAL CARE

- Fetal maturity assessment: LNMP, serial ultrasound measurements, and possibly amniocentesis for L/S ratio
- Determination of fetal lie, presentation, and station
- Assessment of cervical readiness for labor: effacement, dilatation, position, and consistency (Bishop's scoring may be used)
- Cervical ripening agents (PGE$_2$ gel, dynoprostone, or misoprostol) may be used to soften the cervix prior to oxytocin induction
- AROM (artificial rupture of membranes) may stimulate contractions
- Continuous EFM; intravenous oxytocin (Pitocin) piggybacked to a mainline IV via an infusion pump; dilution of pitocin is per order. Pitocin is titrated to labor pattern and fetal tolerance

COMMON NURSING DIAGNOSES

 ### See BASIC CARE PLAN: LABOR AND VAGINAL BIRTH

ADDITIONAL NURSING DIAGNOSES

 ### See RISK FOR INJURY: MATERNAL/FETAL

Related to: Effects of drugs used to induce or augment labor.

Defining Characteristics: None, as this is a potential diagnosis.

Goal: Client and fetus will not experience any injury related to the use of drugs used to induce or augment labor by (date/time to evaluate).

Outcome Criteria

✔ Contraction frequency not less than q 2–3 minutes, not more than 60 second duration, and adequate resting tone between contractions.
✔ FHR remains reassuring with no late decelerations.

NOC: *Risk Control*

INTERVENTIONS	RATIONALES
Obtain baseline maternal v/s. Assess fetal presentation, position, station, and cervical effacement and dilatation. Position client on left side if tolerated.	Assessment provides baseline data prior to induction or augmentation. Position facilitates placental perfusion.

(continues)

(continued)

INTERVENTIONS	RATIONALES
Apply EFM and obtain a 20-minute strip prior to beginning induction. Assess baseline FHR, variability, and periodic and nonperiodic changes. If FHR are nonreassuring, notify provider without starting oxytocin.	Assessment provides data about fetal well-being prior to beginning oxytocin. Increased intensity of contractions might be harmful to an already stressed fetus.
Assess uterine activity by palpation or IUPC before starting induction.	Assessment provides baseline data about contractions and resting tone. Contractions may be adequate without oxytocin.
Explain induction or augmentation rationale and procedure to client and significant other before starting. Allow time for questions.	Explanation decreases client and significant other's anxiety about the procedure and reason for it.
If cervical ripening agent is to be used, follow agency protocol for IV access, placement, length of time to remain supine, and how long to wait before beginning oxytocin (specify).	Cervical ripening preparations have different requirements for placement and timing. Agency protocol may require a heparin lock or KVO IV.
If uterine hyperstimulation or nonreassuring FHT develop, remove the ripening agent, turn client to left side, provide humidified oxygen at 8–12 L/min via facemask, and notify physician. Administer a tocolytic as ordered.	Cervical ripening agents may cause uterine hyperstimulation and decreased uteroplacental perfusion causing fetal hypoxia. Tocolytics decrease uterine activity.
Start mainline IV as ordered by care provider (specify which fluids and rate) with an 18-gauge (or larger) catheter on nondominant arm or hand, avoiding use of armboard.	Mainline IV provides venous access should oxytocin need to be discontinued. 18-gauge or larger needle is indicated if client might need blood; placement allows client use of her hand.
Mix oxytocin in IV solution as ordered by care provider (specify fluid type, amount, and how many units of oxytocin).	Oxytocin has an antidiuretic effect by causing retention of free water. Caregiver may choose an electrolyte fluid (rather than dextrose and water) to ↓ this effect. Dilution determines the volume for each milliunit (mU).
Thread oxytocin IV tubing through an infusion pump. Piggyback oxytocin to mainline IV at a distal port. Begin infusion as ordered (specify: e.g., 0.5 mU/min or 1 mU/min).	Pump ensures correct dosage is given. Piggybacking the drug maintains IV access if oxytocin needs to be discontinued. Using a distal port allows oxytocin to be discontinued without additional drug infusing through excess tubing.

INTERVENTIONS	RATIONALES
Assess maternal BP, P, R, and assess fetal baseline heart rate, variability, periodic, and non-periodic changes q 30 min or before increasing oxytocin infusion rate.	Assessment provides information about complications of oxytocin: fluid excess, ruptured uterus, fetal distress.
Assess uterine contractions for frequency, duration, intensity, and resting tone by palpation or IUPC q 15–30 min or before increasing oxytocin.	Assessment provides information about effects of oxytocin needed for titration of the drug.
Titrate oxytocin as ordered to obtain contractions q 2–3 min, of 60 second duration, and moderate intensity with adequate resting tone. Once active labor is established, the oxytocin dose may be decreased.	Most clients will have adequate contractions with 10 mU/min or less of pitocin.
Decrease or discontinue oxytocin if contractions are closer than q 2 min or last >90 seconds or there is an ↑ in resting tone (>20 mm Hg with IUPC). Observe client for unusual discomfort.	Uterine hyperstimulation may result in ↓ placental perfusion causing fetal hypoxia or uterine rupture.
Notify physician if hypertonus continues after oxytocin has been discontinued. Administer tocolytics as ordered (specify, drug, dose, and route).	Oxytocin has a short half-life (3–5 min). Continued hypertonus may indicate the need for tocolytics to relax the uterus and increase placental perfusion. (Action of drug.)
Discontinue oxytocin if a nonreassuring fetal heart rate pattern develops. Position client on her left side, increase mainline IVF, provide humidified oxygen at 8–12 L/min via facemask. Notify physician of fetal heart rate pattern, actions taken, and result. Document notification.	Oxytocin may cause uterine hyperstimulation or increased resting tone, which interferes with placental perfusion. Interventions increase placental perfusion and oxygen available to the fetus.
Encourage client to void q 2h. Monitor hourly intake and output.	Oxytocin has a slight antidiuretic effect. Interventions prevent bladder distention and provide information about fluid balance.
Perform sterile vaginal exams as needed to monitor progress of labor.	Vaginal exams provide information about effectiveness of induction or augmentation.
Keep client and significant other informed of labor progress and any changes in the plan of care.	Information promotes understanding and decreases anxiety, which may slow labor progress.

NIC: *Labor Induction*

Evaluation

(Date/time of evaluation of goal)

(Has goal been met? not met? partially met?)

(Describe contraction frequency, duration, and intensity and uterine resting tone. Describe baseline FHR, variability, periodic and nonperiodic changes.)

(Revisions to care plan? D/C care plan? Continue care plan?)

RISK FOR EXCESS FLUID VOLUME

Related to: Water intoxication secondary to antidiuretic effect of oxytocin and administration of intravenous fluids.

Defining Characteristics: None, as this is a potential diagnosis.

Goal: Client will not experience fluid volume excess.

Outcome Criteria

✔ Client's urine output = intake.

✔ Client does not experience altered level of consciousness, or convulsions.

NOC: *Fluid Balance*

INTERVENTIONS	RATIONALES
Monitor hourly intake and output while oxytocin is infusing.	Urine output may ↓ as oxytocin causes the kidneys to reabsorb free water.
Observe client for signs of water intoxication including subtle changes in mental status, confusion, lethargy, nausea, and/or convulsions. Discontinue oxytocin and ↓ mainline to KVO; notify physician.	Oxytocin dosage >20 mU/min is associated with ↓ urine output. Excessive retention of free water causes a hyponatremic, hypoosmotic state, resulting in cerebral edema.
Monitor lab values as obtained.	Serum sodium <120 mEq/L or plasma osmolality ≤240 mOsm/kg indicate eminent water intoxication.
Collaborate with caregiver to mix oxytocin in an electrolyte solution rather than dextrose and water.	With large doses of oxytocin, the risk of water intoxication is greater if oxytocin is mixed with electrolyte-free water and dextrose.

INTERVENTIONS	RATIONALES
When oxytocin needs to be infused at >20 mU/min for several hours, increase the strength of the infusion rather than the volume (e.g., mix 10 U oxytocin in 500 cc fluid so that 3 cc/hr = 1 mU/min or 10 U oxytocin in 250 cc fluid so that 1.5 cc/hr = 1 mU/min).	Strengthening the solution decreases the volume that needs to infuse.
Assess mainline IV rate each hour. As oxytocin infusion is increased, decrease mainline IV rate to provide IVF at ordered rate (specify: e.g., 125 cc/hr).	Mainline may be periodically opened up for maternal hypotension or fetal distress. Intervention avoids infusing large amounts of fluid as oxytocin is increased.
If labor is not established after 8 hours, collaborate with caregiver to discontinue the infusion until the next day.	Intervention promotes client rest and decreases the risk of water intoxication from high doses of oxytocin.

NIC: *Fluid Management*

Evaluation

(Date/time of evaluation of goal)

(Has goal been met? not met? partially met?)

(What is urine output? Is client's level of consciousness appropriate? Has client had any convulsions?)

(Revisions to care plan? D/C care plan? Continue care plan?)

RISK FOR IMPAIRED GAS EXCHANGE: FETAL

Related to: Cord compression secondary to AROM and prolapse of the umbilical cord.

Defining Characteristics: None, as this is a potential diagnosis.

Goal: Fetus will not experience impaired gas exchange after AROM.

Outcome Criteria

✔ FHT remain reassuring (specify) after AROM. Prolapsed cord is not palpated on vaginal exam after AROM.

NOC: *Electrolyte and Acid–Base Balance*

INTERVENTIONS	RATIONALES
Assess baseline FHR before membranes are ruptured. Note variability and presence of accelerations or decelerations.	Assessment provides information about individual fetal baseline heart rate and well-being.
Explain AROM procedure to client including expected benefits and sensations she may feel (warm, wet, no pain, possible ↑ contractions).	Explanation decreases anxiety about procedure and ensures client understanding and cooperation.
Encourage client to breathe deeply and relax during procedure.	Client relaxation facilitates vaginal exam and amniotomy.
Assess fetal presentation, position and station prior to AROM. Notify caregiver of findings.	Fetus should be cephalic or frank breech and well-engaged with presenting part against the cervix to prevent prolapsed cord.
Position client on chux or pads and assist caregiver to perform AROM by opening amnihook and applying gentle fundal pressure if requested.	Dry pads will absorb excess fluid. Light fundal pressure may be needed to expel fluid and move the presenting part against the cervix to prevent prolapsed cord.
(If RN is to perform AROM, obtain order, ensure that presenting part is cephalic and well-engaged against the cervix. If not, notify caregiver of findings and do not perform AROM. Perform procedure according to agency protocol. Palpate for a prolapsed cord after fluid has escaped.)	Many boards of nursing do not allow staff nurses to perform AROM or may require extra competency instruction and certification. The RN is responsible for knowing what the state board defines as the scope of practice, and performing the procedure safely.
Assess FHR immediately after amniotomy and through the next few contractions.	Assessment provides information about fetal oxygenation. Prolapsed cord may be obvious or occult.
Note date and time of AROM on EFM strip and in chart.	Documentation provides information about activities affecting fetal condition during labor.
Observe color, amount, and odor of amniotic fluid at time of AROM and during each subsequent vaginal exam.	Assessments provide information about fetal well-being: meconium indicates stress unless fetus is breech, blood may indicate abruption, an unpleasant odor may indicate infection.

INTERVENTIONS	RATIONALES
Provide a dry chux or pad after AROM. Change pads frequently throughout duration of labor.	Dry pads keep client comfortable and decrease the warm, wet environment favored by microorganisms.
Assess client's temp q 2h after membranes have ruptured until birth.	Assessment provides information about possible development of infection.
If nonreassuring variable decelerations develop, change maternal position, provide oxygen at 8–12 L/min via facemask, and perform vaginal exam to rule out prolapsed cord. Notify caregiver of severe variable decelerations, interventions, and fetal response.	Decreased amniotic fluid may cause cord compression resulting in variable decelerations. Maternal position change may relieve the pressure on the cord.
Provide for amnioinfusion as ordered per agency protocol (specify).	Amnioinfusion may be initiated to reduce pressure on the cord.
Prepare client for emergency cesarean if ordered for prolapsed cord or fetal distress.	Obstruction of fetal gas exchange may require emergency cesarean birth.

NIC: *Acid–Base Management*

Evaluation

(Date/time of evaluation of goal)

(Has goal been met? not met? partially met?)

(Is FHR reassuring? Describe FHR: baseline, variability, periodic, and nonperiodic changes. Does vaginal exam rule out prolapsed cord after AROM?)

(Revisions to care plan? D/C care plan? Continue care plan?)

INDUCTION AND AUGMENTATION

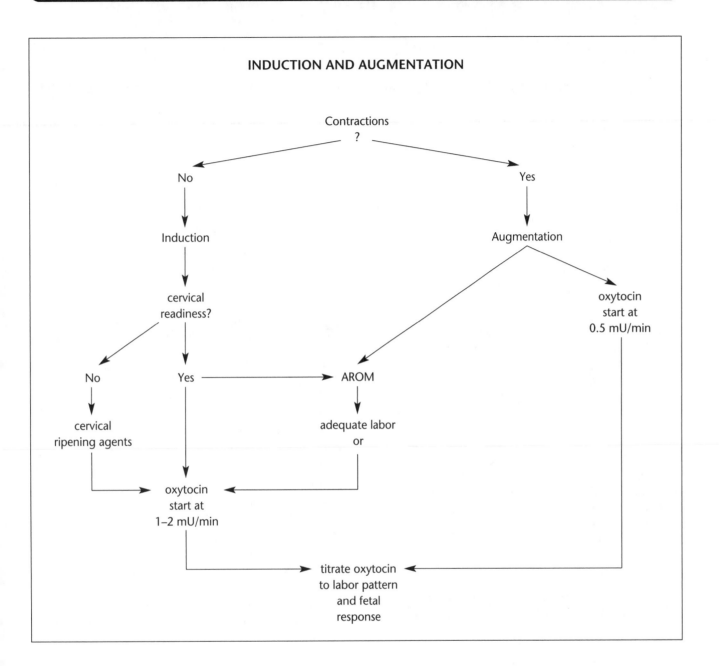

CHAPTER 2.5

REGIONAL ANALGESIA

Pain relief measures that affect a specific body area are termed regional analgesia or anesthesia. The drugs (usually a local anesthetic and/or narcotic analgesic) are injected near specific nerves. Local anesthetics interrupt the transmission of impulses for pain, motor, and sensory nerves. Narcotics bind to opioid receptors and decrease pain perception only. Commonly used local anesthetics in obstetrics are lidocaine, bupivicaine hydrochloride, and 2-chloroprocaine hydrochloride. Commonly used narcotics are fentanyl, sufentanil, and morphine.

The most common regional anesthesia used in childbirth is local perineal infiltration for episiotomy. Another common usage in the United States is epidural analgesia/anesthesia employed for labor pain and cesarean birth. Epidurals may employ local anesthetics alone or be combined with narcotics. Intrathecal analgesia is injection of a narcotic into the subarachnoid space. This provides pain relief without motor, sympathetic, or sensory block. Other types of regional analgesia sometimes used in childbirth include pudendal, and spinal blocks.

COMPLICATIONS

Epidural using local anesthetics:

- maternal hypotension from sympathetic block causing vasodilation and pooling of blood in the legs; may result in nonreassuring FHR patterns
- may interfere with labor pattern causing prolonged labor; may lead to cesarean birth
- may block maternal urge to push; may be associated with increased use of forceps
- high block or complete block may result in respiratory arrest
- post dural-puncture headaches
- systemic toxicity resulting in convulsions, cardiac depression, and dysrhythmias

Epidural or Intrathecal narcotics:

- respiratory depression
- urinary retention, bladder distension
- pruritis, nausea, and vomiting

MEDICAL CARE

- Regional analgesia and anesthesia (excluding local infiltration) should be provided by a qualified, credentialed, licensed anesthesia care provider who injects the drugs, stabilizes the client, and is available to adjust dosage and treat complications
- Contraindications may include hypovolemia, coagulation defects or anticoagulant therapy, and local infection
- IV of a balanced salt solution (e.g., lactated Ringer's) with a bolus of 500–1000 cc given prior to epidural placement to avoid hypotension
- After aspiration to avoid injecting the drug into a blood vessel, a test dose is given to rule out sensitivity
- Drugs may be given by single injection or a catheter may be placed for repeated or continuous epidural analgesia

COMMON NURSING DIAGNOSES

See RISK FOR INFECTION

Related to: Site for organism invasion secondary to presence of epidural catheter.

See RISK FOR PERIOPERATIVE-POSITIONING INJURY

Related to: Loss of usual sensory protective responses.

ADDITIONAL NURSING DIAGNOSES

ACUTE PAIN

Related to: Uterine contractions and perineal stretching during labor.

Defining Characteristics: Client reports pain/discomfort (specify rating on a scale of 1 to 10 with 1 being least, 10 most) and requests relief measures (specify: e.g., "Can I have my epidural now?"). Client is grimacing, crying, and so forth (specify).

Goal: Client will experience a decrease in pain by (date/time to evaluate).

Outcome Criteria

✔ Client will report a decrease in pain (specify: e.g., <5 on a scale of 1 to 10).

✔ Client will not be crying or grimacing (specify for individual response).

NOC: *Pain Control*

INTERVENTIONS	RATIONALES
Assess client for pain every hour during labor. Note verbal and nonverbal cues. Assess location and character. Ask client to rate pain on a scale from 1 to 10 with 1 being least, and 10 being the most pain.	Assessment provides information about etiology of pain (e.g., contractions, perineal stretching, or uterine rupture). Rating allows objective quantitative reassessment.
Accept the client's interpretation of pain and avoid cultural stereotyping.	Pain is a personal experience. The expression of pain is influenced by cultural norms.
Explain the physiology of the discomfort the client is experiencing (e.g., back labor and OP position, cervical dilatation, pressure during descent).	Explanations decrease fear of the unknown and assist the client to cope with discomfort.
Reinforce client's use of breathing and relaxation techniques learned in childbirth classes. Support coaching from significant other.	Support assists the client and significant other to use techniques learned in childbirth education classes.
Assist client and significant other with suggestions and implementation of nonpharmacological pain relief measures if desired (specify: e.g., position changes, back rub, massage, whirlpool, etc.).	Client may wish to have an unmedicated birth and only need support rather than drugs to cope with the discomfort of labor and birth.

INTERVENTIONS	RATIONALES
Explain the medical pain relief options available to the client (specify: IV narcotics, epidural, intratheal, etc.). Briefly discuss advantages and disadvantages of each option.	Information empowers the client to decide between the available options to meet her individual needs.
Administer systemic analgesia as ordered (specify: drug, dose, route, and time).	(Specify action and side effects for each drug.)
Notify anesthesia care provider if client is to have regional analgesia.	Early notification promotes timely pain relief if anesthesia provider is not readily available.
Monitor maternal and fetal response to medication; observe for adverse effects (specify for drug).	(Specify for drugs given: e.g., IV narcotics may cause ↓ FHR variability.)
Reevaluate client's perception of pain after drug has taken effect (specify time frame for drug given) using a scale of 1 to 10.	Timing of pain relief varies with different drugs and routes.
Notify caregiver or anesthesia provider if measures aren't effective in decreasing client's perception of pain.	Pain relief measures need to be individualized. Client may respond better to a different drug or higher dosage.

NIC: *Analgesic Administration*

Evaluation

(Date/time of evaluation of goal)

(Has goal been met? not met? partially met?)

(What does client rate pain on a scale of 1 to 10? Is client crying or grimacing? Describe activity.)

(Revisions to care plan? D/C care plan? Continue care plan?)

RISK FOR INJURY: MATERNAL AND FETAL

Related to: Effects of drugs used for pain relief during labor and birth.

Defining Characteristics: None, as this is a potential diagnosis.

Goal: Client and fetus will not experience any injury from medications used during labor by (date/time to evaluate).

Outcome Criteria

✔ Client's BP, P, R remain within normal limits (specify a range for client).

✔ FHT remain reassuring and newborn exhibits spontaneous respirations at birth.

NOC: *Symptom Control*

INTERVENTIONS	RATIONALES
Assess client's baseline vital signs before analgesia administration.	Assessment provides information about individual baseline to help identify any adverse drug effects.
Assess fetal well-being (FHR, variability, accelerations, or decelerations) before providing analgesia.	Assessment provides information about baseline fetal status to help identify any adverse drug effects.
Start an IV if ordered (specify fluid and rate: e.g., for epidural, give bolus of 500–1000 cc if ordered).	An IV provides venous access for hydration and treatment of complications.
Administer IV push analgesia slowly during a contraction (specify: drug, dose, and time).	Intervention prevents a large bolus of drug from crossing the placenta.
Raise side rails, place call bell within reach and instruct client not to get out of bed after receiving narcotic or epidural analgesia.	Interventions promote safety by preventing maternal falls while sedated.
Reassess client's BP, P, and R and fetal well-being at expected peak of drug action (specify for drug).	Assessment provides information about client's physiologic response to drug and fetal effects.
Time systemic narcotics to avoid respiratory depression in the newborn (specify for individual drug).	Narcotics given to the mother should wear off before or peak after birth to avoid respiratory depression in the newborn.
If client is to receive an epidural encourage the client to void before the procedure.	Epidural analgesia may ↓ the sensation of a full bladder and the ability to void easily.
Apply continuous EFM for clients receiving regional analgesia. Document assessments of fetal well-being per agency protocol.	Continuous EFM provides information about effects of analgesia on the fetus.
Ensure that oxygen, suction, and resuscitation drugs and equipment including bag and mask are readily available.	Systemic effects of regional analgesia may result in life-threatening complications (respiratory arrest, cardiac dysrhythmias, etc.).

INTERVENTIONS	RATIONALES
Assist anesthesia care provider to provide epidural or intrathecal analgesia by obtaining supplies and positioning client as indicated.	Assistance facilitates epidural placement.
Assess client for dizziness, slurred speech, numbness, tinnitus, or convulsions after epidural test dose is given.	Assessment after test dose provides early indications of central nervous system toxicity.
After dose is given, assist with repositioning client and assess maternal v/s and fetal status per protocol (specify: e.g., q 5″ × 20″ etc.).	Repositioning the client facilitates therapeutic effects of the epidural drugs. Epidurals may cause hypotension resulting from sympathetic block and pooling of blood in legs.
If client develops hypotension or nonreassuring FHT, position on left side, provide a bolus of IVF, and administer humidified oxygen at 8–12 L/min. If improvement not noted, notify anesthesia provider.	Maternal hypotension decreases placental blood flow leading to late decelerations. Interventions should ↑ blood volume, oxygen saturation, and placental flow.
Assess bladder and encourage voiding q 2h. Catheterize as ordered if bladder is distended and client is unable to void.	Interventions prevent bladder distension, which may obstruct labor and result in bladder injury and infection.
Palpate contractions and assist client to push during second stage if needed.	Epidural may interfere with the urge to push during second stage.
Assess and support newborn's respiratory effort at birth. Have neonatal naloxone and resuscitation equipment ready for all births.	Labor analgesia may cause neonatal respiratory depression. Naloxone is a narcotic antagonist.
Ensure that entire epidural catheter is removed after delivery by noting mark on the tip.	Mark indicates entire catheter has been removed and hasn't broken off.

NIC: *Electronic Fetal Monitoring: Intrapartum*

Evaluation

(Date/time of evaluation of goal)

(Has goal been met? not met? partially met?)

(What are client's BP, P, and R? Did FHT remain reassuring? Did newborn exhibit spontaneous respirations?)

(Revisions to care plan? D/C care plan? Continue care plan?)

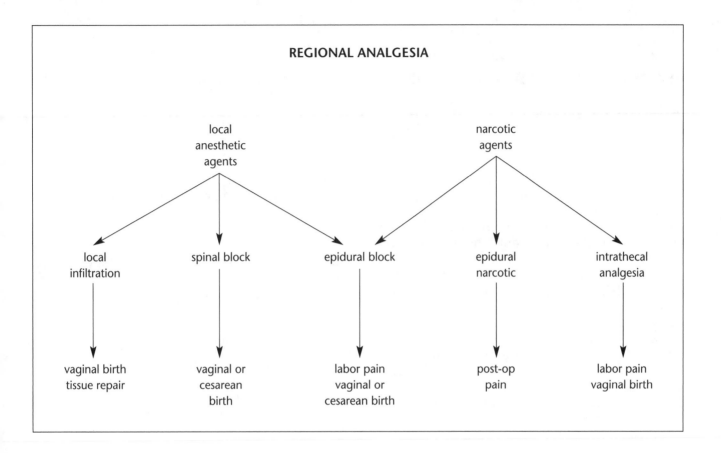

CHAPTER 2.6

FETAL DISTRESS

Fetal well-being during labor is assessed by evaluation of the FHR pattern. The healthy fetus is able to compensate for the normal interruption of oxygen delivery during the peak of contractions. A reassuring FHR pattern includes a stable individual baseline rate (usually between 110–160), presence of variability (notably STV; assessment terminology varies), presence of accelerations and absence of variable or late decelerations.

When the oxygen supply is inadequate to meet fetal needs, changes in the FHR pattern indicate fetal distress. Common causes are placental insufficiency, cord compression, and anemia. Signs of fetal distress include decreased fetal movement, nonreassuring or ominous FHR patterns, and meconium in the amniotic fluid (unless fetus is a breech presentation).

RISK FACTORS

- PIH
- Diabetes mellitus
- Uterine hypertonus
- Hemorrhage
- Infection
- Maternal hypotension
- Maternal or fetal anemia
- Oligohydramnios
- Cord entanglement/prolapse
- Preterm or IUGR fetus

MEDICAL CARE

- Continuous EFM with scalp electrode; IVF, discontinue oxytocin, change maternal position, give humidified oxygen at 8–12 L/min.
- Fetal scalp sampling
- Amnioinfusion

- Delivery by forceps, vacuum extraction, or cesarean section if indicated

COMMON NURSING DIAGNOSES

See ANXIETY

Related to: Threat to fetal well-being, perceived possible fetal loss or injury.

Defining Characteristics: Client expresses anxiety (specify using quotes: e.g., "I'm scared. Is my baby going to be all right?"). Client exhibits physiological signs of anxiety (specify: e.g., tension, pallor, tachycardia, etc.).

ADDITIONAL NURSING DIAGNOSES

IMPAIRED GAS EXCHANGE: FETAL

Related to: Inadequate oxygen supply secondary to (specify: placental insufficiency, cord compression, or anemia).

Defining Characteristics: (Specify details of nonreassuring or ominous FHR pattern, BPP findings, laboratory values: e.g., maternal Hgb, fetal scalp pH, O_2 and CO_2 if available).

Goal: Fetus will experience improved gas exchange by (date/time to evaluate).

Outcome Criteria

- ✔ FHR returns to individual baseline rate with a reassuring pattern: present STV, no late or severe variable decelerations.
- ✔ APGAR score is >7 at 1 and 5 minutes.

NOC: *Electrolyte and Acid–Base Balance*

INTERVENTIONS	RATIONALES
Monitor FHR, contractions, and resting tone continuously by EFM and palpation. Apply scalp electrode if possible.	Monitoring provides continuous information about fetal oxygenation. Internal scalp electrode provides the most accurate FHR information.
Assess FHR systematically q 15 min during 1st stage and q 5 min during 2nd stage of labor.	Frequent assessment for high-risk clients provides information about fetal well-being and response to interventions.
Evaluate color, amount, and odor of amniotic fluid when membranes rupture and hourly thereafter.	Provides information about passage of meconium, bleeding, possible oligohydramnios, or development of infection.
Monitor for vaginal bleeding, abdominal tenderness, or ↑ abdominal girth.	Assessment provides information about possible placental abruption.
Assess maternal BP, P, and R on same schedule as FHR; assess temp q 2h after ROM.	Assessment provides information about maternal homeostasis and possible development of chorioamnionitis.
Discontinue oxytocin if infusing and the fetus shows signs of distress.	Oxytocin may cause uterine hypertonus, which interferes with placental perfusion and fetal oxygenation.
Ensure adequate maternal hydration. Increase rate of IV or start IV as ordered (specify: fluid, site, rate).	Maternal dehydration and hypovolemia ↓ placental perfusion and fetal oxygen supply.
Administer humidified oxygen at 8–12 L/min via facemask. Explain rationale to client and significant others.	Intervention provides ↑ oxygen saturation of maternal blood perfusing placenta.
Position client on left side. If severe variable decelerations occur, try alternative positions: left, right sides, knee–chest, and so forth. Explain purpose to client and significant others.	Positioning the client on her left side facilitates placental perfusion. Alternative positions may relieve cord compression indicated by variable decelerations. Explanations promote client compliance.
Perform sterile vaginal exam if indicated to rule out prolapsed cord and evaluate labor progress.	Vaginal exam provides information about possible causes of distress. Compression of a prolapsed cord interferes with oxygen delivery to the fetus. Rapid fetal descent may cause a prolonged deceleration.
If prolapsed cord is felt or suspected (severe variable decelerations or bradycardia), keep hand in vagina and apply	Contraction pressure causes the prolapsed cord to be occluded causing fetal distress or death. Interventions help relieve

INTERVENTIONS	RATIONALES
pressure to hold presenting part off the cord. Position client in knee–chest or Trendelenburg and call for help.	pressure of the cord until fetus can be delivered by cesarean.
Administer tocolytic medication as ordered (specify: e.g., terbutaline 0.25 mg SC).	Tocolytics ↓ uterine activity and improve fetal oxygenation if uterine hypertonus or a prolapsed cord is causing distress.
Evaluate and document fetal response to interventions.	Evaluation provides information about effectiveness of interventions.
Notify caregiver of FHR pattern, interventions, and fetal response.	Notification provides caregiver with information about fetal status.
Offer calm explanations and reassurance to client and significant others while providing care.	Interventions for fetal distress may be frightening to client and her family.
Implement amnioinfusion as ordered (specify: fluid, rate, warmer, etc.).	Amnioinfusion may ↓ cord compression and dilute thick meconium to prevent fetal or neonatal meconium aspiration.
Assist caregiver with fetal scalp sampling if needed.	Assistance helps obtain a sample of fetal blood used to determine acid–base status.
Prepare client for delivery if indicated (specify: forceps, vacuum extractor, or cesarean).	Preparation facilitates emergency delivery of the distressed fetus who has not responded to intrauterine resuscitation efforts.
Notify neonatal caregivers (specify: pediatrician, neonatologist, NICU) of fetal distress and expected birth route and time.	Notification ensures that caregivers are prepared to resuscitate the newborn at birth.
Provide additional equipment as needed for birth (specify: e.g., forceps, vacuum extractor, Delee mucus trap, etc.).	Preparation avoids delay when delivery is needed for fetal distress. Thick meconium should be suctioned from the pharynx after birth of the head.
Ensure that neonatal resuscitation equipment is ready and in working order and preheat warmer before every birth.	Interventions avoid delays after infant is born. Warmer prevents cold stress that further compromises oxygenation in the newborn.
Implement or assist with neonatal resuscitation at birth: dry infant quickly, clear airway (intratracheal suctioning for thick meconium), stimulate crying, assess respiration, HR, and color.	Nurses present at delivery should be prepared to resuscitate the newborn until medical assistance is available. A person skilled at intubation should be present at all births.

(continues)

(continued)

INTERVENTIONS	RATIONALES
Provide oxygen, PPV, chest compressions, and drugs as indicated/ordered.	Interventions promote neonatal oxygenation.
Assess APGAR score at 1 and 5 minutes after birth (continue q 5 min until score is greater than 6).	APGAR assessment provides quantitative measurement of fetal oxygen and neurological status.
Allow parents to see and touch infant before transfer to the nursery or NICU.	Intervention promotes attachment and bonding.
Discuss events with client and significant other after infant is transferred.	Discussion promotes client understanding of unfamiliar events.

NIC: *Acid–Base Management*

Evaluation

(Date/time of evaluation of goal)

(Has goal been met? not met? partially met?)

(Describe FHR pattern after interventions. What was Apgar score at 1 and 5 minutes?)

(Revisions to care plan? D/C care plan? Continue care plan?)

FETAL DISTRESS

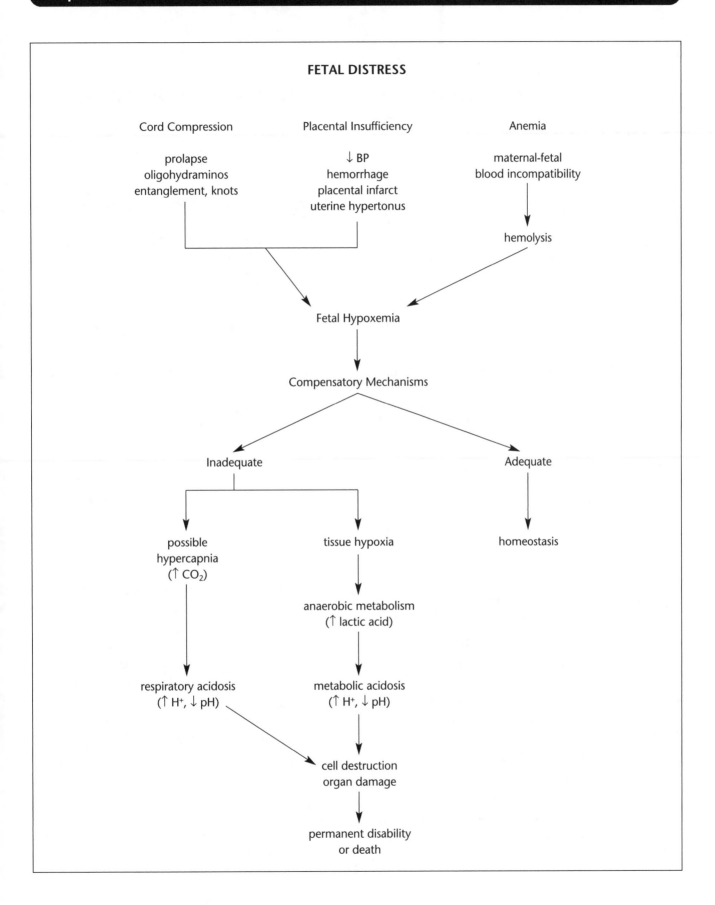

Cord Compression

prolapse
oligohydraminos
entanglement, knots

Placental Insufficiency

$\downarrow$ BP
hemorrhage
placental infarct
uterine hypertonus

Anemia

maternal-fetal
blood incompatibility

hemolysis

Fetal Hypoxemia

Compensatory Mechanisms

Inadequate

Adequate

possible
hypercapnia
($\uparrow$ CO$_2$)

tissue hypoxia

homeostasis

anaerobic metabolism
($\uparrow$ lactic acid)

respiratory acidosis
($\uparrow$ H$^+$, $\downarrow$ pH)

metabolic acidosis
($\uparrow$ H$^+$, $\downarrow$ pH)

cell destruction
organ damage

permanent disability
or death

CHAPTER 2.7

ABRUPTIO PLACENTAE

Placental abruption is the separation of a normally implanted placenta before birth of the baby. The separation may be partial or complete. A marginal abruption describes detachment of the edges of the placenta. Partial separation may also occur in the center of the placenta. With a total placental abruption the entire placenta detaches.

Hemorrhage from the exposed surfaces may be obvious or occult. The amount can vary from mild with a marginal abruption to torrential with a total separation. Classic symptoms of abruption are abdominal tenderness and board-like abdominal rigidity with or without vaginal bleeding. Fetal prognosis is poor if >50% of the placenta detaches. Maternal complications include development of DIC, hypovolemic shock, kidney or heart failure, and increased risk for post partum hemorrhage. The cause is unknown but abruptio placentae is associated with hypertensive disorders, maternal cocaine use, abdominal trauma, and uterine overdistention.

MEDICAL CARE

- Ultrasound examination of the placenta

- IV fluid and electrolyte replacement; blood transfusion as needed

- Laboratory studies to rule out DIC: platelets, fibrinogen, fibrin degradation products, PT, and PTT

- Cesarean delivery if the fetus exhibits distress

- Vaginal delivery may be preferred for a fetal demise of if the fetus is tolerating a partial abruption

- Close observation may be employed if the abruption is small, the fetus is immature, and appears stable

COMMON NURSING DIAGNOSES

 See RISK FOR DEFICIENT FLUID VOLUME

Related to: Excessive losses secondary to premature placental separation.

 See IMPAIRED GAS EXCHANGE: FETAL

Related to: Insufficient oxygen supply secondary to premature separation of the placenta.

Defining Characteristics: Signs of fetal distress (specify: loss of variability, late decelerations, tachycardia, or bradycardia, etc.).

 See FEAR

Related to: Perceived or actual grave threat to body integrity secondary to excessive bleeding, and threat to fetal survival.

Defining Characteristics: Client verbalizes fear (specify using quotes). Client exhibits physiologic sympathetic responses (specify: e.g., dry mouth, pallor, tachycardia, nausea, etc.).

ADDITIONAL NURSING DIAGNOSES

 INEFFECTIVE TISSUE PERFUSION (PLACENTAL, RENAL, CEREBRAL, PERIPHERAL)

Related to: Excessive blood loss secondary to premature placental separation.

Defining Characteristics: (Specify: estimated blood loss, FHR pattern, BP compared to baseline, pulse, severe abdominal pain and rigidity, pallor, changes in LOC, ↓ urine output, etc.).

Goal: Client will maintain adequate tissue perfusion by (date/time to evaluate).

Outcome Criteria

✔ Client will maintain BP and pulse (specify for client: e.g., >100/60, pulse between 60–90), skin warm, pink, and dry.

✔ Urine output >30 cc/hr.

✔ Client will remain alert and oriented. FHR pattern remains reassuring.

NOC: *Vital Sign Status*

INTERVENTIONS	RATIONALES
Assess client's SaO$_2$, BP, P, and R (specify frequency).	Assessment provides information about client's tissue perfusion. Hypovolemia causes ↓ BP with ↑ P and ↑ R as compensatory mechanisms for ↓ perfusion and hypoxemia.
Monitor for restlessness, anxiety, "air hunger," and changes in level of consciousness.	Intervention provides information of developing indications of inadequate cerebral tissue perfusion.
Monitor all intake and output (insert Foley catheter as ordered). Evaluate blood loss by weighing peri pads or chux (1 gm = 1 cc). (Specify frequency of documentation.) Notify caregiver of ↑ losses.	Monitoring provides information about renal perfusion and function and the extent of blood loss. Partial abruption may progress rapidly to complete abruption.
Continuously monitor FHR pattern and compare to baseline data from prenatal record. Inform caregiver of nonreassuring changes.	The fetus may initially respond to ↓ placental perfusion by raising the FHR above the normal baseline. Nonreassuring FHR is an indication for delivery.
Assess for uterine irritability, abdominal pain, rigidity, and increasing abdominal girth (measure abdomen at umbilicus). (Specify frequency.)	Assessment provides information about severity of placental abruption. Bleeding may be occult causing abdominal rigidity and pain.

INTERVENTIONS	RATIONALES
Assess client's skin color, temperature, moisture, turgor, and capillary refill (specify frequency).	Assessment provides information about peripheral tissue perfusion. Hypovolemia results in shunting of blood away from the peripheral circulation to the brain and vital organs.
Initiate IV access with 18-gauge (or larger) catheter and provide fluids, blood products, or blood as ordered (specify fluids and rate).	Intervention provides venous access to replace fluids. Size 18-gauge or larger is preferred to transfuse blood.
Monitor laboratory values as obtained (e.g., Hgb, Hct, clotting studies).	Laboratory studies provide information about extent of blood loss and signs of impending DIC.
Observe client for signs of spontaneous bleeding (e.g., bruising, epistaxis, seeping from puncture sites, hematuria, etc.).	Observation provides information about the depletion of clotting factors and development of DIC.
Keep client and significant other informed of condition and plan of care.	Information promotes understanding and cooperation.
Notify caregivers and prepare for immediate delivery and neonatal resuscitation if maternal or fetal	Continued blood loss or development of DIC may lead to maternal or fetal injury or death.

NIC: *Shock Management*

Evaluation

(Date/time of evaluation of goal)

(Has goal been met? not met? partially met?)

(What is client's BP and P? Is skin warm, pink, and dry? Is urine output >30 cc/hr? Is client alert and oriented? Describe FHR pattern.)

(Revisions to care plan? D/C care plan? Continue care plan?)

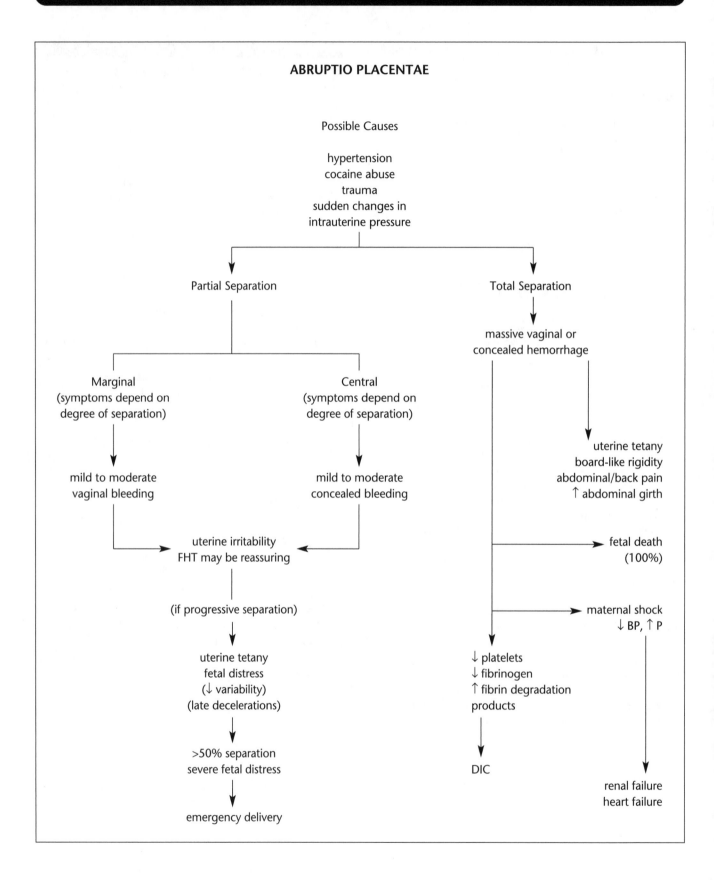

ABRUPTIO PLACENTAE

Possible Causes

hypertension
cocaine abuse
trauma
sudden changes in
intrauterine pressure

Partial Separation

Total Separation

massive vaginal or
concealed hemorrhage

Marginal
(symptoms depend on
degree of separation)

Central
(symptoms depend on
degree of separation)

uterine tetany
board-like rigidity
abdominal/back pain
↑ abdominal girth

mild to moderate
vaginal bleeding

mild to moderate
concealed bleeding

uterine irritability
FHT may be reassuring

fetal death
(100%)

(if progressive separation)

maternal shock
↓ BP, ↑ P

uterine tetany
fetal distress
(↓ variability)
(late decelerations)

↓ platelets
↓ fibrinogen
↑ fibrin degradation
products

>50% separation
severe fetal distress

DIC

renal failure
heart failure

emergency delivery

CHAPTER 2.8

PROLAPSED CORD

Prolapse of the umbilical cord may occur when the membranes rupture and the presenting part is not well-engaged and seated against the cervix. The cord is then washed down in front of the presenting part. Pressure from contractions compresses the cord against the presenting part resulting in fetal distress or death from hypoxia. An occult prolapse occurs when the cord is wedged between the presenting part and the cervix but cannot be seen or felt by the examiner. Severe variable decelerations and fetal bradycardia after ROM are signs of a prolapsed cord; either occult or palpable/visible.

RISK FACTORS

- Small fetus (preterm or IUGR)
- Contracted pelvis
- Transverse lie, complete, or footling breech presentation
- Multiple gestation
- Hydraminos
- Labor with an unengaged fetus; grand multiparity
- AROM

MEDICAL CARE

- Prevention: bed rest with bulging or ruptured membranes and an unengaged fetus
- Pressure is applied to the presenting part to hold it off the cord until birth
- Client may be placed in knee–chest or Trendelenburg position to relieve cold compression until birth. These measures are often implemented by nurses who are the first to identify the emergency.
- If the cord is pulsating and the fetus is alive, rapid cesarean delivery is indicated

COMMON NURSING DIAGNOSES

 ### See IMPAIRED GAS EXCHANGE: FETAL

Related to: Insufficient oxygen delivery secondary to cord occlusion.

Defining Characteristics: Signs of fetal distress (specify: severe variable decelerations, loss of variability, etc.).

ADDITIONAL NURSING DIAGNOSES

 ### FEAR

Related to: Perceived grave danger to fetus and self from obstetric emergency.

Defining Characteristics: Client states (Specify: e.g., "I'm scared; This can't be happening!" etc.). Client is crying, confused, appears pale, $\uparrow$ P and R, dry mouth, and so forth (specify).

Goal: Client will cope with fear during emergency.

Outcome Criteria

✔ Client and significant other can identify the threat.
✔ Client is able to cooperate with instructions from caregivers.

NOC: *Fear Control*

INTERVENTIONS	RATIONALES
Inform client and significant other of a problem as soon as it is identified. Speak slowly and calmly.	Calm information decreases client and significant other's fear. It is more frightening to "sense" that something is wrong than to know what it is.

(continues)

(continued)

INTERVENTIONS	RATIONALES
Describe the problem in simple terms and what interventions might be expected (specify: e.g., for prolapsed cord the nurse will hold the baby up until a cesarean can be done).	Simple explanations are less frightening than complicated physiology or medical terminology the client may not understand.
Explain all equipment and procedures as they're being done (specify: e.g., Foley catheter, IV, etc.).	Explanation promotes understanding of unfamiliar interventions and decreases fear of the unknown.
Inform client and significant other of things they can do to help (specify: e.g., position changes; keep oxygen mask on; significant other can support client breathing and relaxation, etc.).	Information promotes a sense of control over frightening events by allowing client and significant others to be involved in the solutions.
Observe client and significant other for signs of distress: pallor, trembling, crying, and so forth.	The "fight or flight" sympathetic response may indicate ↑ fear. Significant other may need attention.
Provide emotional support; validate fears. Encourage significant other to remain with client during birth if possible.	Emotional support and validation helps client and significant other to cope with fears.
Inform client and significant other of infant's condition at birth.	Information increases a sense of control and ability to cope.

INTERVENTIONS	RATIONALES
Allow client and significant other to hold infant as soon as it is born. Defer nonessential newborn care (if condition allows).	Intervention provides reassurance that the baby is all right and promotes parent–child attachment and bonding.
Praise client and significant other for their cooperation and coping during a stressful birth.	Praise enhances self-esteem. Intervention shows that the client's abilities are valued.
Visit client after birth (specify when: e.g., 1st or 2nd PP day) to discuss events surrounding birth. Clarify any misconceptions about the emergency.	Discussion provides an opportunity for client and significant other to relive the experience and fill in any gaps in understanding before discharge.

NIC: *Coping Enhancement*

Evaluation

(Date/time of evaluation of goal)

(Has goal been met? not met? partially met?)

(Did client and significant other verbalize correct understanding of the emergency? Was client able to cooperate with instructions? Specify.)

(Revisions to care plan? D/C care plan? Continue care plan?)

PROLAPSED CORD

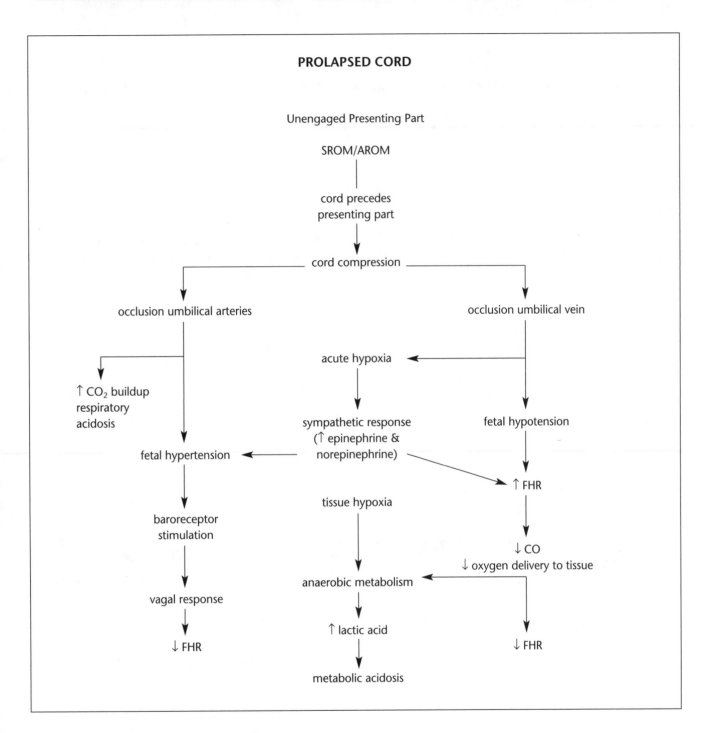

Unengaged Presenting Part

SROM/AROM

cord precedes
presenting part

cord compression

occlusion umbilical arteries   occlusion umbilical vein

↑ CO_2 buildup
respiratory
acidosis

acute hypoxia

sympathetic response
(↑ epinephrine &
norepinephrine)   fetal hypotension

fetal hypertension

↑ FHR

baroreceptor
stimulation

tissue hypoxia

↓ CO
↓ oxygen delivery to tissue

vagal response

anaerobic metabolism

↓ FHR

↑ lactic acid

↓ FHR

metabolic acidosis

CHAPTER 2.9

POSTTERM BIRTH

A pregnancy that continues to 42 weeks or more after the LNMP with fertilization two weeks later, is considered to be postterm. The postterm fetus is at higher than normal risk for hypoxia, birth injury, meconium aspiration, and hyperbilirubinemia in the neonatal period. The cause of prolonged pregnancy is unknown though some congenital anomalies are associated with postterm birth including anencephaly and congenital adrenal hypoplasia.

Sometimes the date of the LNMP is hard to determine, or the woman may have had a long menstrual cycle in which case the fetus really isn't postterm even at 42+ weeks. Confirmation of dates is important to prevent induction of a premature infant.

The truly postterm neonate has a characteristic appearance. The infant appears wide-eyed and alert, is long and thin with abundant scalp hair and long fingernails. The skin may be meconium stained, loose, dry and peeling, with little subcutaneous fat. No vernix or lanugo are present.

COMPLICATIONS

- Fetal macrosomia, birth trauma, shoulder dystocia, cesarean birth
- Oligohydramnios: dry, cracked skin; cord compression and acute hypoxia
- Placental aging with ↓ exchange of oxygen and nutrients: chronic hypoxia; fetal loss of subcutaneous tissue: appears long and thin
- Passage of meconium because of hypoxia; meconium staining
- Risk for aspiration
- Polycythemia

MEDICAL CARE

- Careful determination of dates: LNMP, fundal height, serial ultrasound measurements

- Daily fetal movement counts by client after 40 weeks
- Weekly cervical exam, NST and ultrasound for amount of amniotic fluid; may be 2 times per week after 41 weeks
- Other fetal testing possible: BPP or OCT (CST)
- Induction at 42 weeks if dates are accurate and cervix is favorable
- Uncertain dates: close surveillance with induction if ↓ amniotic fluid or signs of compromise
- Fetal monitoring during labor with scalp electrode and possibly IUPC; possible amnioinfusion
- Cesarean birth for unsuccessful induction
- Suctioning of oropharynx after birth of the head and before birth of the chest, tracheal suctioning before infant is stimulated for the first breath if meconium present

COMMON NURSING DIAGNOSES

 ### See IMPAIRED GAS EXCHANGE: FETAL

Related to: Aging placenta, oligohydramnios and cord compression.

Defining Characteristics: Signs of fetal distress (specify: e.g., decreased variability, late decelerations in labor).

 ### See RISK FOR INJURY: MATERNAL AND FETAL

Related to: Fetal macrosomia, risk for shoulder dystocia.

 ### See ANXIETY

Related to: Prolonged pregnancy and threat to fetal well-being.

Defining Characteristics: Client expresses concern about prolonged pregnancy (specify using quotes). Client states she is worried about the baby (specify).

ADDITIONAL NURSING DIAGNOSES

 ### RISK FOR ASPIRATION: FETAL/NEONATAL

Related to: Passage of thick meconium in the amniotic fluid prior to birth.

Defining Characteristics: None, as this is a potential diagnosis.

Goal: Infant will not aspirate meconium at birth.

Outcome Criteria

✔ Infant does not experience aspiration of meconium.

✔ Airway is clear, respirations at birth are 40–60

NOC: *Risk Control*

INTERVENTIONS	RATIONALES
Assess color and character of amniotic fluid when membranes rupture and each hour thereafter and during each vaginal exam.	Assessment provides information about passage of meconium and whether it is thin or thick. Thick meconium is more likely to cause meconium aspiration syndrome.
Notify primary caregiver if fluid is meconium stained and fetus is not breech presentation.	Notification allows caregiver to consider amnioinfusion and plan for suctioning at birth. A breech may pass meconium because of pressure, not hypoxia.
Initiate amnioinfusion with sterile normal saline via IUPC and an infusion pump (specify rate and agency policy for warming fluid) per physician orders.	Amnioinfusion may dilute thick meconium, reducing the risk of aspiration during birth. Normal saline is isotonic and sterile technique prevents introduction of nosocomial pathogens.
Monitor fetus continuously during labor. Note nonreassuring patterns and notify caregiver. Apply scalp electrode to determine STV if indicated.	A postterm fetus may experience chronic or acute hypoxia caused by aging of the placenta or oligohydramnios.
Ensure that a caregiver skilled at tracheal suctioning and intubation is present at every delivery.	Presence of a skilled caregiver allows for smooth and prompt suctioning of meconium below the vocal cords before the first breath is taken.

INTERVENTIONS	RATIONALES
Ensure that all infant emergency equipment is ready at birth. Arrange laryngoscope, suction, and catheter for immediate use. Preheat overhead warmer.	Preparation avoids delay in tracheal suctioning after infant is born. Maintaining warmth ↓ infant's metabolic needs and oxygen requirements.
Instruct client that she will need to stop pushing after the head has been born so that meconium may be suctioned before the baby breathes.	Instruction ensures maternal cooperation while the pharynx is being suctioned.
When the head is delivered, assist client to avoid pushing by panting or blowing.	Panting or blowing keeps the glottis open and ↓ maternal bearing-down efforts.
After the caregiver has suctioned the oropharynx and nasopharynx, gently carry infant to warmer, fold warm blanket over baby and assist with tracheal suctioning. Do not stimulate infant until after tracheal suctioning.	Interventions allow the mouth and nose to be cleared of meconium, and the trachea to be visualized and suctioned before the infant is stimulated and takes its first breath.
Auscultate the infant's breath sounds and note respiratory rate and effort (specify how frequently).	Assessments provide information about success of interventions.
Document and notify nursery personnel of meconium fluid and interventions at delivery.	Notification, in addition to documentation, ensures continuity of care.

NIC: *Aspiration Precautions*

Evaluation

(Date/time of evaluation of goal)

(Has goal been met? not met? partially met?)

(Did infant aspirate meconium? Was any meconium suctioned from the pharynx or trachea? Is airway clear? What is respiratory rate?)

(Revisions to care plan? D/C care plan? Continue care plan?)

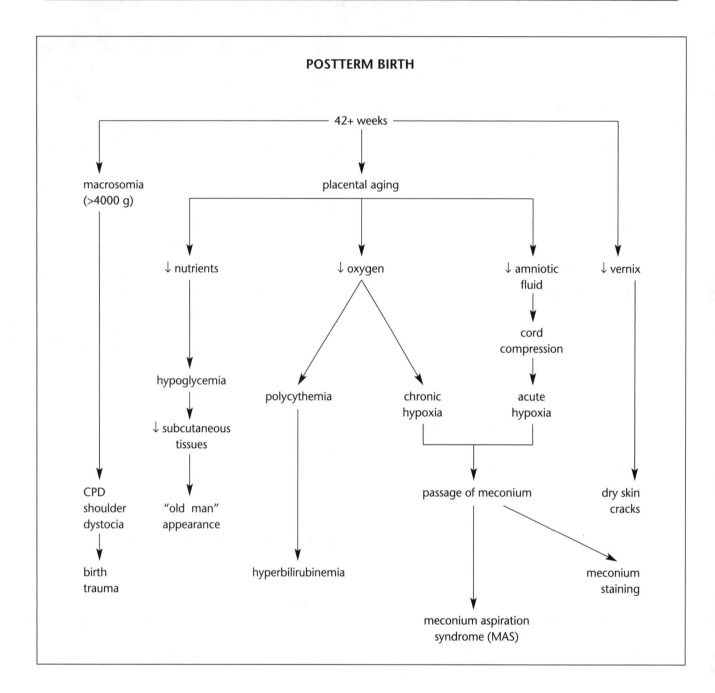

POSTTERM BIRTH

CHAPTER 2.10

INCOMPETENT CERVIX

Painless dilatation of the cervix without noticeable uterine contractions during the second trimester is the hallmark of an incompetent cervix. Generally the client presents with bulging or ruptured membranes and an inevitable abortion of an immature fetus. The events repeat in subsequent pregnancies if treatment is not initiated. The cause is not well-established but previous cervical trauma may be a risk factor.

MEDICAL TREATMENT

- Cervical cerclage: surgical reinforcement of the cervix with a purse-string suture during the early second trimester: MacDonald or Shirodkar procedures.
- The suture is cut at term to permit vaginal delivery or a cesarean birth is planned to avoid removing the suture.

COMMON NURSING DIAGNOSES

 ### See FEAR

Related to: Anticipated loss of second-trimester pregnancy.

Defining Characteristics: Specify for client (e.g., client expresses feeling afraid, use quotes; specify physiologic signs of fear: tachycardia, tachypnea, nausea, etc.).

 ### See ANTICIPATORY GRIEVING

Related to: Probable birth of nonviable fetus.

Defining Characteristics: Expressed feelings of grief (specify e.g., verbal or nonverbal indications of denial, anger, guilt, bargaining, or depression).

ADDITIONAL NURSING DIAGNOSES

 ### DEFICIENT KNOWLEDGE: CERVICAL CERCLAGE

Related to: Surgical procedure to reinforce the incompetent cervix.

Defining Characteristics: Client states (specify) lack of knowledge about incompetent cervix and cervical cerclage procedures.

Goal: Client will obtain knowledge about cervical cerclage by (date/time to evaluate).

Outcome Criteria

✔ Client describes how (specify for type chosen by caregiver) cerclage is performed.
✔ Client verbalizes risks and benefits of the (specify for type chosen by caregiver) procedure.

NOC: *Knowledge: Treatment Regimen*

INTERVENTIONS	RATIONALES
Ask client and s/o to describe current understanding of cervical incompetence.	Allows nurse to correct any misconceptions the client may have.
Describe the physiology of incompetent cervix in simple terms (e.g., the cervix is weakened and unable to support the weight of the growing pregnancy).	Explanation provides information in terms the client can understand.
Explain the proposed cerclage procedure (specify MacDonald or Shirodkar procedures) to client, including timing of procedure (specify) and associated risks: anesthesia and surgical risk, preterm labor, hemorrhage, and infection. Encourage questions.	Provides client and s/o with complete information about the procedure and risks.

(continues)

(continued)

INTERVENTIONS	RATIONALES
Describe delivery plans (specify whether the suture will be clipped to allow for vaginal birth or if the client will be scheduled for a cesarean). Elicit client's feelings about plans.	The client should be involved in decisions regarding her care.
Ask client to verbalize understanding of the proposed procedure by describing how it works and what potential risks are involved in it. Correct any misconceptions.	Provides additional opportunity to provide correct information to client & s/o.
Provide written materials about the designated procedure (specify).	

NIC: *Teaching, Perioperative*

Evaluation

(Date/time of evaluation of goal)

(Was goal met? Not met? Partially met?)

(Did client correctly describe how cerclage is performed?)

(Did client verbalize risks and benefits of the procedure? Provide quotes)

 ## INEFFECTIVE PROTECTION: FETAL

Related to: Decreased strength of cervical sphincter and fetal immaturity.

Defining Characteristics: Specify for client (e.g., history of previous second-trimester fetal loss; painless dilatation of the cervix at 16 weeks).

Goal: Fetus will remain in the protected uterine environment until viability.

Outcome Criteria

✔ Fetus will not be born before 36 weeks gestation.

NOC: *Endurance*

INTERVENTIONS	RATIONALES
Assess client's history for risk factors for incompetent cervix: cervical trauma, DES exposure, previous second trimester fetal losses.	Provides information about client's risk for incompetent cervix.

INTERVENTIONS	RATIONALES
Describe signs of cervical dilatation the client may notice such as: ↑ vaginal discharge, pelvic pressure, and lower back pain. Advise client to seek medical care for these symptoms.	Early identification of cervical change may prevent complete dilatation and abortion.
Explain the use of serial transvaginal ultrasound examinations to evaluate cervical length of clients at risk for an incompetent cervix.	Decreased cervical length in the second trimester is an indication that the cervix is incompetent.
Provide information and rationales about the medical plan of care. (Specify: e.g., bed rest, or MacDonald or Shirodkar cervical cerclage.)	Information helps the client and s/o to comply with the plan of care.
Administer medications as ordered (specify with drug, dose, route, and times: e.g., tocolytics, antibiotics).	Provide information about the action of the specific drugs ordered.
Maintain client on bed rest with hips elevated on a pillow and tilted to left.	Relieves pressure on the cervix and promotes uteroplacental perfusion.
Document ongoing evaluation of gestational age using fundal height, LNMP, and U/S.	Provides information about fetal growth and viability.
Monitor fetal well-being by auscultation or EFM (specify frequency; NST).	Ensures that uterus continues to be a safe environment that promotes fetal well-being.
Provide information about planned delivery method and when client should seek medical care (specify whether client is to have cerclage removed or deliver by cesarean).	Information allows client to participate in self-care and seek assistance as needed.

NIC: *Surgical Precautions*

Evaluation

(Date/time of evaluation of goal)

(Was goal met? Not met?)

(What was gestational age at delivery?)

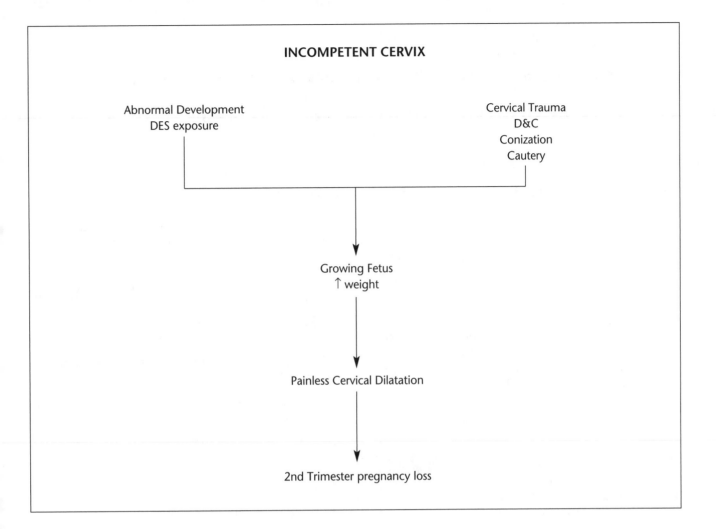

INCOMPETENT CERVIX

Abnormal Development   Cervical Trauma
DES exposure   D&C
                              Conization
                              Cautery

Growing Fetus
↑ weight

Painless Cervical Dilatation

2nd Trimester pregnancy loss

CHAPTER 2.11

PRECIPITOUS LABOR AND BIRTH

Precipitous labor is defined as a labor that lasts three hours or less from start to finish. Precipitous birth is any birth that happens much faster than is normally anticipated. This may result in an unattended birth. The fetus may suffer head trauma from rapid descent through the birth canal. When the contractions are very intense or tumultuous, the mother is at risk for lacerations: cervical, vaginal, perineal, periurethral, or even uterine rupture. This type of rapid intense labor may also be associated with amniotic fluid embolus or postpartum hemorrhage.

Clients who are at risk for precipitous labor and birth are those who have had a previous precipitous labor/birth; clients with a large pelvis or a small fetus; and clients with uterine hypertonus.

MEDICAL CARE

- Close observation of clients with risk factors; client may be asked to stay close to the hospital as she reaches term gestation
- Client may be induced if she lives far from the hospital
- Tocolytics may be used to decrease the intensity of contractions.

COMMON NURSING DIAGNOSES

See PAIN

Related to: Tumultuous labor contractions and maternal tension.

Defining Characteristics: Client verbalizes acute pain (specify using quotes or a pain scale). Client is (specify: crying, grimacing, etc.).

See FEAR

Related to: Perceived threat to self and fetus secondary to rapid labor progress, possibility of unattended birth.

Defining Characteristics: Client verbalizes fear (specify using quotes). Client exhibits physiologic signs of sympathetic response (specify: e.g., tachycardia, tachypnea, dry mouth, pallor, tremors, etc.).

ADDITIONAL NURSING DIAGNOSES

RISK FOR IMPAIRED TISSUE INTEGRITY

Related to: Mechanical trauma from uterine hypertonus and rapid fetal descent.

Defining Characteristics: None, as this is a potential diagnosis.

Goal: Client will not experience tissue injury during birth.

Outcome Criteria

✔ Perineum is intact after delivery.

NOC: *Tissue Integrity: Skin and Mucous Membranes*

INTERVENTIONS	RATIONALES
Palpate contractions for frequency, duration, intensity, and resting tone (specify frequency). Assess FHR per agency protocol (specify).	Assessments provide information about hypertonic uterine activity and fetal well-being.
Notify caregiver if uterine resting tone lasts less than 60 seconds between contractions.	Notification provides information about fetal risk. The caregiver may elect to use tocolytics to ↑ resting tone to improve placental perfusion.
Stay with the client experiencing tumultuous contractions. Provide reassurance.	Staying with the client avoids an unattended birth. Client may be frightened by the intensity of the contractions.

INTERVENTIONS	RATIONALES
Obtain precip. supplies. Notify caregiver of rapid progress. Wash hands, open precip. pack; don sterile gloves if birth appears imminent.	Preparation allows a sterile controlled birth by caregiver. Sterile technique prevents the introduction of microorganisms during birth.
Encourage client to blow or pant if the urge to push occurs before complete cervical dilatation.	Intervention may help avoid cervical or vaginal lacerations.
Support the client's perineum as the head crowns. Ask client to blow as the head delivers. Suction the infant's nose then mouth. Check for a nuchal cord and slip over the head or double-clamp and cut the cord.	Gentle counter pressure and a slow delivery of the head help prevent rapid expulsion and tearing of the perineum.
Guide infant's body down to slide the anterior shoulder under the symphysis pubis, then up to deliver the posterior shoulder.	Guidance during birth helps prevent perineal or vaginal tears during delivery of the infant's shoulders.
Observe client for signs of placental separation. Ask her to push to expel the placenta.	As the placenta separates, there may be an ↑ in bleeding, the cord may lengthen, the fundus changes shape. Maternal pushing facilitates delivery of the placenta.

INTERVENTIONS	RATIONALES
After the placenta and membranes completely deliver, massage the uterus, put the infant to breast, and/or administer oxytocin per standing orders (specify: drug, dose, and route).	Interventions help prevent excessive postpartum bleeding by stimulating contraction of the uterus via mechanical and endogenous or exogenous oxytocin.
Assess perineum for lacerations, hematomas, or ↑ vaginal bleeding.	Assessment provides information about possible tissue injury.
Provide routine postdelivery care to mother and infant per protocol until caregiver arrives.	Post delivery care promotes attachment and helps prevent complications.

NIC: *Wound Care*

Evaluation

(Date/time of evaluation of goal)

(Has goal been met? not met? partially met?)

(Were any lacerations noted after delivery?)

(Revisions to care plan? D/C care plan? Continue care plan?)

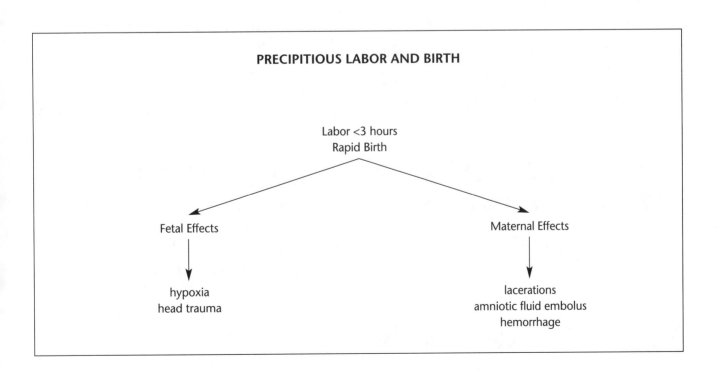

PRECIPITIOUS LABOR AND BIRTH

Labor <3 hours
Rapid Birth

Fetal Effects

hypoxia
head trauma

Maternal Effects

lacerations
amniotic fluid embolus
hemorrhage

CHAPTER 2.12

HELLP/DIC

HELLP is a complication of PIH that may or may not be associated with disseminated intravascular coagulation (DIC). HELLP stands for Hemolysis, Elevated Liver enzymes (AST & ALT), and Low Platelets. The underlying pathology is vasospasm that results in damage to the endothelial layer of small blood vessels. Platelets adhere to the vessel lesions (resulting in low serum platelet levels), fibrin is deposited, and red blood cells are damaged (hemolysis) as they are forced through the narrowed vessel. Microemboli clog the vasculature of organs resulting in ischemia and tissue damage (elevated liver enzymes). The treatment is delivery and resolution of PIH.

Disseminated Intravascular Coagulation (DIC) is also known as consumptive coagulopathy. The normal coagulation process is overstimulated and the coagulation factors are depleted. This places the client at risk for hemorrhage. The underlying pathology may be endothelial damage as in HELLP, or tissue damage resulting in release of thromboplastin. DIC may be associated with abruptio placentae, chorioamnionitis, sepsis, fetal demise, or retained products of conception. Subtle signs of DIC include bleeding from injection sites, spontaneous bleeding from the nose or gums, bruises, and petechiae. The treatment is delivery and correction of the underlying cause.

LAB VALUE CHANGES

	HELLP	DIC
Fibrinogen	↓	↓
Fibrin degradation products (FDP, FSP)	↑	↑
Platelets	↓	↓
PT and PTT	WNL	prolonged

MEDICAL CARE

- HELLP: Stabilization of PIH (MgSO$_4$) induction, and delivery either vaginal or cesarean

- DIC: Stabilization and delivery, preferably vaginal without an episiotomy
- IV fluids with a 16- or 18-gauge cannula, Foley catheter, intake and output
- Transfusions with packed RBCs
- Fresh frozen plasma (FFP) to replace fibrinogen and clotting factors
- Cryoprecipitate to replace fibrinogen

COMMON NURSING DIAGNOSES

 ### See RISK FOR DEFICIENT FLUID VOLUME

Related to: Excessive losses secondary to inadequate protective mechanisms.

 ### See IMPAIRED GAS EXCHANGE: FETAL

Related to: Maternal microangiopathic hemolytic anemia secondary to coagulopathy.

Defining Characteristics: Signs of fetal distress (specify: e.g., loss of FHR variability, late decelerations, tachycardia, or bradycardia).

 ### See INEFFECTIVE TISSUE PERFUSION (PLACENTAL, RENAL, CEREBRAL, HEPATIC)

Related to: Vascular occlusion by microemboli secondary to consumptive coagulopathy.

Defining Characteristics: (Specify: e.g., fetal IUGR, oliguria, BUN and creatinine, changes in LOC, liver enzymes, etc.).

 ### See FEAR

Related to: Threat to physiologic integrity of client and fetus secondary to serious complication of pregnancy.

Defining Characteristics: Client and family express fear (specify using quotes). Client exhibits signs of fear (specify: e.g., crying, withdrawn, tremors, pallor, etc.).

ADDITIONAL NURSING DIAGNOSES

INEFFECTIVE PROTECTION

Related to: Abnormal blood profile: thrombocytopenia, anemia, decreased clotting factors.

Defining Characteristics: Altered clotting (specify: e.g., platelets <50,000/µL, fibrinogen <300 mg/dL, ↑ fibrin degradation products, prolonged PT and PTT, ↓ Hct, etc.). Bleeding from nose, gums, and injection sites. Petechiae, bruising, and so forth (specify).

Goal: Client will regain intrinsic protection mechanisms by (date/time to evaluate).

Outcome Criteria

✔ Client does not exhibit bleeding from injection sites, gums, etc. (specify for client).

✔ Clotting factors increased to (specify for client: e.g., platelets ≥ 150,000/µL, fibrinogen ≥ 300 mg/dL).

NOC: *Abuse Protection*

INTERVENTIONS	RATIONALES
Assess client for signs of abnormal bleeding from injection sites, oozing from IV, mucous membranes, bruising, or petechiae.	Assessment provides information about subtle signs of bleeding related to clotting deficiencies.
Start and maintain IV access with a 16- or 18-gauge cannula (specify fluids and rate as ordered).	IV access allows rapid medication administration and replacement of fluids, blood, and blood products. Large bore IV cannulas are needed for RBC replacement.
Administer PRBCs, FFP, and/or cryoprecipitate IV as ordered per agency protocol (specify: product, amount, and time).	Intervention provides replacement of blood and clotting factor losses.
Monitor for transfusion reactions: changes in v/s, chills, fever, urticaria, rashes, dyspnea, and diaphoresis throughout transfusion per agency protocol.	Monitoring allows prompt recognition and treatment of transfusion reactions.

INTERVENTIONS	RATIONALES
Gently insert and anchor a Foley catheter. Monitor hourly intake and output. Notify physician if output <30 cc/hr.	Gentle insertion prevents trauma and bleeding. Renal vascular occlusion may occur leading to ischemia and necrosis.
Monitor laboratory values as obtained for improvement or worsening of condition.	Laboratory values may provide information about clotting profile, renal and hepatic function. Monitors the effect of treatment on condition.
Pad sides of bed with bath blankets. Avoid any trauma or breaks in the client's skin (e.g., injections). If injection is necessary, apply pressure for 5 full minutes after needle is removed.	Padding prevents bruising/bleeding from mechanical trauma. Avoiding breaks in the skin maintains vascular integrity to prevent hemorrhage.
Position client on her left side and monitor fetus continuously using soft EFM belts.	Position promotes placental perfusion. Tight belts may cause bruising.
Take manual BP rather than electronic. Wrap cuff gently around extremity without wrinkles.	Electronic BP machines may inflate the cuff too tightly and cause bleeding/bruising.
Explain clotting deficiency and treatment to client and significant other. Offer reassurance and support.	Client and significant other may be confused and frightened by unfamiliar interventions.

NIC: *Surveillance, Safety*

Evaluation

(Date/time of evaluation of goal.)

(Has goal been met? not met? partially met?)

(Does client exhibit any bleeding? What are clotting factor lab values?)

(Revisions to care plan? D/C care plan? Continue care plan?)

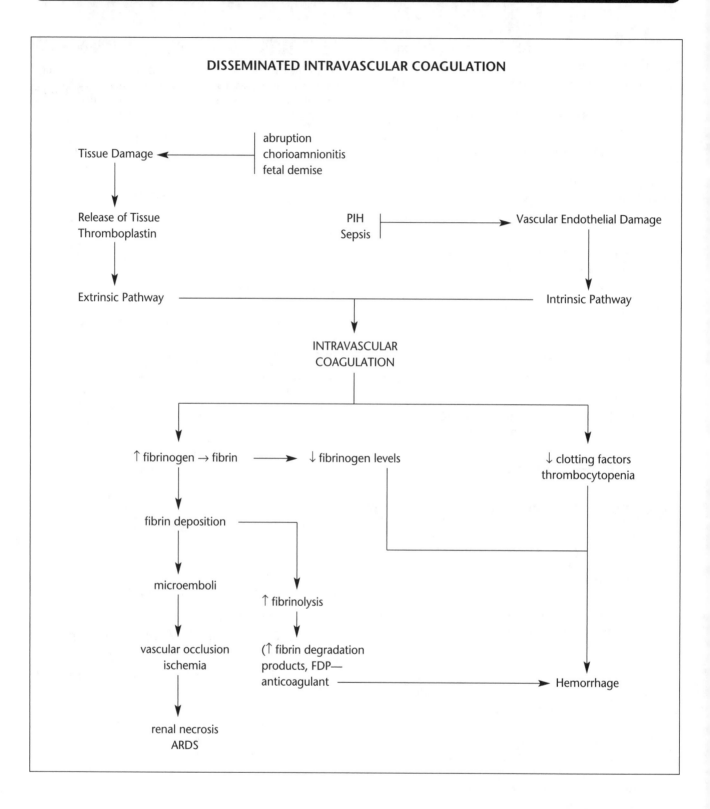

DISSEMINATED INTRAVASCULAR COAGULATION

Tissue Damage ← {abruption, chorioamnionitis, fetal demise}

Release of Tissue Thromboplastin

Extrinsic Pathway

PIH / Sepsis → Vascular Endothelial Damage

Intrinsic Pathway

INTRAVASCULAR COAGULATION

↑ fibrinogen → fibrin → ↓ fibrinogen levels

↓ clotting factors thrombocytopenia

fibrin deposition

microemboli

↑ fibrinolysis

vascular occlusion ischemia

(↑ fibrin degradation products, FDP— anticoagulant

Hemorrhage

renal necrosis ARDS

CHAPTER 2.13

HIV-POSITIVE CLIENT IN LABOR

Acquired immunodeficiency syndrome (AIDS) is increasingly affecting women of childbearing age and their infants. The human immunodeficiency virus (HIV) is transmitted through contact with infected blood or body fluids such as semen, vaginal secretions, amniotic fluid, and breast milk. Most infected women will develop AIDS within 10 years of infection with the virus. Infants of HIV-positive mothers will test positive at birth as a result of maternal antibodies that have crossed the placenta. Infants who are not infected will test negative by 18 months of age.

Most women who are HIV positive were infected by means of heterosexual transmission and their numbers are increasing in the United States. Many infants who are infected with HIV were exposed to the virus during birth. There is a decreased rate of neonatal infection when HIV-positive women receive prophylactic ZDT (zidovudine) during pregnancy and labor. Cesarean birth decreases the neonatal infection rate to less than 1%.

MEDICAL CARE

- ELISA testing for HIV followed by Western Blot assay to confirm diagnosis
- Counseling services
- Prevention and early treatment of infection
- Oral ZDT (zidovudine) during pregnancy and IV during labor and birth
- Other antiretroviral medications
- Lab tests: CD4+ T-lymphocyte counts, CBC with differential, sedimentation rate, platelets

COMMON NURSING DIAGNOSES

 See DECISIONAL CONFLICT: PREGNANCY TERMINATION

Related to: HIV-positive mother.

Defining Characteristics: Specify for client (verbalizes uncertainty about continuing the pregnancy; delays making a decision; states she is afraid of what her family/significant other will do, etc.).

 See ANTICIPATORY GRIEVING

Related to: Realization that the HIV+ mother may not live to raise the child; realization that the fetus may contract HIV.

Defining Characteristics: Specify for client (client states she is afraid her baby will get HIV; client cries, states she will miss her child's wedding, etc.).

ADDITIONAL NURSING DIAGNOSES

RISK FOR INFECTION: MATERNAL AND FETAL

Related to: Compromised maternal immune defenses.

Defining Characteristics: Specify data for client (e.g., 12-week pregnant client tested HIV positive on [date, type of test]; current CD4+ T-lymphocyte count; history of opportunistic infections, etc.).

Goal: Client and fetus will not exhibit signs of infection by (date and time to reevaluate this diagnosis).

Outcome Criteria

✔ Client's temperature remains <100.4° F.
✔ Fetal growth is appropriate for gestational age.
✔ Client identifies (specify how many: e.g., 2 or 3) ways to decrease risk of infection.

NOC: *Immune Status*

INTERVENTIONS	RATIONALES
Use universal precautions with all clients: wear gloves and protective barriers when contact with blood or body fluids is likely; dispose of needles and sharps in appropriate containers—never re-cap needles; practice meticulous hand-washing between clients.	Universal precautions prevent transmission of blood-borne pathogens.
Assess client's vital signs at each visit and interview for subtle signs of infection. Instruct client to monitor herself for fever, weight loss, diarrhea, cough, yeast infections, skin lesions, and any other nonspecific indications of infection and to report any of these to the caregiver.	Nonspecific symptoms may indicate early signs of an opportunistic infection.
Evaluate client's immunization history and provide immunizations as ordered.	Hepatitis B, influenza, and pneumococcal vaccines are not contraindicated and may prevent serious illness.
Monitor lab work as obtained: CBC, CD4+ T-lymphocyte (T4) count, sedimentation rate.	Changes may indicate early signs of infection: ↑ sed. rate, ↓ T4 lymphocytes, ↓ Hgb.
Monitor fetal well-being throughout pregnancy: U/S, fundal height, NSTs.	Signs of transplacental infection include fetal growth restriction.
Teach client to take ZDT (zidovudine) and other antiretroviral medications used for prophylaxis during pregnancy as ordered by caregiver.	These drugs do not cure HIV but may decrease the risk of opportunistic infection.
Inform client that she will receive ZDT by intravenous infusion during her labor and her infant will be given the drug after birth.	Teaching allows the client to participate in self-care and encourages compliance with medical plan of care. Prophylactic ZDT has been shown to ↓ the transmission of HIV to the fetus.
Teach the client to avoid people with infections, get adequate rest, and eat a well-balanced, nutritious diet (specify for client). Ask client to verbalize ways to avoid infection.	Rest and adequate nutrients are necessary to prevent infection and promote healing.
Inform client that she will be able to care for her infant but should avoid breast-feeding.	HIV may be transmitted in breast milk.

INTERVENTIONS	RATIONALES
Instruct client to avoid spreading the virus by not sharing toothbrushes or razors, avoiding sexual contact or using latex condoms with spermicide, and cleaning up any blood or body fluid spills with a 10% bleach solution. Ask client to verbalize ways to prevent spreading infection.	Information helps the client protect her family from the virus.
Refer client as needed (specify for client e.g., dietician, social services, counseling services, etc.).	

NIC: *Infection Protection*

Evaluation

(Date/time of evaluation of goal)

(Was goal met? Not met? Partially met?)

(What is client's temperature?)

(Is fetal growth appropriate for gestational age?)

(Specify what the client says are ways to decrease risk of infection. Use quotes.)

 ## COMPROMISED FAMILY COPING

Related to: Temporary family disorganization and stress secondary to multiple stressors of pregnancy and a terminal illness.

Defining Characteristics: Specify for client (client states that her significant other/family are unable to be supportive to her at this time. Family members and/or significant other report difficulty supporting client's decision to continue with pregnancy, etc.).

Goal: Client and family will demonstrate adequate coping.

Outcome Criteria

✔ Client and family will identify current stressors.

✔ Client and family will plan (specify how many: e.g., 2 or 3) strategies to decrease stress.

NOC: *Family Coping*

INTERVENTIONS	RATIONALES
Establish a therapeutic relationship with the client and her family. Provide privacy and allow time for discussion.	Trust is necessary for disclosure of personal information to the nurse.
Encourage client and family to list the stressors they are currently experiencing.	Identification of stressors is needed before the family can cope effectively.
Assist client and family to explore ways to reduce the impact of stressors on the family. (Specify some suggestions, e.g., does the family need some additional counseling? would household help relieve the burden some?)	The family needs to develop their own coping mechanisms. The nurse facilitates the process by offering suggestions.
Offer praise and positive feedback to the family as they work through the process of developing new coping mechanisms.	The nurse reflects the positive movement of family processes as a way of supporting the family's coping.

INTERVENTIONS	RATIONALES
Refer the family to community support services (specify for the client's community) as indicated.	Support services help the family adapt to the current stressors.

NIC: *Family Involvement*

Evaluation

(Date/time of evaluation of goal)

(Was goal met? Not met? Partially met?)

(Did client and family identify current stressors? What are they?)

(Specify strategies the client and family developed to decrease stress.)

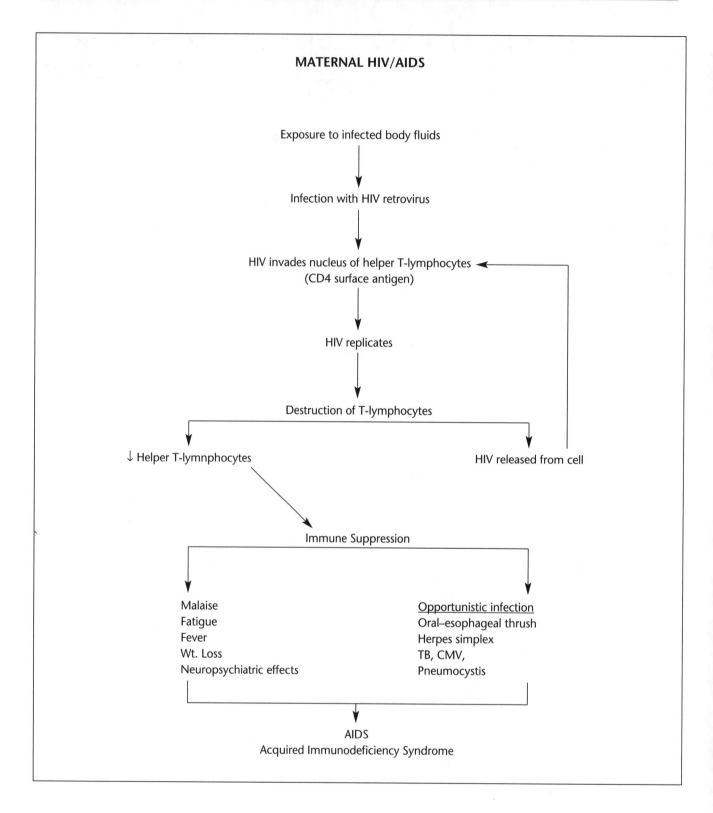

MATERNAL HIV/AIDS

Exposure to infected body fluids

Infection with HIV retrovirus

HIV invades nucleus of helper T-lymphocytes
(CD4 surface antigen)

HIV replicates

Destruction of T-lymphocytes

↓ Helper T-lymnphocytes   HIV released from cell

Immune Suppression

Malaise   Opportunistic infection
Fatigue   Oral–esophageal thrush
Fever   Herpes simplex
Wt. Loss   TB, CMV,
Neuropsychiatric effects   Pneumocystis

AIDS
Acquired Immunodeficiency Syndrome

CHAPTER 2.14

FETAL DEMISE

Fetal death after 20 weeks gestation is often referred to as an Intrauterine Fetal Demise (IUFD) or still-birth. Causes of fetal demise may be related to complications of pregnancy such as PIH, diabetes, hemorrhage, a cord accident, or fetal anomalies. No apparent cause is found in approximately 25% of cases.

The mother may notice a lack of fetal movement and decreased breast size. Fundal height may not correlate with expected gestational age. Frequently the first sign is an absence of FHT on auscultation. Fetal death is confirmed by real-time ultrasound. 90% of women will spontaneously labor and deliver within three weeks of fetal death. When the pregnancy continues beyond a month, the mother is at risk for developing DIC from the release of tissue thromboplastin.

The attachment process begins early in pregnancy. Fetal demise represents an emotionally devastating tragedy for the mother and family. Normal grief responses that may be noted during labor include denial, anger, bargaining, and depression. The birth of a subsequent baby may be accompanied by renewed grief for the lost child.

MEDICAL CARE

- May wait 2 to 3 weeks if client desires, to see if labor begins spontaneously
- Monitoring of blood clotting factors to avoid DIC
- Induction with oxytocin if near term and cervix is favorable
- Use of cervical ripening agents followed by oxytocin if cervix is unfavorable
- Prostaglandin E_2 suppositories may be used before 28 weeks to induce labor
- Analgesia and sedation is often ordered
- EFM may be applied with the toco only or an IUPC inserted
- Autopsy to determine cause of death

COMMON NURSING DIAGNOSES

Intrapartum care is the same as for any laboring client with the exception of measures designed to ensure fetal well-being. The Basic Care Plan: Labor and Birth should be adapted for the client experiencing a still-birth.

ADDITIONAL NURSING DIAGNOSES

RISK FOR INJURY

Related to: Effects of suppository medications used to terminate pregnancy with IUFD before 28 weeks.

Defining Characteristics: None, as this is a potential diagnosis.

Goal: Client will not experience any injury during labor or birth.

Outcome Criteria

- ✔ Client's vital signs remain stable (specify for client, give ranges for temperature, BP, P, and R).
- ✔ EBL <500 cc after birth.

NOC: *Safety Status: Physical Injury*

INTERVENTIONS	RATIONALES
Assess TPR, BP, and contraction status prior to insertion of suppository. May place toco only if fetal monitor in place or use palpation to assess contractions.	Assessment provides baseline information about maternal homeostasis and uterine activity.
Explain procedure and expected outcome to client (specify: e.g., vaginal suppositories initiate contractions; birth is usually accomplished within 24 hours).	Explanations help the client and significant other to anticipate what will happen next. Facilitates coping with unfamiliar experience.

(continues)

(continued)

INTERVENTIONS	RATIONALES
Position client supine for 10–15 minutes after suppository is inserted.	Positioning facilitates absorption of drug and prevents expulsion.
Administer acetaminophen, antidiarrheal, and antiemetic drugs as ordered (specify drug, dose, route, and times).	Prophylactic medications help ↓ adverse effects of drug. PGE₂ causes fever, nausea, vomiting, and diarrhea in most clients.
Monitor vital signs during induction per protocol (specify: e.g., BP, P, R q 30 min, temp q 2h, etc.).	Vital signs provide information about complications of induction and adverse effects of medications. Fever is a normal response to PGE₂.
Monitor client for cramping or contractions. Notify physician if pain or vaginal bleeding appears excessive. Count or weigh pads for more than expected amounts of bleeding.	Drug may cause intense contractions that could result in uterine rupture. Pad count or weighing helps estimate EBL (1 gm = 1 cc).
Provide pain medication as needed (specify: drug, dose, route, and time).	Describe action of specific drug.
Notify caregiver if cramping subsides without sufficient cervical softening and dilatation.	Drug does may need to be repeated after 6 hours up to 3 doses.
Perform vaginal exams only as needed. Observe client for signs of second stage expulsive efforts.	Client's labor may progress more rapidly than usual.
Initiate oxytocin induction as ordered and per protocol.	Once cervix is softened, oxytocin may be effective in inducing labor.

NIC: Labor Induction

Evaluation

(Date/time of evaluation of goal)

(Has goal been met? not met? partially met?)

(What are client's vital signs? What is EBL after delivery?)

(Revisions to care plan? D/C care plan? Continue care plan?)

ANTICIPATORY GRIEVING

Related to: Intrauterine fetal loss.

Defining Characteristics: Client and significant other express distress about loss (specify for client: e.g., "This can't be happening"). Client and significant other exhibit (specify denial: "The baby is still moving, I can feel her"; anger at staff; or guilt "I shouldn't have done . . ."; etc.).

Goal: Client and significant other will begin the grieving process by (date/time to evaluate).

Outcome Criteria

✔ Client and significant other are able to express their grief in a culturally acceptable manner.

✔ Client and family are able to share their grief with each other.

NOC: Family Coping

INTERVENTIONS	RATIONALES
Assess the client and significant other's response to the expected loss: denial, anger, bargaining, depression, and so forth.	Client and significant other may present to the hospital in any phase of the grief process. Client may move in and out of the stages.
Provide support without offering false hopes (specify for client: e.g., if in denial, don't force acceptance of loss; explain that denial is a normal coping mechanism).	Coping mechanisms assist the client to gradually face the loss. Knowledge assists the client and family to move through their grief.
Ensure that all caregivers and auxiliary staff are aware of the client's loss (e.g., sign on door).	Intervention prevents anguish from well-intentioned comments about the baby.
Support cultural grief behavior of client and family (e.g., screaming, tearing clothes, etc.). Provide for privacy if needed and remain nonjudgmental.	Grieving is an individual process influenced by cultural norms that may be very different from the nurse's.
Provide clear explanations and instructions. May need to repeat information.	Client and significant other may be distracted and have trouble concentrating on information.
Encourage parents to talk about the baby and their feelings about the loss. Use touch as culturally appropriate.	Encouragement provides permission to grieve together openly. The use of touch has cultural implications.
Allow visitors as client and significant other desire.	Intervention promotes family support for client and significant other while protecting them from unwanted guests.
Encourage parents to name the baby if not already done. Refer to the baby by name.	Naming the baby validates the existence and loss of the child.

INTERVENTIONS	RATIONALES
Encourage client and significant other to see and hold the baby. Clean and wrap infant in warm blanket (may apply lotion or powder to infant). Prepare parents for how the baby will look and feel (e.g., bruising, cold, etc.). Point out attractive characteristics of the baby. Allow parents to bathe and dress baby if desired.	Seeing and holding the baby validates the birth of a unique individual and the loss. The infant generally doesn't look as bad as the parents might imagine it does. Bathing and dressing the baby provides an opportunity to parent the infant before giving it up.
Prepare a memory packet for the parents. Include pictures of the baby, footprints, a lock of hair if requested, and so forth. If client refuses packet, file it safely for future requests.	Memory items provide tangible evidence of the reality of the baby. Clients may initially reject the packet and then want it later (e.g., on the anniversary of the birth).
Assist parents to make decisions regarding disposal of the remains, transfer to a postpartum or gyn room, and early discharge if possible.	The hospital may be prepared to dispose of remains if under 20 weeks. Some funeral homes do not charge for the services to couples who have a stillborn.
Provide information about the normal grief process (written and verbal).	Information assists client to understand feelings that may be overwhelming at times.
Discuss gender differences in grieving (e.g., the mother has usually formed a longer attachment to the fetus than the father has).	Discussion facilitates open communication between parents to prevent anger or guilty feelings about differences in grieving.
Provide age-appropriate information about helping siblings to cope with their grief.	Understanding of death varies with age. Ensures that siblings are not forgotten.
Refer client and significant other to a grief support group (specify for area).	Support groups may help client and significant other to cope with loss.

NIC: *Grief-Work Facilitation: Perinatal Death*

Evaluation

(Date/time of evaluation of goal)

(Has goal been met? not met? partially met?)

(Give example of how client, significant other, and family expressed and shared their grief with each other.)

(Revisions to care plan? D/C care plan? Continue care plan?)

SPIRITUAL DISTRESS

Related to: Perinatal loss.

Defining Characteristics: Client expresses feelings of rejection, of disturbance in spiritual belief system (specify: e.g., "How could God do this?").

Goal: Client will experience relief from spiritual distress by (date/time to evaluate).

Outcome Criteria

✔ Client will be able to express feelings about belief system and pregnancy loss.

✔ Client verbalizes that spiritual needs are being met.

NOC: *Anxiety Control*

INTERVENTIONS	RATIONALES
Assess client's usual means of expressing spiritual beliefs (e.g., church, synagogue, temple, meditation, etc.). Avoid making assumptions about beliefs.	Assessment provides information about the client's beliefs and gives "permission" to talk about these matters.
Encourage client and significant other to express feelings about spirituality related to perinatal loss: anger, doubt, or failure to find comfort.	Client and significant other may feel that it is inappropriate to discuss these feelings. Encouragement facilitates identification of feelings.
Reassure client and significant other that anger and doubt are a common reaction to loss.	Client and significant other may feel guilty about being angry or having doubts.
Offer to pray or meditate with client (or ask another caregiver to do this) if desired.	Prayer or meditation may help the client to seek spiritual assistance.
Ask client and family if there are spiritual rituals that may be done for the parents or infant (e.g., infant baptism).	Baptism may provide comfort for clients belonging to certain religions. Rituals may include bathing the infant, chanting, and so forth.
Contact the client's spiritual advisor or pastoral care department if client desires.	A spiritual advisor may offer support and comfort to the client and family.

NIC: *Spiritual Support*

Evaluation

(Date/time of evaluation of goal)

(Has goal been met? not met? partially met?)

(Is client able to express feelings about belief system? Does client indicate that spiritual needs are being met? Specify: e.g., talked with pastor, memorial service planned, etc.).

(Revisions to care plan? D/C care plan? Continue care plan?)

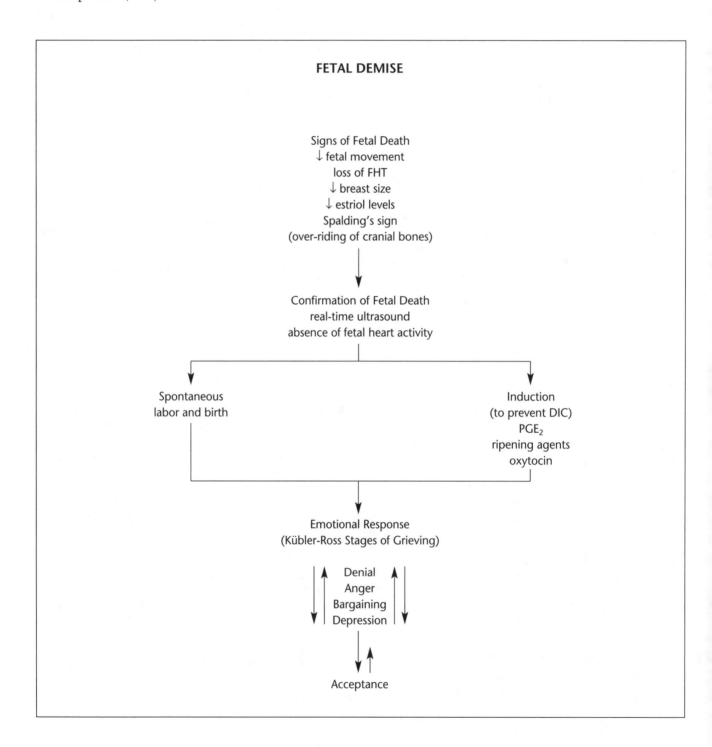

FETAL DEMISE

Signs of Fetal Death
↓ fetal movement
loss of FHT
↓ breast size
↓ estriol levels
Spalding's sign
(over-riding of cranial bones)

Confirmation of Fetal Death
real-time ultrasound
absence of fetal heart activity

Spontaneous
labor and birth

Induction
(to prevent DIC)
PGE₂
ripening agents
oxytocin

Emotional Response
(Kübler-Ross Stages of Grieving)

Denial
Anger
Bargaining
Depression

Acceptance

UNIT 3

POSTPARTUM

CHAPTER 3.0

HEALTHY PUERPERIUM

The puerperium, or postpartum period, begins physiologically with the birth of the baby and lasts for approximately six weeks. During this time the maternal reproductive organs recover from pregnancy and ovulation may return in nonbreast-feeding mothers. Psychological adjustment to the birth of a new baby certainly may take longer than six weeks. Sometimes a "fourth trimester" is described to include mental and emotional adaptation as well as the physiologic recovery from childbirth.

PHYSICAL CHANGES

- Uterine Involution: The uterus contracts after expulsion of the placenta to prevent hemorrhage from the placental site. After the first 24 hours, the uterine fundus ↓ 1 cm/day until it is no longer palpable above the symphysis pubis at 10 days.
- Endometrial Regeneration: Restoration of the endometrium takes 3 weeks except at the placental site, which takes up to 6 weeks.
- Lochia: rubra (2–3 days), serosa (7–10 days), and alba (1–2 weeks, or up to 6 weeks).
- Perineum: Usually redness and edema are present after birth. May have an episiotomy, lacerations, bruising, or hematomas. The urethra may be edematous.
- Breasts: Engorgement (venous and lymphatic congestion) occurs on about the third day after delivery. Secretions change from colostrum to milk on about the third to fifth day after birth.
- Fluid Balance: Client exhibits characteristic diuresis and diaphoresis as fluid moves from the extravascular spaces back into circulation.
- Cardiovascular: Loss of <500 cc blood for vaginal birth, <800 cc for cesarean birth is compensated for by loss of placental circulation and ↓ uterine circu-

lation. An ↑ CO caused by the fluid shift may cause ↓ pulse. BP should remain WNL.
- GI: Hunger and thirst are common after birth. Decreased GI motility, perineal or hemorrhoid discomfort may lead to constipation.

TABLE 3.1 Lab Value Changes

	AT BIRTH	RETURN TO NORMAL
Hgb/Hct	↑	4–6 weeks
WBC	↑	2 weeks
Clotting Factors	↑	4–5 weeks

PSYCHOLOGICAL CHANGES

- Attachment and bonding behaviors: eye contact, touch, enfolding, talking/smiling, and identification process.
- Taking-In Phase: Mother relives birth experience, focuses on own physical needs, dependency on others.
- Taking-Hold Phase: Client is more independent, focuses on caring for self and infant, needs education and reassurance that she is capable.
- Maternal Role Attainment: Client moves from the idealized fantasies during pregnancy to trying to care for infant as others advise, to independent decisions regarding parenting.
- Up to 80% of new mothers experience "Postpartum Blues": depression and emotional lability associated with unexpected crying, feeling overwhelmed. Occurs within the first week and lasts no more than 2–3 days. Should be differentiated from postpartum depression.

CULTURAL DIVERSITY

All cultures have beliefs related to maternal/infant care after childbirth. The nurse should ask the client about her individual cultural beliefs to avoid stereo-typing. Assessment of the following areas may reveal cultural prescriptions and prohibitions. Some of these are listed below:

Activity/Rest
- no activity restriction, rooming-in desirable, rest when the baby does, father helps at home, PP exercises
- avoid rooming-in, someone else cares for baby while mother rests and regains her strength
- bed rest under several blankets for 7 days to 3 months
- female relatives or hired women help with baby
- activity may be restricted up to 40 days

Nutrition
- increase calories and calcium for lactation; otherwise, lose weight gained during pregnancy
- eat and drink only foods/liquids considered "hot" and avoid those considered "cold" (not necessarily related to temperature or spices)
- special traditional foods may be indicated (e.g., seaweed soup, steak dinner)

Hygiene
- shower and hair washing as soon as possible
- avoid cold air or water; no showers
- avoid bathing until lochia stops
- don't wash hair for one week; wear head covering for warmth

Safety
- infant car seat; infant sleeps in crib, not with mother
- avoidance of evil influences: no praise of infant, don't touch infant's head, use of talismans/protective objects
- infant sleeps with mother, carried close to body

Spirituality
- infant Baptism/Christening, Bris
- naming ceremony (may be named after someone special)
- rituals performed by father
- burial/burning of placenta

Infant Care
Breast-Feeding
- breast offered at birth, feed on demand, avoid formula supplements
- colostrum discarded, infant fed sugar-water or honey and water until milk comes in (3–5 days)
- infant dressed in diaper and shirt, loose blanket
- infant tightly wrapped, belly-binder applied

Other
- cigars, flowers, balloons, announcements
- men are excluded from birth or contact with lochia
- desired visitors include family, friends, neighbors
- freely ask for pain medication and information
- avoid complaining or showing pain, avoid eye contact
- avoid asking questions and bothering the staff

TABLE 3.2   Postpartum Care Path: Vaginal Birth

BIRTH	ASSESSMENTS	TEACHING	MEDS/TX	OTHER

1st hour	TPR, BP
	OB √ q 15″ × 4 BP, P,
	  fundus, lochia, perineum
	  hemorrhoids
	  breast assessment
	bladder √
	epidural catheter removed
	bonding: eye contact/
	touch
		normal newborn
		
		holding infant
		bulb syringe
		
		breast-feeding: position,
		  latch, suck, swallow,
		  removal
		
		infant security
		answer all questions
			IV pitocin
			
			ice pack to perineum
			× 8 hr
			
			analgesics prn
				diet as tolerated with
				snacks
				
				mother/baby ID

4 hours	TPR, BP
	OB √ q 30″ × 2
	  then q 1 hr × 2
	
	empty bladder q 4 hr
	(void/catheter)
	leg movement & sensation
	
	infant handling
	  attachment
	nipple soreness
		handwashing
		pericare
		peri meds
		fundus/lochia
		
		nursing:
		breast care
		nutrition
		↑ fluids
		
		bottle feeding: burping,
		positioning
		breast care
			D/C IV prn
			
			Tucks, peri-spray
				ambulate with assistance
				to BR
				
				OB Gift Pack

8 hours	TPR, BP, Homan's sign, breast assessment & OB √ q shift if WNL bladder √ after void × 2 or until WNL	self-care nutrition activity/rest elimination	stool softener PNV sitz bath heat	activity as tolerated shower prn lactation specialist prn
1st PP day	Hgb & Hct bowel movement	infant care: cord, bathing, circ. care, safety, immunizations	RhoGAM Rubella prn	social services WIC prn
Discharge	VS, OB √ WNL elimination WNL infant/self-care adequate	Unit phone # and written instructions given warning s/s reviewed infant & self-care reviewed contraception, PP exercises, PKU, & immunizations reviewed	prescriptions given enema or stool softener prn	car seat mother/baby appointments referral for home visit

TABLE 3.3 Postpartum Care Path: Cesarean

BIRTH	ASSESSMENTS	TEACHING	MEDS/TX	OTHER

1st hour	IV, Foley
	temp, LOC, pain,
	I&O
	BP, P, R, SaC$_2$
	dsg CD&I
	fundus/lochia
	  q 5" × 4
	  q 15" × 2
	  q 30" × 2
	  q 1h × 2
	bonding: eye
	contact/touch
		pain relief
		TCDB, splinting
		
		normal newborn
		
		answer all questions
			IV with pitocin
			
			    pain relief:
			    duramorph
			    PCA pump
			    IM/IV
			
			pericare
				mother/baby ID

4 hours	BP, T, P, R, dsg CD&I fundus/lochia q 4h × 2 LOC, MAEe bowel sounds I&O	holding infant bulb syringe handwashing pericare fundus/lochia infant security		sips & chips or DAT with snacks
8 hours	BP, T, P, R, fundus/lochia dsg CD&I bowel sounds Homan's sign, breast assessment and bonding q 8h I&O	breast-feeding: position, latch, suck, swallow, removal bottle feeding: positioning, burping, breast care		up with assistance
1st PP day	bladder √ q 4h (catheterize prn) Hgb & Hct	self-care: nutrition, body mechanics activity/rest elimination	D/C IV prn D/C Foley prn	Cl liquids or DAT with snacks ambulate with assistance lactation specialist prn
2nd PP day	bladder √ after void × 2 or until WNL assess for BM	infant care: cord care bathing, circ care, safety, immunizations	po pain meds RhoGAM Rubella prn	regular diet with snacks ambulate w/o assistance
3rd PP day	assess infant and self-care	incision care review infant and self-care	remove dsg prn staples removed Steri-Strips	shower prn
Discharge	V/S, OB √ WNL incision CD&I elimination WNL infant/self-care adequate	Unit phone # and written instructions given warning s/s reviewed infant/self-care, contraception, PKU, and immunizations reviewed	prescriptions given enema or stool softener prn	car seat mother/baby appointments referral for home visit

CHAPTER 3.1

BASIC CARE PLAN: VAGINAL BIRTH

The nursing care plan is based on a thorough review of the prenatal record, labor and delivery summary, and continuing postpartum assessments. Individual data should be inserted whenever possible.

COMMON NURSING DIAGNOSES

 See RISK FOR INFECTION

Related to: Site for invasion of microorganisms (specify: e.g., episiotomy, lacerations, catheterization, etc.).

 See PAIN

Related to: Tissue trauma and edema after childbirth, uterine contractions (after-pains), engorged breasts, etc.

Defining Characteristics: Client reports pain (specify site and type of pain, rating on a scale of 1 to 10 with 1 being least, 10 most). Client is (specify: e.g., grimacing, crying, guarding, requesting pain meds, etc.).

ADDITIONAL NURSING DIAGNOSES

 RISK FOR DEFICIENT FLUID VOLUME

Related to: Active losses after childbirth (vaginal or cesarean), inadequate intake.

Defining Characteristics: None, as this is a potential diagnosis.

Goal: Client will not experience deficient fluid volume by (date/time to evaluate).

Outcome Criteria

✔ Client's pulse is <100, BP > (specify for client), mucous membranes moist and pink, fundus is firm with moderate-small amount of lochia.

NOC: *Risk Control*

INTERVENTIONS	RATIONALES
Assess client's hx for risk factors for hemorrhage (e.g., long labor, use of pitocin, overdistended uterus, clotting problems, etc.).	Assessment provides information about client's risk for puerperal hemorrhage.
Assess client's BP, P, and R (specify frequency).	Hypovolemia results in ↓ BP; the body compensates by vasoconstriction and ↑ P. ↓ volume leads to less available oxygen and ↑ R.
Assess uterine tone, position, and color and amount of lochia; observe for hematomas and integrity of incisions or dressings (specify frequency).	Assessments provide information about uterine displacement and tone, vaginal blood loss, occult bleeding, and wound dehiscence.
Massage the uterus if boggy, guarding over the symphysis pubis. Do not overstimulate.	Massage stimulates uterine contraction. Guarding prevents uterine prolapse. Overstimulation may cause uterine relaxation and hemorrhage.
Administer uterotonic drugs as ordered (specify: drug, dose, route, time).	Specify action of drug ordered (e.g., oxytocin, ergotrates, and prostaglandins).
Encourage frequent emptying of the bladder at least q 4h (catheterize prn as ordered).	Bladder distension may displace the uterus up and to a side causing ↓ tone and ↑ bleeding.
Estimate blood loss by counting or weighing peri-pads. Soaked pad in 15 min is excessive. 1 gm = 1 cc if weighing pads.	The degree of blood loss may not be apparent from appearance of vaginal discharge. Estimate helps determine replacement requirements.
Assess intake and output (specify frequency).	Assessment of intake and output provides information about fluid balance.
Assess skin color, temp, turgor, and moisture of lips/mucous membranes (specify frequency).	Pale, cool skin, poor skin turgor, and dry lips or membranes may indicate fluid loss/dehydration.
Monitor lab results as obtained (specify: e.g., Hgb, Hct, urine sp. gravity, clotting studies, etc.).	Monitoring provides information about fluid loss. Increased urine specific gravity may indicate ↓ fluid. Hgb and Hct indicate the extent of blood loss. Clotting

INTERVENTIONS	RATIONALES
	studies indicate the client at ↑ risk for hemorrhage.
Inform caregiver of any signs of unusual bleeding (e.g., from injection sites, gums, epistaxis, or petechiae).	Bleeding from unusual sites may indicate a clotting abnormality.
Initiate and maintain IV fluids and blood products as ordered (specify fluids and rate).	Intervention provides replacement of fluid or blood losses.
Encourage p.o. fluid intake (specify culturally appropriate types and amounts) if allowed.	Encouragement promotes fluid replacement for losses. Some cultures prefer hot liquids after childbirth and may avoid cold drinks.
Notify care giver if bleeding continues after nursing interventions.	Continued blood loss may indicate retained placental fragments or a cervical laceration requiring medical treatment.

NIC: *Hypovolemia Management*

Evaluation

(Date/time of evaluation of goal)

(Has goal been met? not met? partially met?)

(What is client's pulse? BP? Are mucous membranes moist and pink, fundus firm with moderate-small amount of lochia? Specify findings.)

(Revisions to care plan? D/C care plan? Continue care plan?)

 ## READINESS FOR ENHANCED SPIRITUAL WELL-BEING

Related to: Life-affirming experience of childbirth and motherhood.

Defining Characteristics: Client reports spiritual well-being (specify: e.g., "There must be a God," "This gives meaning to my life," etc.—does not need to be religious in nature). Client exhibits a sense of awareness, inner peace, and trust in relationships with infant and family (provide examples). Client offers prayers of thanksgiving.

Goal: Client will continue to experience spiritual well-being by (date/time to evaluate).

Outcome Criteria

✔ Client expresses continued feelings of spiritual well-being.

✔ Client exhibits nurturing behaviors towards infant.

NOC: *Spiritual Well-Being*

INTERVENTIONS	RATIONALES
Assess client's perceptions about the experience of giving birth.	Assessment provides information about client's perceptions.
Offer accurate information if client has questions about the experience.	Information assists the client to construct an accurate birth story.
Assess client's religious preferences or any desired spiritual practices that are related to childbirth.	Assessment provides information about the client's spiritual needs.
Facilitate religious or spiritual practices as indicated (specify for client).	Client and family may have special requests (e.g., a time/place for a ceremony, the placenta for burial, etc.).
Contact clients' spiritual advisor or hospital pastoral care if client wishes.	Intervention ensures that client has access to a spiritual advisor if she wishes.
Observe client's nurturing behaviors towards infant.	Spiritual well-being promotes love and commitment towards others.
Offer assistance and explanations as needed about caring for the infant.	Inexperienced clients may need assistance with infant-care skills.
Praise client for her nurturing and skill with infant care.	Praise reinforces nurturing of the infant and enhances client's self-esteem.

NIC: *Spiritual Support*

Evaluation

(Date/time of evaluation of goal)

(Has goal been met? not met? partially met?)

(Does client report feelings of spiritual well-being? Does client nurture her infant? Specify client's activities.)

(Revisions to care plan? D/C care plan? Continue care plan?)

DEFICIENT KNOWLEDGE: INFANT AND SELF-CARE

Related to: Limited experience and skill in providing infant care and self-care after giving birth.

Defining Characteristics: Client is a primipara (or first time to breast-feed, etc.). Client expresses need for information about self- or infant care (specify). Client reports inaccurate perceptions about self- or infant care (specify).

Goal: Client will gain cognitive knowledge and psychomotor skills needed for self- and infant care by (date/time to evaluate).

Outcome Criteria

✔ Client verbalizes understanding of self-care and infant care instruction.

✔ Client demonstrates psychomotor skills needed for infant and self-care.

NOC: *Knowledge: Postpartum*

INTERVENTIONS	RATIONALES
Assess client's previous experience with childbirth or caring for a newborn infant.	Assessment provides information about client's current knowledge base and experience.
For clients who have experienced childbirth before, ask if they have any questions about infant or self-care. Review current information with client.	Clients may have had difficulty in prior experiences with infant or self-care. Reviewing material with multiparous clients ensures that accurate information is provided.
Teach client as nursing care is provided and reinforce with videos, follow-up instruction, and written materials (if client if literate). Obtain the services of an interpreter as needed. Include significant other and family in teaching.	Varied teaching methods facilitate learning by addressing client's individual learning style. Repetition and inclusion of the family may be helpful as the client experiences increased sensory input during the puerperium.
Teach client about uterine involution, fundal tone, and lochia. Instruct in perineal care, hand-washing, use of peri-bottle, wiping from front to back, correct application of pads, avoiding sex, tampons, or douches per caregiver instructions.	Instruction aids the client in gaining skills and knowledge needed for self-care. Interventions remove pathogens from the hands, cleanse the perineum, and prevent trauma and fecal contamination of perineum.

INTERVENTIONS	RATIONALES
Teach cesarean clients to care for incision per caregiver instructions (specify). Teach signs and symptoms of infection to report.	Information assists the client to care for incision, prevent infection, and promote healing.
Teach client to care for infant: demonstrate use of bulb syringe, safety and nurturing for the infant and holding, feeding, burping, diapering, circumcision care (if indicated), cord care, bathing, how to take a temperature, and when to call the doctor. Observe client as she cares for infant and reinforce positive attempts.	Instruction promotes confidence for the mother as she gains skills. Observation and reinforcement ensure appropriate technique.
Instruct client in breast care. For nonnursing mothers teach to wear a snug bra, avoid stimulation of the breasts and to use ice packs (frozen peas) and mild analgesics as ordered for discomfort. Reassure client that discomfort should subside in a day or two.	Information helps the client to avoid activities that may stimulate the breasts and cause increased discomfort from engorgement.
Teach breast-feeding mothers to wash their hands before feeding, wash their breasts without soap, and inspect the nipples for pain or sores after each feeding.	Information helps the client to avoid mastitis.
Teach client to continue PNV, drink 8–10 glasses of water/day, and eat a nutritious diet. Use the food guide pyramid to plan a culturally acceptable diet including fresh fruits and vegetables, fiber, protein, and vitamin C. Provide information for breast-feeding mothers about extra fluids and dairy products needed (specify).	Information helps the client to plan for adequate nutrition for recovery from childbirth. Fresh fruits, vegetables, and added fiber help prevent constipation. Protein and vitamin C enhance tissue healing. Nursing mothers require extra calories and fluids to produce milk and meet their own needs.
Teach client to avoid strenuous activity or exercise for six weeks. Provide information from caregiver about postpartum period period exercises.	Strenuous exercise may cause postpartum hemorrhage before the placental site is healed. Exercise helps the client's body return to its prepregnancy shape.
Encourage client to obtain adequate rest during the puerperium. Teach her that activity that leads to an increase in the flow of lochia is a sign that she needs to slow down.	Client may try to do too much, delaying healing and risking exhaustion. Client may need "permission" to rest.

INTERVENTIONS	RATIONALES
Demonstrate respect for client's cultural prescriptions and prohibitions regarding postpartum care.	Cultural respect avoids conflicts about care that may make the client feel guilty.
Teach client about the return of menstruation and ovulation. Inform about the possibility of becoming pregnant and assist her to make contraceptive choices.	Knowledge helps the client to understand how her body works and to make personal decisions about family planning.
Teach client about any medications that are prescribed for her after discharge. Instruct breastfeeding moms to avoid taking medications without checking with the baby's caregiver first.	Specify action, dose, route, and indications for any prescribed medications. Most drugs distributed by the blood are also found in the breast milk.
Provide information about and phone numbers for local support groups (specify: e.g., La Leche League, Mothers of Twins, etc.).	Support groups may offer increased information about topics of special interest to the client.
Teach client about use of infant car seat, need for follow-up PKU, and infant immunizations.	Information promotes infant safety.
Provide written and verbal information about danger signs to call the primary caregiver: fever, chills, ↑ bleeding, foul smelling lochia, ↑ incision, breast or leg pain, wound dehiscence, or burning on urination.	Information assists the client to seek immediate care for puerperal complications.
Observe client's self-care and infant care ability during hospitalization. Refer client for additional assistance as needed (specify: e.g., home visit).	Observation provides information about client's ability to care for herself and her baby after discharge. Referral provides additional education.

INTERVENTIONS	RATIONALES
Discuss the need for Rh immune globulin (RhoGAM) with Rh negative clients. Provide blood type card.	Rh-negative clients should understand the need for Rh immune globulin after miscarriage or birth of an Rh-positive baby to prevent isoimmunization of future infants.
Inform nonimmune client of the advisability for rubella immunization and to avoid pregnancy for at least 3 months.	Information helps the nonimmune client avoid teratogenic effects of rubella in future pregnancies. Rubella is a live vaccine and should not be given during pregnancy
Review and reinforce all teaching at discharge. Provide client with a phone number to call for questions after she gets home.	Intervention promotes access to continued information after client is discharged.

NIC: *Teaching, Infant Care*

Evaluation

(Date/time of evaluation of goal)

(Has goal been met? not met? partially met?)

(Does client verbalize understanding of self-care and infant care information? Does client demonstrate psychomotor skills needed for self- and infant care? Specify.)

(Revisions to care plan? D/C care plan? Continue care plan?)

CHAPTER 3.2

BASIC CARE PLAN: CESAREAN BIRTH

The nursing care plan is based on a thorough review of the prenatal record, labor and delivery summary, operative records, and a continual postpartum assessment. Individualized data should be inserted wherever possible.

COMMON NURSING DIAGNOSES

 ### See RISK FOR DEFICIENT FLUID VOLUME

Related to: Excessive fluid losses secondary to operative delivery. Inadequate intake for needs.

 ### See READINESS FOR ENHANCED SPIRITUAL WELL-BEING

Related to: Life-affirming experience of giving birth.

Defining Characteristics: Describe client and significant other's response to birth (e.g., quotes related to spiritual dimension of the experience). Specify nurturing and loving behaviors of client and significant other towards infant.

 ### See DEFICIENT KNOWLEDGE: INFANT AND SELF-CARE

Related to: Limited experience with infant and self-care (specify: e.g., first baby, first cesarean birth, etc.).

Defining Characteristics: Client expresses lack of knowledge about self- and infant care after birth (specify). Client verbalizes incorrect information about self- or infant care (specify).

ADDITIONAL NURSING DIAGNOSES

 ### RISK FOR INFECTION

Related to: Site for microorganism invasion secondary to childbirth and/or surgical interventions.

Defining Characteristics: None, as this is a potential diagnosis.

Goal: Client will not experience signs of infection by (date/time to evaluate).

Outcome Criteria

✔ Client's temperature is <100.4° F, P <100, incision is dry and intact, edges well-approximated without redness or edema, no foul-smelling lochia or pelvic pain.

NOC: *Risk Control*

INTERVENTIONS	RATIONALES
Wash hands before and after caring for client; use gloves when indicated; don't share equipment with other units.	Interventions help prevent the spread of pathogens between staff and patients.
Assess client's temperature, BP, P, and R (specify frequency). Notify caregiver if temp is >100.4° F after the first 24 hours, or if pulse is consistently >100.	Assessment provides information about developing infection: temperature may be slightly ↑ early caused by dehydration from labor. Slight ↓ P is common after birth and tachycardia may indicate infection.
Teach surgical clients to TCDB and encourage ambulation. Instruct in leg exercises while in bed.	Teaching helps gain client compliance to prevent pulmonary stasis that may lead to infection.
Assess dressings or incisions (specify frequency) noting if dressing is clean, dry, and intact, if incisions exhibit redness, edema, ecchymosis, drainage, and approximation (REEDA).	Assessment provides information about developing infection: Local inflammatory effects cause redness and edema. This may be followed by purulent drainage and wound dehiscence.
Assess client for increased abdominal tenderness during fundal checks. Instruct client to report continuous pelvic pain.	Assessment provides information about inflammation of the endometrium.

INTERVENTIONS	RATIONALES
Note color, odor, and consistency of lochia. Instruct client to report foul-smelling lochia.	Foul smelling or purulent lochia signals infectious processes. Lochia has a characteristic odor somewhat like menstrual discharge.
Provide catheter care per agency protocol. Keep catheter bag below the level of the bladder and off the floor. Use aseptic technique to obtain specimens.	Interventions keep the opening to the urethra clean, prevent urine backflow and contamination of catheter bag.
Teach client to perform peri care after elimination and to change peripads frequently, applying pads from front to back.	Teaching helps client keep the perineum clean and dry. Warm, moist environment facilitates the growth of microorganisms.
Encourage client to void every 4 hours. Assess bladder emptying (specify frequency). Catheterize only as needed employing sterile technique. Instruct client to report any burning or pain with urination.	Postpartum diuresis may cause over-distention or incomplete emptying of the bladder. Urinary stasis provides a medium for growth of microorganisms. Burning and pain are signs of inflammation associated with UTI.
Obtain specimens as ordered (specify: e.g., urine specimens, wound cultures). Monitor lab results.	Laboratory examination of specimens is indicated to determine the causative organisms and their sensitivity to antibiotics.
Inspect IV sites per agency protocol. Note redness, warmth, pain, or edema. Discontinue or change site as indicated.	Inspection provides information about the development of inflammation and infection at invasive sites.
Administer antibiotics as ordered (specify: drug, dose, route, times).	Specify action of each drug given.
Encourage clients with an episiotomy to take sitz baths as ordered (specify). Ensure that tub is cleaned before each use or use individual disposable tubs.	The moist heat from a sitz bath increases circulation to the perineum and facilitates healing. Cleaning or individual tubs prevent cross-contamination.
Maintain a clean environment. Ensure that client's room and bathroom are cleaned frequently and appropriately.	A clean environment may discourage the growth of microorganisms.

NIC: *Infection Control*

Evaluation

(Date/time of evaluation of goal)

(Has goal been met? not met? partially met?)

(What is client's temperature? pulse? Are incisions dry and intact, edges well-approximated, without redness or edema, no foul-smelling lochia or pelvic pain?)

(Revisions to care plan? D/C care plan? Continue care plan?)

ACUTE PAIN

Related to: Tissue trauma secondary to surgery, perineal trauma from vaginal birth, uterine involution; engorged breasts.

Defining Characteristics: Client complains of pain (specify using quotes). Client rates pain on a scale of 1 to 10 (specify). Client is grimacing, guarding painful area, etc. (specify).

Goal: Client will experience a decrease in pain by (date/time to evaluate).

Outcome Criteria

✔ Client rates pain as less than (specify) on a scale of 1 to 10 with 1 being least, 10 being most.

✔ Client appears calm, no grimacing or guarding of area.

NOC: *Pain Control*

INTERVENTIONS	RATIONALES
Assess client's pain using a scale of 1 to 10 with 1 being least, 10 being most (specify frequency).	Assessment provides objective measurement of the client's perception of pain.
Observe client for nonverbal signs of pain: grimacing, guarding, pallor, withdrawal, etc. (specify frequency).	Observation helps identify discomfort when the client doesn't ask for help. Cultural variations may govern the expression of pain.
Assess location and character of pain each time the client reports discomfort. Notify caregiver if unusual pain develops.	Assessment provides information about the cause of pain. Unusual pain may indicate complications.
Instruct client to use an ice pack for 8 hours after birth as ordered. Keep pack 2/3 full of ice.	Application of ice decreases edema and provides a local anesthetic effect.
Administer appropriate pain medication as ordered (specify: drug, dose, route, times).	Specify action of specific drug and rationale for choice.
Assess client for pain relief within an appropriate time after medication administration (specify for drug).	Assessment provides information about client's response to peak levels of drug.

(continues)

(continued)

INTERVENTIONS	RATIONALES
Observe client for adverse effects of drug (specify for drug given).	Observation allows early detection and treatment of adverse effects.
Instruct clients receiving regular pain medication to ask for the drug before pain becomes unbearable.	Pain medication is more effective and lower doses are needed if given before pain becomes severe.
Teach client about the physiology of her discomfort (specify for client: e.g., after-pains when breast-feeding are caused by stimulation of oxytocin release and uterine contraction).	Knowledge may ↓ the anxiety associated with unfamiliar pain.
Teach client nonpharmacologic pain relief measures: positioning to avoid pressure on painful areas; splinting of incision; tightening buttocks before sitting to prevent traction on perineum; wearing a snug bra, if nonnursing; ensuring the infant is latched on and removed from the breast correctly if breast-feeding, and so forth.	Teaching provides the client with information about self-care activities to decrease pain. Interventions decrease pressure on painful areas and incisions. Painful nipples may be caused by inadequate latching-on.
Assist client to take a sitz bath if ordered (specify type available and method to use). Instruct client to use the sitz for approximately 20 minutes 3–4 times a day.	Moist heat from the sitz bath promotes comfort and healing by increasing circulation to the perineum.
Teach client to perform Kegel exercises (suggest frequency).	Kegel exercises promote perineal circulation and healing.
Teach client correct use of products ordered for relief of episiotomy or hemorrhoid pain (specify: e.g., anesthetic ointments, sprays, or witch hazel pads).	Specify action of medications ordered.

INTERVENTIONS	RATIONALES
Teach client to eat fresh fruits and vegetables, and whole grains daily and to drink 8–10 glasses of water. Administer stool softeners as ordered (specify).	Teaching provides information the client needs to make diet decisions that will help prevent constipation. Stool softeners help decrease pain from bowel movements when client has a 4th degree laceration or episiotomy.
Encourage ambulation as soon as possible after birth. Evaluate client for development of pain in the lower extremities (Homan's sign).	Ambulation decreases venous stasis. Venous stasis and ↑ platelets at birth lead to potential development of thrombophlebitis.
Encourage client to plan frequent rest periods in the first few postpartum weeks. Teach relaxation techniques as needed.	Fatigue may add to perceptions of pain and distress.

NIC: *Pain Management*

Evaluation

(Date/time of evaluation of goal)

(Has goal been met? not met? partially met?)

(What does client rate pain on a scale of 1 to 10? Does client appear calm? Is client grimacing or guarding body areas?)

(Revisions to care plan? D/C care plan? Continue care plan?)

CHAPTER 3.3

BASIC CARE PLAN: POSTPARTUM HOME VISIT

The postpartum home visit enables the client to receive additional assessment and instruction in the comfort and reality of her own home. Many questions about self- and infant care arise once the mother has been discharged. The care plan is based on a thorough review of the client's records and assessments made in the home.

COMMON NURSING DIAGNOSES

 See DEFICIENT KNOWLEDGE: INFANT AND SELF-CARE

Related to: Inexperience and limited information about infant and self-care after childbirth.

Defining Characteristics: Client verbalizes lack of knowledge or misunderstanding about infant and/or self-care (specify using quotes). Client exhibits incorrect self- or infant care techniques (specify).

ADDITIONAL NURSING DIAGNOSES

 READINESS FOR ENHANCED FAMILY COPING

Related to: Adaptation of family to new family member.

Defining Characteristics: Family members are involved in care of the mother and newborn. Family members verbalize positive reactions to addition of a new family member (specify).

Goal: Family will continue to experience growth in coping with the stresses of a new baby by (date/time to evaluate).

Outcome Criteria

✔ Family members express positive feelings about their new baby and new roles in the family (other specifics as indicated).

NOC: *Family Coping*

INTERVENTIONS	RATIONALES
Identify family structure and encourage members' participation in home visit.	Family may include grandparents or friends in addition to the nuclear family.
Assess family members' verbal and nonverbal responses to the new baby.	Birth of a new family member alters each member's role in the family.
Assess the infant's sleeping and eating patterns and how these affect family members.	Frequent infant feeding and lack of sleep are stressors for new families.
Praise effective coping mechanisms used by the family (specify).	Praise reinforces the family's effective coping with the stress of a new baby.
Discuss infant growth and development with the family. Point out infant reflexes and attachment behaviors.	Discussion provides anticipatory guidance for family to facilitate infant growth and development.
Refer family to support groups as indicated (specify).	Support groups may reinforce positive coping.

NIC: *Family Involvement Promotion*

Evaluation

(Date/time of evaluation of goal)

(Has goal been met? not met? partially met?)

(Do family members report positive feelings about their new baby and their changed roles in the family? Specify.)

(Revisions to care plan? D/C care plan? Continue care plan?)

 FATIGUE

Related to: Demands of caring for newborn while recovering from childbirth.

Defining Characteristics: Client states she is exhausted (specify). Client states she doesn't have enough energy to accomplish desired tasks (specify: e.g., fix dinner, care for other children, etc.). Client appears lethargic, has dark circles under eyes, and so forth (physical signs of fatigue).

Goal: Client will experience less fatigue by (date/time to evaluate).

Outcome Criteria

✔ Client identifies priority activities that she will focus on during the postpartum period.

✔ Client and family identify tasks that family members will be responsible for.

NOC: *Energy Conservation*

INTERVENTIONS	RATIONALES
Assess client's current rest and activity patterns.	Assessment provides information about adequacy of client's rest and activity pattern.
Assist client to identify primary cause of fatigue (e.g., worry, lack of sleep at night, etc.).	Client may be too tired to identify primary problem without some assistance.
Discuss physiologic factors that increase fatigue during the puerperium: long labor, cesarean birth, episiotomy pain, and anemia.	Understanding the physiologic basis of fatigue helps the client plan self-care activities to ↓ fatigue.
Assess client for postpartum complications; excessive bleeding or signs of infection: fever, malaise, redness, edema, purulent drainage from incisions, pelvic pain or foul-smelling lochia. Notify caregiver.	Excessive bleeding may cause anemia and fatigue related to insufficient hemoglobin. Signs of infection also include fatigue.
Help client express frustration related to infant care and fatigue. Provide emotional support and reassurance.	Facilitating expression of feelings validates the client's experience.

INTERVENTIONS	RATIONALES
Assess client for signs of postpartum "blues" or depression. Discuss hormonal changes, role changes, and exhaustion as precipitating factors.	A short-lived period of depression accompanied by emotional fragility is common in the first few weeks postpartum. Continued depression needs further investigation.
Discuss situational factors that increase fatigue (e.g., small children to care for, lack of social support system, beliefs about housekeeping, difficult-to-console infant, etc.).	Discussion helps client and family identify factors that increase fatigue.
Assist client and family to identify strengths they can use to cope with current increased demands. Reassure family that expressed feelings are common and that most families adjust by 6 weeks postpartum.	The family may have unexpected resources and strengths. Reassurance helps decrease anxiety and associated fatigue.
Assist client and family to identify priority activities (e.g., mother and infant care, eating, sleeping) and those which may be delayed (e.g., cleaning, social responsibilities).	Identification of priorities helps the family to determine essential and nonessential tasks.
Assist client and family to identify tasks that each member can be responsible for (specify for ages of children).	Delegation allows the client to focus only on essential activities.
Encourage the client to rest or sleep when the infant is sleeping.	Encouragement gives the client permission to nap frequently.
Teach relaxation techniques, mental imagery, or meditation to help cope with tension.	Anxiety produces increased psychological demands and reduces energy.
Assess current diet and encourage client to ingest recommended amounts of calories, protein, vitamin C, and fluids.	Poor nutrition and dehydration add to feelings of fatigue. Protein and vitamin C are needed for tissue regeneration after childbirth.
Refer client for additional assistance as indicated (e.g., WIC, counseling, community services, etc.).	Client may have inadequate financial means or support system to cope with postpartum stresses.

NIC: *Energy Management*

Evaluation

(Date/time of evaluation of goal)

(Has goal been met? not met? partially met?)

(What are the priority tasks the client identified? Which tasks did client and family identify that family members will be responsible for?)

(Revisions to care plan? D/C care plan? Continue care plan?)

IMBALANCED NUTRITION: MORE THAN BODY REQUIREMENTS

Related to: Intake in excess of that required for metabolic needs.

Defining Characteristics: Client verbalizes a desire to lose excessive weight gained during pregnancy (specify client's current weight and prepregnancy weight or ideal weight). Client reports eating habits that are in excess of current needs (specify: e.g., high in calories and fat, low in fruits and vegetables).

Goal: Client will ingest an appropriate diet by (date/time to evaluate).

Outcome Criteria

✔ Client identifies excess in current diet.

✔ Client plans a diet to meet nutritional and metabolic needs.

NOC: *Weight Control*

INTERVENTIONS	RATIONALES
Assess client's weight. Compare to prepregnancy weight and ideal weight for height and build.	Assessment provides information about appropriate weight for individual client and evaluation of possible excessive weight gain during pregnancy.
Encourage client to continue taking PNV as ordered during puerperium.	Supplements replenish vitamin and iron supplies decreased by pregnancy and birth.
Describe normal weight loss after childbirth: the average mother loses 10–12 Lb at birth followed by average weight loss of 1 to 1½ Lb/week during the following 6 weeks.	Client may have unrealistic expectations about weight loss after giving birth.
Inform the client that she should not attempt to diet while breastfeeding. Nursing clients will usually lose weight faster because of metabolic needs of lactation.	Nursing mothers require increased calories to produce milk. Breast-feeding increases metabolism and usually weight loss as well.

INTERVENTIONS	RATIONALES
Assist client to review current eating habits using a 24-hour diet recall and a copy of the food guide pyramid.	Review provides information about current intake compared to nutritional needs.
Provide client with a copy of the food guide pyramid and suggested diets for weight loss after childbirth.	Visual aids and reading materials provide the client with a source of continued information at home.
Assist client to plan a nutritious diet for her family that incorporates cultural preferences and financial ability. Help client to plan how to reduce her own calories by 300/day. Include necessary nutrients without added fats or empty calories.	Assistance ensures that correct foods are chosen while empowering the client to make her own plan. Generic diets may not be affordable, include culturally preferred foods, or be appropriate for the whole family.
Discuss the need for exercise as well as dietary modification to lose weight. Encourage client to begin with daily walking and exercise program with advice of her caregiver.	Walking is generally an appropriate postpartum exercise. The client should avoid strenuous exercise until the placental site has healed at approximately 6 weeks.
Refer client to a dietitian as indicated (specify: e.g., diabetic moms, clients with unusual diets or special needs).	A dietitian is specifically prepared to advise clients with numerous or unusual nutrition questions.

NIC: *Nutrition Management*

Evaluation

(Date/time of evaluation of goal)

(Has goal been met? not met? partially met?)

(What excesses did the client identify in her diet? What diet plan did the client make to meet nutritional and metabolic needs?)

(Revisions to care plan? D/C care plan? Continue care plan?)

INEFFECTIVE SEXUALITY PATTERNS

Related to: Effects of childbirth on sexual behavior.

Defining Characteristics: Client reports negative perceptions about sexuality after childbirth (specify: e.g., "My husband is hounding me to have sex and I don't want to" or "I'm really afraid that it's going to hurt"). Client reports lack of interest in sexuality. Client reports concern about sexual feelings during breast-feeding (specify).

Goal: Client and partner will report satisfactory patterns of sexuality by (date/time to evaluate).

Outcome Criteria

✔ Client and partner will verbalize understanding of postpartum physiologic changes affecting sexuality.

✔ Client and partner will identify ways to meet sexual needs during the puerperium.

NOC: *Role Performance*

INTERVENTIONS	RATIONALES
Establish rapport with the client and partner (if available). Provide privacy for discussion of sexuality.	Client and partner may feel uncomfortable discussing sexual concerns in front of anyone else (e.g., children).
Offer general information about reproductive concerns and sexuality after childbirth. Elicit questions.	Offering general information allows the client and partner to ask questions they may have been too shy to bring up.
Identify the need to abstain from sexual intercourse (as advised by caregiver) until the placental site has healed (lochia has stopped and perineal incisions or lacerations are healed: usually 3–4 weeks for vaginal birth) to avoid infection or trauma.	Client and partner may not understand the rationale for abstinence in the immediate postpartum period. Many couples resume sexual relations before the six-week postpartum visit.
Discuss postpartum physiology that may interfere with sexuality: fatigue, vaginal and perineal soreness, lack of lubrication until ovulation recommences, and breast tenderness.	Information decreases unwarranted anxiety about altered sexuality related to physiologic changes during the puerperium.

INTERVENTIONS	RATIONALES
Assist client and partner to identify ways to meet sexual needs during the puerperium (suggest other forms of expression of affection, varied positions, use of water-soluble lubricants, etc.).	Assistance empowers client and partner to adapt to transient physiologic changes while providing information about possible solutions.
Reinforce the understanding that subsequent pregnancy is possible even before the first postpartum menses begin.	Client may believe that she can't get pregnant if she's breast-feeding or until menstruation returns.
Provide contraceptive counseling as indicated.	Client may need information about contraceptive options.
Reassure nursing clients that pleasurable pelvic sensations associated with breast-feeding are a normal result of uterine contraction stimulated by the release of oxytocin.	Reassurance validates the client's perceptions and allays guilt feelings that may be present when breast-feeding results in pleasurable sensations.
Refer client to caregiver for unusual signs of pain on intercourse or sexual dysfunction.	Unusual pain or dysfunction may be the result of physical or psychological complications.

NIC: *Sexual Counseling*

Evaluation

(Date/time of evaluation of goal)

(Has goal been met? not met? partially met?)

(Did client and partner verbalize understanding of postpartum physiologic changes affecting sexuality? Have client and partner identified ways to meet sexual needs during the puerperium?)

(Revisions to care plan? D/C care plan? Continue care plan?)

CHAPTER 3.4

BREAST-FEEDING

Lactation is a normal physiologic process that provides optimum nutrition for the infant. The hormones of pregnancy prepare the breasts for lactation. The process is completed when the placenta separates and there is an abrupt drop in estrogen and progesterone. This allows the unobstructed influence of pituitary prolactin to stimulate milk production. Oxytocin is released by the posterior pituitary gland in response to suckling. This hormone causes contraction of the uterus (enhances involution) and the myoepithelial cells in the breast alveoli. Milk is then released into the ducts and sinuses and ejected from the nipples. This is known as the "let-down reflex." The infant's cry or even just thinking about the infant may stimulate the reflex. If the mother is very tense and anxious, the let-down reflex may be inhibited causing frustration for both infant and mother.

Colostrum is a clear yellow secretion produced by the breasts during the third trimester of pregnancy and for the first few days after birth. It is gradually replaced by production of mature breast milk. Colostrum contains antibodies that may protect the infant from pathogens. In some cultures colostrum is thought to be unhealthy for the newborn and is discarded.

On the 3rd or 4th day after birth the mother may notice breast discomfort associated with venous and lymphatic engorgement accompanying the start of lactation. This usually subsides within 24–48 hours. Frequency of nursing has a direct effect on the level of prolactin released and therefore on the amount of milk produced. Most women will be discharged from the hospital before milk production begins. Anticipatory guidance and follow-up may be needed to ensure success.

CONTRAINDICATIONS

- Maternal cytomegalovirus, chronic hepatitis B, or HIV infection

- Maternal need for medications that may adversely affect the infant (the mother may pump her breasts for the duration of drug therapy and resume breast-feeding later).

ADVANTAGES

- human milk is 95% efficiently used by the human infant: breast-fed infants experience less constipation and gas than bottle-fed infants
- nursing accelerates uterine involution and loss of weight gained during pregnancy
- children who were breast-fed have higher IQ scores
- breast-fed infants have fewer allergies
- breast milk is free, warm, sterile, and always available

DISADVANTAGES

- the mother may feel "tied to the infant" in the early puerperium while supply is being established
- leaking breasts
- need to plan ahead to pump breasts when the mother will not be available for feedings

COMMON NURSING DIAGNOSES

 See READINESS FOR ENHANCED SPIRITUAL WELL-BEING

Related to: Life-affirming experience of successfully breast-feeding a newborn infant.

Defining Characteristics: Client reports feeling spiritual well being (describe).

ADDITIONAL NURSING DIAGNOSES

EFFECTIVE BREAST-FEEDING

Related to: Maternal–infant dyad satisfaction and success with breast-feeding process.

Defining Characteristics: Client reports satisfaction with the breast-feeding process (specify: e.g., "I always breast-feed my babies, it's so easy"). Client positions infant to ensure good latch-on at the breast. Infant exhibits regular sucking and swallowing, appears content after feeding.

Goal: Maternal–infant dyad continues to experience effective breast-feeding by (date/time to evaluate).

Outcome Criteria

✔ Client reports continued satisfaction with breast-feeding.

✔ Client demonstrates skill with breast-feeding. Infant appears content after feeding.

NOC: *Breast-Feeding Maintenance*

INTERVENTIONS	RATIONALES
Promote breast-feeding as soon as possible after birth, if client wishes. Delay nonessential nursing care for 1–2 hours (e.g., weighing, footprints, eye prophylaxis, vitamin K injection, etc.).	Early breast-feeding takes advantage of the first period of reactivity, promotes maternal homeostasis, and provides comfort for the infant after birth.
Demonstrate respect for cultural variations in breast-feeding practices (e.g., some cultures discard the colostrum and feed the infant sugar-water until the milk comes in).	Deeply held cultural beliefs are not likely to be changed by disapproval. Respect for variances promotes self-esteem and cultural integrity.
Encourage skin-to-skin contact for mother and infant. Place a warm blanket over mother and baby.	Skin-to-skin contact provides tactile stimulation, promotes attachment, and maintains the infant's temperature.
Assess client's previous experiences, knowledge, and skill (positioning, latch-on, removal, etc.) with breast-feeding. Elicit questions or concerns. Share current research findings as appropriate.	Assessment provides information about knowledge and skills. Client may benefit from current research findings.

INTERVENTIONS	RATIONALES
Ask client to share any tips she may have for others about breast-feeding (e.g., relieving engorgement, promoting "let-down" reflex, pumping, working, etc.).	Intervention promotes client's self-esteem and provides anecdotal information about successful breast-feeding techniques.
Facilitate client's breast-feeding by not offering supplements to the infant, promoting rooming-in, etc. as client desires.	Interventions promote infant's interest in nursing and allow frequent stimulation of the breasts.
Praise client and infant for effective breast-feeding activity.	Praise reinforces effective breast-feeding.

NIC: *Lactation Counseling*

Evaluation

(Date/time of evaluation of goal)

(Has goal been met? not met? partially met?)

(Does client report continued satisfaction with breast-feeding? Does client demonstrate skill with breast-feeding? [Specify: e.g., positioning, latch-on, removal, etc.] Does infant appear content after feeding?)

(Revisions to care plan? D/C care plan? Continue care plan?)

IMBALANCED NUTRITION: LESS THAN BODY REQUIREMENTS

Related to: Increased caloric and nutrient demands secondary to breast-feeding.

Defining Characteristics: Client is breast-feeding her infant and reports, or is observed, eating less than the recommended daily allowance of calories and/or nutrients for effective lactation (specify for client).

Goal: Client will ingest adequate calories and nutrients to promote effective lactation by (date/time to evaluate).

Outcome Criteria

✔ Client verbalizes the caloric and food guide pyramid requirements for good nutrition while breast-feeding her baby.

✔ Client plans to eat appropriate nutrients.

NOC: *Nutritional Status: Nutrient Intake*

INTERVENTIONS	RATIONALES
Assess client's weight, weight gain during pregnancy, and ideal weight. Calculate caloric requirements for lactation (usually 500 kcal over regular dietary needs).	Assessment provides information about client's weight and individual caloric needs (2500 to 3000 calories for lactation).
Assess client's usual intake using 24-hour diet recall.	Assessment provides information about current intake.
Provide client with written and verbal information about daily nutrient and caloric needs during lactation: PNV, 4 servings protein, 5 servings dairy (1 quart milk), 2–3 servings fruit (2 vitamin C-rich), 2–3 servings vegetables (1+ green leafy), 2–3 quarts fluids.	Written instruction allows client to review material once she is discharged. For illiterate clients, materials may be in picture format. Individual instruction promotes compliance.
Assist client to compare usual diet with needs for lactation. Explore food preferences and cultural prescriptions.	Assistance empowers the client to evaluate her intake compared to needs for lactation.
Assist client to plan daily food choices to meet lactation needs while allowing for cultural/personal preferences and financial ability. Provide time to problem solve with client.	Client is most likely to adhere to a plan of her own devising. Preprinted diets often are not culturally sensitive, contain disliked foods (e.g., liver), and are too expensive.
Suggest that client have fluids accessible during breast-feeding sessions.	Breast-feeding stimulates thirst. This is a good time to include additional fluids.
Refer client for financial or nutritional assistance as needed (specify: e.g., social services, WIC, dietitian).	Referral helps clients with financial or unusual nutritional needs (e.g., diabetic or PKU mothers).

NIC: *Nutrition Management*

Evaluation

(Date/time of evaluation of goal)

(Has goal been met? not met? partially met?)

(Did client verbalize the caloric and food guide pyramid requirements for good nutrition while breast-feeding her baby? Did client plan to eat appropriate nutrients? Specify.)

(Revisions to care plan? D/C care plan? Continue care plan?)

INEFFECTIVE BREAST-FEEDING

Related to: Specify (e.g., maternal anxiety/insecurity/ambivalence, or discomfort, ineffective infant

sucking/swallowing secondary to prematurity, cleft lip/palate, etc.)

Defining Characteristics: Specify (e.g., infant not latched-on to breast correctly, nonsustained suckling, maternal perception of insufficient milk production, reports to "let-down" reflex, extremely sore nipples, etc.).

Goal: Client and infant will demonstrate effective breast-feeding by (date/time to evaluate).

Outcome Criteria

✔ Client will identify actions to promote effective breast-feeding.

✔ Infant will latch-on correctly and nurse for 10 minutes.

NOC: *Breast-Feeding Establishment: Maternal*

INTERVENTIONS	RATIONALES
Offer to assist client with breast-feeding.	Offering assistance obtains permission to assist client.
Assess client's beliefs, previous experience, knowledge, and role models for breast-feeding.	Assessment provides information to help plan assistance. Lack of knowledge or support for breast-feeding may interfere with client's ability to succeed.
Provide for privacy and a calm, relaxed atmosphere. Reassure client that breast-feeding is a natural activity in which her body is prepared to engage.	Anxiety and embarrassment interfere with learning. Reassurance helps client to believe in the wisdom of her body.
Teach client that relaxation is necessary for effective breast-feeding. Describe how the infant's behavior and the "let-down" reflex are affected by her emotions.	Teaching helps client understand that infants respond to their mother's emotional state and tension level. Maternal tension and emotional upset inhibit the "let-down" reflex causing frustration for the infant.
Instruct client about comfortable positions for breast-feeding. Suggest she keep a glass of water close by and use pillows for support.	Comfort promotes relaxation. Nursing stimulates thirst and the client shouldn't interrupt feeding to go get a drink. Pillows may help support client's arms to avoid discomfort or fatigue.
Describe the feedback loop of milk production and suckling. Inform client that infant will need to nurse often (q 1 to 3 hr) at first in order to build up milk	Understanding the relationship between milk supply and infant's suckling empowers the client to evaluate frequency of breast-feeding. Anticipatory guidance

(continues)

(continued)

INTERVENTIONS	RATIONALES
supply. The infant may need to nurse more frequently later during growth spurts at 2 and 6 weeks, then again at 3, 4, and 6 months of age.	related to growth spurts helps the client feel secure about her milk supply.
Teach client that the infant will empty a breast within 10–15 minutes. The client may choose to alternate breasts once or more often during each feeding. The "hind milk" or last milk in the breast contains ↑ fat content to promote growth.	Understanding the physiology of breast-feeding promotes self-confidence and decision making about method for breast-feeding.
Describe and demonstrate her infant's reflexes that facilitate breast-feeding (rooting, latching-on).	Demonstration increases client's understanding of infant reflexes that promote effective nursing.
Assist client to get herself and infant into a comfortable position for nursing with infant's body flat against hers: "tummy-to-tummy."	Client may benefit from suggestions about infant and self-positioning to avoid fatigue and promote correct latching-on.
Teach client that the infant needs to have most of the areola in his mouth in order to empty the milk sinuses and avoid nipple soreness.	Teaching provides information about breast-feeding technique to avoid complications.
Encourage client to stimulate infant's rooting reflex and help the infant to latch-on while his mouth is open.	Encouragement and assistance help the client to develop needed skills for initiating nursing her infant.
Show client how to hold her fingers in a "C" around the breast while nursing to ensure the infant's nose is not covered.	Demonstration facilitates maternal understanding. Newborns are obligate nose-breathers and will detach from the breast if unable to breathe.
Teach the client how to break the suction by slipping a finger into the infant's mouth before removing him from the breast	Teaching correct way to remove infant from the breast helps client avoid sore nipples.
Praise client for skill development and nurturing behaviors. Reinforce that breast-feeding is a natural process.	Praise increases self-worth and promotes confidence in abilities.
Instruct client in breast care: wash hands before nursing; wash nipples with warm water and no soap, allow to air dry; may rub some colostrum or milk into nipples after feeding.	Instruction promotes self-care. Handwashing prevents the spread of pathogens; soap may dry the nipples causing cracks; colostrum and milk have healing properties.

INTERVENTIONS	RATIONALES
Describe what client will feel when her milk "comes in" (breast engorgement) and what she can do to ease discomfort: suggest warm showers, application of warm, moist cabbage leaves for 15 min, ↑ frequency of breast-feeding or expression of milk, mild analgesics (acetaminophen) as ordered by caregiver.	Anticipatory guidance and suggestions decrease anxiety and promotes effective self-care. Moist heat causes vasodilatation and decreases venous and lymphatic congestion; cabbage leaves are anecdotally reported to be effective, emptying the breasts decreases feelings of fullness.
For nipple soreness, teach client to ensure the infant has the whole areola in his mouth; begin with nontender side first; apply warm, moist compresses (breast pads or tea bags) to nipples after feeding. Rub milk into nipples and allow them to air-dry. Avoid using nipple shields.	Interventions promote nipple integrity and healing; the hungry infant may suck more vigorously on the first side; moist heat promotes dilation and healing; milk has healing properties. Nipple shields have been shown to ↓ the amount of milk the infant can obtain.
Teach client that infants are usually alert in the first hour after birth and again at 12 to 18 hours, but otherwise are often very sleepy. The baby will wake up when he is hungry.	Teaching the mother to respond to her infant's hunger cues promotes self-confidence and success. New mothers often feel that they have failed if their infant is sleepy and doesn't nurse well in the hospital.
Reassure client that the baby is getting enough milk if he gains weight, wets 6 or more diapers per day, and appears content for an hour or more after eating.	Mothers are sometimes concerned when they can't measure how much milk the infant has received. Six wet diapers indicate adequate fluid intake.
Encourage client to explore her feelings about breast-feeding. Discuss client concerns about modesty, working, and so forth.	Client may have concerns that increase anxiety and interfere with successful breast-feeding.
Praise client's attempts and successes. Reinforce the benefits of breast-feeding if only for the first few weeks or months.	Praise helps bolster self-confidence and intent to continue breast-feeding.
Refer client as indicated (specify: e.g., to a lactation specialist, other mothers breast-feeding multiple infants, books on breast-feeding, or La Leche League, etc.).	Referral provides additional information and assistance. A lactation specialist may be needed for continued difficulty or special needs. La Leche League provides information and support for breast-feeding mothers.

NIC: *Breast-Feeding Assistance*

Evaluation

(Date/time of evaluation of goal)

(Has goal been met? not met? partially met?)

(Did client identify actions to promote effective breast-feeding? Specify. Did infant latch-on correctly and nurse for 10 minutes?)

(Revisions to care plan? D/C care plan? Continue care plan?)

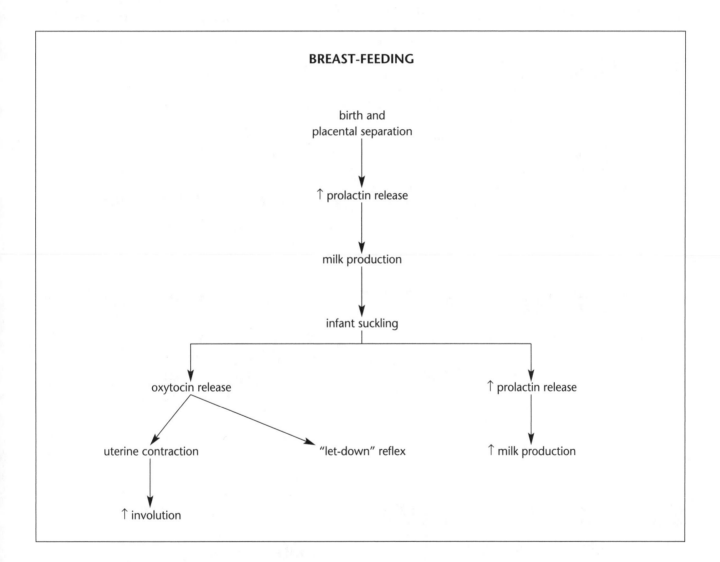

BREAST-FEEDING

birth and
placental separation

↑ prolactin release

milk production

infant suckling

oxytocin release   ↑ prolactin release

uterine contraction   "let-down" reflex   ↑ milk production

↑ involution

CHAPTER 3.5

EPISIOTOMY AND LACERATIONS

Episiotomy is an intentional incision into the perineum designed to facilitate birth and avoid perineal lacerations. Midline episiotomy is the most common procedure in the United States.

Mediolateral episiotomy is an incision from the midline of the posterior vagina and extends at a 45° angle to either left or right. Mediolateral episiotomies provide more room without danger of extension into the rectum. They bleed more and cause greater discomfort postpartum than midline episiotomies.

Lacerations of the perineum or vagina may occur during birth. This is more common in nulliparas and young clients, when an episiotomy has been done (extension), or the client has a vacume extractor or forceps-assisted birth.

CLASSIFICATION

- 1st degree: laceration through the skin and mucous membrane only
- 2nd degree: continues into the underlying fascia and muscles of the perineal body
- 3rd degree: continues through to the anal sphincter
- 4th degree: extends through the rectal mucosa

MEDICAL CARE

- Surgical repair under local or regional anesthesia
- Mild analgesics, anesthetic sprays or cream, stool softeners; clients with epidurals may receive intrathecal narcotics for 4th degree lacerations/ extensions
- Application of ice packs for the first 8 hours followed by sitz baths (warm or cool) 3 or 4 times per day

COMMON NURSING DIAGNOSES

See PAIN

Related to: Tissue trauma secondary to (specify: e.g., operative obstetrics, vaginal birth).

Defining Characteristics: Client reports pain (specify location and severity based on a scale of 1 to 10). Client exhibits grimacing, crying, reluctance to move affected area, etc. (specify).

See RISK FOR INFECTION

Related to: Site for organism invasion secondary to (specify: e.g., episiotomy, lacerations, etc.).

ADDITIONAL NURSING DIAGNOSES

IMPAIRED URINARY ELIMINATION

Related to: Diminished bladder tone and sensation secondary to (specify: e.g., childbirth trauma; anesthesia; periurethral edema).

Defining Characteristics: Client exhibits bladder distention and inability to completely empty bladder when voiding (specify for client).

Goal: Client will regain normal urinary elimination patterns by (date/time to evaluate).

Outcome Criteria

✔ Client demonstrates ability to empty bladder completely every 2 to 4 hours.
✔ Client verbalizes signs and symptoms of urinary tract infection to report.

 NOC: *Urinary Elimination*

INTERVENTIONS	RATIONALES
Assess for bladder distention whenever fundal height is checked after childbirth.	Assessment provides information about bladder distention.
Encourage client to void every 2 to 3 hours after birth. Provide for privacy, assist client to bathroom if possible, or to sit on bedpan, run water, pour warm water over perineum, and so forth. Measure amount voided until normal pattern is established.	A distended bladder interferes with uterine contraction and may cause hemorrhage (atony). Interventions may stimulate micturition. Client should void at least 100 cc each time.
Monitor intake and output (specify frequency).	Monitoring intake and output provides information about expected diuresis and bladder emptying.
Assess for bladder distention after each voiding until the client demonstrates ability to empty bladder completely.	Assessment provides information about bladder emptying. Bladder tone and sensation may return slowly after childbirth.
Catheterize, using sterile technique, clients who have a distended bladder and are unable to void, or have not voided within 4 hours after birth.	Catheterization relieves bladder distention when client is unable to void. Sterile technique avoids introduction of microorganisms into the bladder.
Reassess client in 2 hours and if still unable to void, insert a retention (Foley) catheter as ordered.	Retention catheter prevents bladder distention in clients who have not regained bladder sensation and tone.
Administer antibiotics as ordered by caregiver (specify: drug, dose, route, and times).	Caregiver may order antibiotics to avoid urinary tract infection. (Specify action of drug.)
Teach client to wash hands before and after using the bathroom and to wipe and apply peripads front to back.	Teaching provides information the client needs to avoid the introduction of pathogens into the urinary tract.
Inform client about postpartum diuresis and diaphoresis. Reassure client that ↑ urine output is expected and that she shouldn't delay voiding.	Information empowers the client to care for self with an understanding of puerperal physiology. Frequent voiding prevents urinary stasis, which provides a medium for infection.
Teach client the signs and symptoms of urinary tract infection to report to caregiver: frequency, urgency, burning or pain with urination.	Teaching ensures that the client will recognize signs of developing infection and seek appropriate medical care.

NIC: Urinary Elimination Management

Evaluation

(Date/time of evaluation of goal)

(Has goal been met? not met? partially met?)

(Does client demonstrate ability to empty bladder every 2 to 4 hours? Does client verbalize signs and symptoms of UTI to report?)

(Revisions to care plan? D/C care plan? Continue care plan?)

RISK FOR CONSTIPATION

Related to: Decreased muscle tone and GI motility after childbirth, dehydration, fear of discomfort secondary to episiotomy, lacerations, or hemorrhoids.

Defining Characteristics: (date, time, type of delivery, date last BM).

Goal: Client will obtain relief from constipation by (date/time to evaluate).

Outcome Criteria

✔ Client has an adequate bowel movement.

✔ Client verbalizes understanding of need for fiber and fluids in her diet.

NOC: Bowel Elimination

INTERVENTIONS	RATIONALES
Assess usual bowel pattern and date of last bowel movement. Assess bowel sounds.	Assessment provides information about normal bowel habits and current peristaltic activity.
Inform client that the bowels tend to be sluggish after childbirth due to hormonal influences, ↓ muscle tone, dehydration, and the lack of food during labor.	Client may be expecting to have a daily bowel movement and become alarmed by any delay.
Reassure client that a bowel movement is not going to disrupt her stitches.	Client may be fearful of damaging perineal incisions or experiencing great pain with passage of stool.
Promote comfort of perineum and hemorrhoids by use of sitz baths, sprays, creams, and so forth as ordered (specify).	Sitz baths promote circulation, comfort, and healing (specify how specific spray, cream, etc. works).
Instruct client to stimulate bowel motility by eating fiber, fresh fruits and vegetables, drinking 8 to 10 glasses of fluids per day, and mild exercises such as walking daily.	Client may be unfamiliar with information. Client may find new motivation to improve diet and exercise in order to prevent constipation.

(continues)

(continued)

INTERVENTIONS	RATIONALES
Administer stool softeners as ordered (specify with nursing measures: e.g., with a full glass of water).	Specify action of ordered drug and rationale for nursing measures.
Evaluate effectiveness of stool softener (specify timing).	Evaluation provides information about success of intervention.
Administer enema or suppository (specify) as needed.	Specify action of particular type of enema or suppository.

NIC: *Constipation Management*

Evaluation

(Date/time of evaluation of goal)

(Has goal been met? not met? partially met?)

(Has client had an adequate bowel movement? Does client verbalize the importance of fiber and fluids in her diet to prevent constipation?)

(Revisions to care plan? D/C care plan? Continue care plan?)

EPISIOTOMY AND LACERATIONS

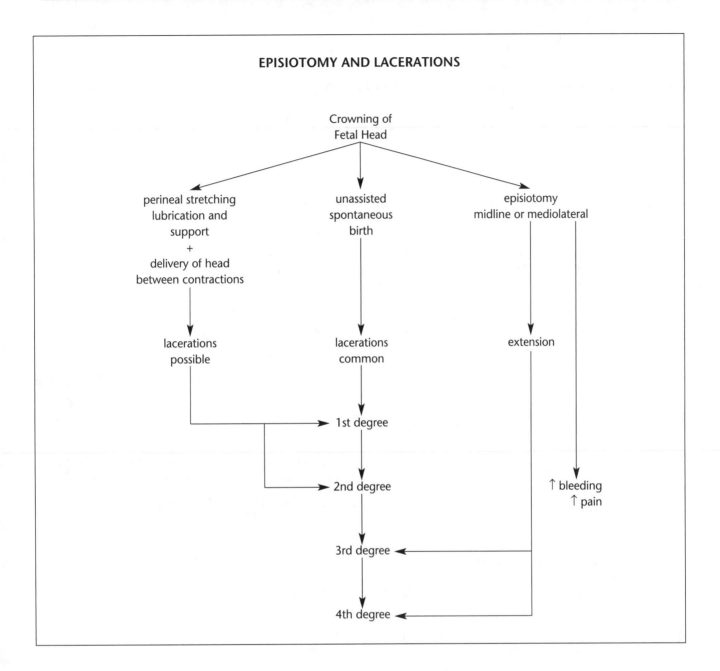

CHAPTER 3.6

POSTPARTUM HEMORRHAGE

Puerperal hemorrhage is classified as early (within the first 24 hours) or late (after the first 24 hours and up to 6 weeks postpartum). The causes of early hemorrhage are uterine relaxation (atony), lacerations, uterine rupture, hematomas, retained placental fragments, and coagulation deficiencies (DIC). Late puerperal hemorrhage may be related to abnormal healing of the placental site or retained placental fragments. The amount of blood lost during a hemorrhage greatly exceeds the usual definition of more than 500 cc.

RISK FACTORS

- Poor general health status: malnutrition, infection, anemia, PIH, clotting deficiencies
- Over-distended uterus during pregnancy: macrosomic infant, hydramnios, multiple gestation, uterine fibroids
- Grand multiparity
- Rapid or prolonged labor, oxytocin induction or augmentation
- Medications: $MgSO_4$, deep general anesthesia (halothane)
- Placental defects: history of previa, abruption, incomplete separation, placenta acreta
- Difficult birth: forceps rotation, intrauterine manipulation

MEDICAL CARE

- Evaluation of the placenta and membranes for completeness followed by intrauterine examination and manual removal of any missing pieces
- Fundal massage or bimanual compression of the uterus
- Uterotonic medications: oxytocin, methylergonovine maleate (Methergine), Ergotrate, or prostaglandins
- Evaluation of the cervix and vagina for lacerations if the fundus is firm and bleeding continues
- IV fluid replacement, initiation of a second IV, and blood transfusion as needed
- Foley catheter to evaluate renal function, oxygen therapy
- Surgical exploration and repair as indicated: laceration repair, hematoma evacuation and ligation of bleeders, possible ligation of uterine arteries or hysterectomy

COMMON NURSING DIAGNOSES

 ### See RISK FOR DEFICIENT FLUID VOLUME

Related to: Excessive losses secondary to complication of birth (specify: e.g., atony, lacerations, etc.).

 ### See RISK FOR INFECTION

Related to: Compromised defenses secondary to decreased circulation, puerperal site for organism invasion.

ADDITIONAL NURSING DIAGNOSES

 ### INEFFECTIVE TISSUE PERFUSION (CEREBRAL, RENAL, PERIPHERAL)

Related to: Excessive blood loss secondary to (specify: e.g., uterine atony, retained placental fragments, lacerations of the birth canal, retroperitoneal hematoma, etc.).

Defining Characteristics: Specify (e.g., EBL, ↓ BP, ↑ P & R, ↓ SaO₂, changes in skin color and temperature, ↓ urine output, ↓ LOC, etc.).

Goal: Client will maintain adequate tissue perfusion by (date/time to evaluate).

Outcome Criteria

✔ Client will maintain BP and pulse (specify for client: e.g., >100/60, pulse between 60–90), skin warm, pink, and dry; urine output >30 cc/hr; client will remain alert and oriented).

NOC: *Tissue Perfusion*

INTERVENTIONS	RATIONALES
Assess client's BP, P, R, and SaO₂, (specify frequency).	Assessment provides information about hypovolemia. Excessive losses cause ↓ BP with ↑ P and ↑ R as compensatory mechanisms.
Assess fundus, perineum, and bleeding. Evaluate blood loss by weighing peri pads or Chux (1 gm = 1 cc). (Specify frequency of documentation.) Notify caregiver of ↑ losses.	Assessment provides information about uterine tone and position, hematoma development, extent of losses.
Insert Foley catheter as ordered. Monitor hourly intake and output.	Interventions provide information about renal perfusion and function. Intake and output evaluates fluid balance.
Monitor for restlessness, anxiety, c/o thirst, "air hunger," and changes in level of consciousness.	Intervention provides indications of inadequate cerebral tissue perfusion.
Administer humidified oxygen at 8–12 L/min via facemask as ordered.	Intervention provides supplemental oxygen for tissues.
Assess client for abdominal pain, rigidity, increasing abdominal girth, vulvar or vulvovaginal hematomas.	Assessment provides information about possible uterine rupture or internal hematoma formation and hidden bleeding.
Assess client's skin color, temperature, moisture, turgor, and capillary refill (specify frequency).	Assessment provides information about peripheral tissue perfusion. Hypovolemia results in shunting of blood away from the peripheral circulation to the brain and ital organs.
Administer medications as ordered (specify: e.g., oxytocin, ergotrates, prostaglandins).	Specify action of drugs.

INTERVENTIONS	RATIONALES
Initiate secondary IV access with 18-gauge (or larger) catheter and provide fluids, blood products, or blood as ordered (specify fluids and rate).	Intervention provides venous access to give medications or replace fluids. Size 18-gauge or larger is preferred to transfuse blood.
Monitor laboratory values as obtained (e.g., Hgb, Hct, clotting studies).	Laboratory values may provide information about extent of losses or impending DIC.
Observe client for signs of spontaneous bleeding (e.g., bruising, epistaxis, seeping from puncture sites hematuria, etc.).	Observation provides information about the depletion of clotting factors and development of DIC.
Keep client and significant other informed of client's condition and current plan of care.	Information promotes understanding and cooperation.
Notify caregiver of all findings and prepare for immediate surgical intervention if ordered.	Surgical intervention may be required if other measures are ineffective in stopping hemorrhage.

NIC: *Circulatory Care*

Evaluation

(Date/time of evaluation of goal)

(Has goal been met? not met? partially met?)

(What are client's BP and P? Is skin warm, pink, and dry? Is urine output >30 cc/hr? Is client alert and oriented?)

(Revisions to care plan? D/C care plan? Continue care plan?)

FEAR

Related to: Perceived grave danger to self or infant secondary to (specify: e.g., postpartum hemorrhage, infant with a congenital anomaly, etc.).

Defining Characteristics: Client or significant other state (specify: e.g., "I'm scared; What's wrong with my baby?" etc.). Client and significant other demonstrate physical signs of fear (specify: e.g., sympathetic response: pale, ↑ P, ↑ R, dry mouth, nausea, etc.).

Goal: Client and significant other will cope with fear while emergency interventions are being employed.

Outcome Criteria

✔ Client and significant other can identify the threat.

✔ Client is able to cooperate with instructions from caregivers.

NOC: *Fear Control*

INTERVENTIONS	RATIONALES
Inform client and significant other of a problem as soon as it is identified. Speak slowly and calmly.	Calm information ↓ fears. It is more frightening to "sense" that something is wrong than to know what it is.
Describe the problem in simple terms and what interventions might be expected (specify: e.g., for hemorrhage the nurse will start another IV, massage the fundus; the neonatologist is resuscitating the baby, etc.).	Simple explanations are less frightening than complicated physiology or medical terminology the client may not understand.
Explain all equipment and procedures as they're being done (specify: e.g., Foley catheter, IV, ambu bag and mask, etc.).	Explanation promotes understanding of unfamiliar interventions.
Inform client and significant other of things they can do to help (specify: e.g., position changes; keep on oxygen mask; significant other can support client, etc.).	Information promotes a sense of control over frightening events to be able to be involved in the solution.
Observe client and significant other for signs of distress: pallor, trembling, crying, etc. Provide emotional support.	The "fight or flight" sympathetic response may indicate ↑ fear. Emotional support helps the client and significant other to cope.

INTERVENTIONS	RATIONALES
Encourage significant other to remain with client.	Significant other provides support during a stressful period. Allows understanding of events.
Allow expression of feelings (helplessness, anger). Support cultural variation in emotional expression.	Intervention shows respect for client's experience and cultural expression of emotion.
Inform client and significant other when crisis has passed. Provide information about what will happen next.	Information allows client and significant other to reevaluate their feelings and consider what to expect next.
Praise client and significant other for their cooperation and coping during a stressful event.	Praise enhances self-esteem. Intervention shows that the client's abilities are valued.
Visit client after birth (specify when: e.g., 1st or 2nd PP day) to discuss events surrounding birth. Clarify any misconceptions about the emergency or complication.	Visiting the client after the crisis has passed provides an opportunity to relive the experience and fill in any gaps in understanding before discharge.

NIC: *Anxiety Reduction*

Evaluation

(Date/time of evaluation of goal)

(Has goal been met? not met? partially met?)

(Did client and significant other verbalize correct understanding of the emergency? Was client able to cooperate with instructions? Specify.)

(Revisions to care plan? D/C care plan? Continue care plan?)

POSTPARTUM HEMORRHAGE

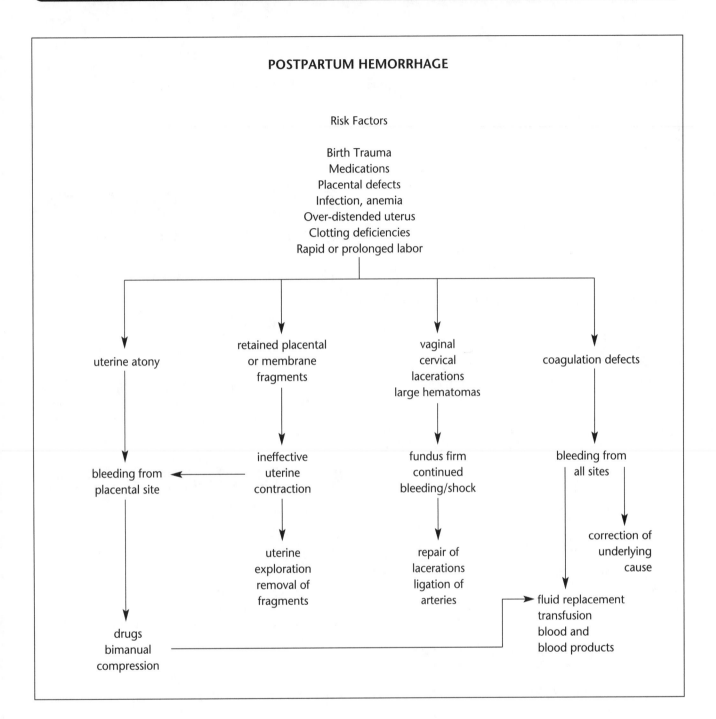

Risk Factors

Birth Trauma
Medications
Placental defects
Infection, anemia
Over-distended uterus
Clotting deficiencies
Rapid or prolonged labor

| uterine atony | retained placental or membrane fragments | vaginal cervical lacerations large hematomas | coagulation defects |

bleeding from placental site ← ineffective uterine contraction

fundus firm continued bleeding/shock

bleeding from all sites

correction of underlying cause

uterine exploration removal of fragments

repair of lacerations ligation of arteries

fluid replacement transfusion blood and blood products

drugs bimanual compression

CHAPTER 3.7

HEMATOMAS

A hematoma forms when injury to a blood vessel allows bleeding into adjacent tissues. Hematomas sustained as a result of birth trauma are usually small but they may be large enough to result in life-threatening hemorrhage. Puerperal hematomas commonly develop in the vulvar, vulvovaginal, vaginal (at the level of the ischial spines), or retroperitoneal areas.

The primary symptom of a hematoma is constant pain that may be severe. Other symptoms include rectal pressure or difficulty voiding. Abdominal pain with increasing girth and unexplained signs of shock may result from a large retroperitoneal hematoma.

RISK FACTORS

- Obstetrical interventions: episiotomy, pudendal block, forceps delivery
- Genital varicose veins
- Precipitous birth
- Prolonged second stage
- Macrosomic infant
- Primipara
- PIH, clotting abnormalities

MEDICAL CARE

- Application of ice packs to perineum after delivery and observation
- Incision, evacuation, and ligation of bleeding vessels if indicated
- Vaginal packing
- Administration of broad spectrum antibiotics
- Administration of blood and clotting factors if indicated
- Laparotomy with ligation of hypogastric artery or possible hysterectomy for severe hemorrhage

COMMON NURSING DIAGNOSES

See RISK FOR DEFICIENT FLUID VOLUME

Related to: Excessive losses secondary to disrupted vasculature.

See PAIN

Related to: Ischemia and edema secondary to blood vessel trauma.

Defining Characteristics: Client reports discomfort (specify location, type, and severity using a pain scale). Client exhibits (specify: e.g., guarding, grimacing, moaning, etc.).

ADDITIONAL NURSING DIAGNOSES

ANXIETY

Related to: Perceived threat to self or infant secondary to (specify: e.g., postpartum or neonatal complication).

Defining Characteristics: Client verbalizes anxiety (specify: e.g., feels physically threatened, afraid, can't sleep, etc.). Client rates anxiety as a (specify) on a scale of 1 to 5 with 1 being no anxiety and 5 being the most.

Goal: Client will demonstrate decreased anxiety by (date and time to evaluate).

Outcome Criteria

- ✔ Client will rate anxiety as a (specify) or less on a scale of 1 to 5 with 1 being least, 5 the most anxiety.
- ✔ Client will appear calm (specify not crying, no tremors, HR <100, etc.).

NOC: *Anxiety Control*

INTERVENTIONS	RATIONALES
Assess for physical signs of anxiety: tremors, palpitations, tachycardia, dry mouth, nausea, or diaphoresis.	Anxiety may cause the "fight or flight" sympathetic response. Some cultures prohibit verbal expression of anxiety.
Assess for mental and emotional signs of anxiety: nervousness, crying, difficulty with concentration or memory, and so forth.	Anxiety may interfere with normal mental and emotional functioning.
Ask client to rate her feelings of anxiety on a scale of 1 to 5.	Rating allows measurement of changes in anxiety level.
Provide reassurance and support: acknowledge anxiety, provide time for discussion, and use touch if culturally appropriate.	Severe anxiety may interfere with the client's ability to take in information. Interventions may help ↓ anxiety levels.
Encourage client to involve significant other(s) in attempts to identify and cope with anxiety.	Significant others are also under stress during complicated pregnancy.
When client is calmer, validate concerns with factual information about postpartum or newborn condition and what will be done to lessen the risks (specify: bedrest, ice packs, sitz baths, antibiotics, consults, etc.).	Client may be overly fearful. Realistic understanding of risks and treatment options empowers the client to participate in her own care.
Ask client how she usually copes with anxiety and if this would be helpful now.	Intervention promotes identification of adaptive coping mechanisms v. maladaptive (e.g., smoking, alcohol, etc.).

INTERVENTIONS	RATIONALES
Assist client to plan coping strategies for anxiety. Suggest possibilities: meditation, breathing and relaxation, creative imagery, music, biofeedback, talking to self, and so forth (suggest others).	Developing a plan to address anxiety promotes a sense of control, which enhances coping ability.
Arrange a tour of the NICU if appropriate, or ask for a consult with appropriate caregivers (specify).	Familiarity and knowledge decrease fear of the unknown.
Provide information about counseling or support groups as appropriate (specify: groups for parents of multiple gestation, congenital anomalies, etc.).	Severe anxiety may require individual counseling. Support groups provide reassurance and coping strategies.

NIC: *Anxiety Reduction*

Evaluation

(Date/time of evaluation of goal)

(Has goal been met? not met? partially met?)

(What does the client rate her anxiety as now? Does client appear calm—specify: not crying, smiling, pulse 72, etc.)

(Revisions to care plan? D/C care plan? Continue care plan?)

HEMATOMAS

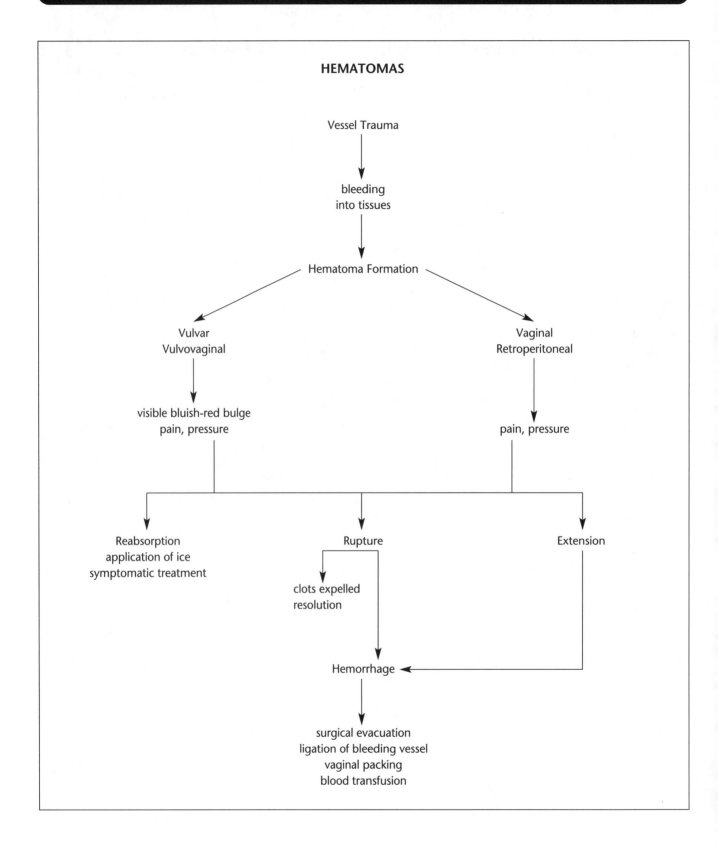

CHAPTER 3.8

PUERPERAL INFECTION

Bacterial infection of the reproductive tract during the postpartum period used to be called "childbed fever." This was the cause of significant maternal mortality and morbidity before the introduction of aseptic techniques and antibiotics. Uterine infection usually occurs at the placental site, the endometrium, and/or the myometrium, though it may spread, resulting in pelvic cellulitis or peritonitis.

The most significant sign of puerperal infection is fever greater than 100.4° F after the first 24 hours after birth. The accepted definition includes that fever is found on any 2 of the first 10 postpartum days, when taken by mouth every 4 hours. The client may also experience malaise, anorexia, chills, abdominal pain, and slowing of involution. Lochia may be profuse, bloody, frothy, with a foul odor, or may be scant and nonoffensive. Elevation of WBCs is normal during the early puerperium.

Fever may also result from respiratory complications, breast engorgement or mastitis, thrombophlebitis, pyelonephritis, and local wound abscesses (cesarean, vaginal, or perineal). When these causes are ruled out, puerperal infection is suspected.

RISK FACTORS

- Cesarean birth
- Extensive vaginal or uterine manipulation
- Multiple vaginal exams
- Long labor, prolonged ruptured membranes
- Intrauterine fetal monitoring
- Chorioamnionitis
- Retained placental fragments

MEDICAL CARE

- Administration of broad-spectrum antibiotics (p.o. or IV)
- CBC with sedimentation rate
- Urinalysis
- Cultures

COMMON NURSING DIAGNOSES

See RISK FOR INFECTION

Related to: Spread of microorganisms from the reproductive tract.

See PAIN

Related to: Inflammation and edema of reproductive tract secondary to invading microorganisms.

Defining Characteristics: Client reports pelvic pain (specify: abdominal tenderness, deep continuous pain, etc.). Client rates pain (specify) on a scale of 1 to 10 with 1 being least, 10 being most. Client is (specify: e.g., crying, grimacing, guarding abdomen, etc.).

ADDITIONAL NURSING DIAGNOSES

RISK FOR IMPAIRED PARENTING

Related to: Delayed attachment secondary to maternal illness or discomfort.

Defining Characteristics: (Specify: mother unable to hold infant; describe interactions).

Goal: Client will exhibit appropriate parenting behaviors (by date/time to evaluate).

Outcome Criteria

✔ Client makes eye contact with infant; strokes, hugs, and talks to infant.
✔ Client states desire to care for infant.

NOC: *Parent–Infant Attachment*

INTERVENTIONS	RATIONALES
Assess attachment behaviors recorded at birth. Note alterations. Validate findings with client (e.g., "You don't seem to have the energy to hold your baby now?").	Assessment provides information about the etiology of altered parenting to distinguish between illness and psychological causes.
Evaluate the possibility of cultural variation related to infant care responsibility (e.g., is Grandmother or sister caring for the baby?).	Evaluation provides information about the family's expectations related to infant care and "parenting" activities as defined by western European culture.
Promote culturally relevant parenting activities through flexible visiting hours and access to infant as desired by parents.	Adjustment of hospital rules and routines should be made to promote family-centered care. The nurse acts as client advocate.
Encourage client to share feelings about disruption of parenting. Offer emotional support and empathy.	Client may experience guilt and depression because she is unable to care for her infant. Support assists client to cope; empathy validates client's feelings.
Promote sleep and rest by scheduling nursing care to avoid interruptions (specify).	Rest is necessary to promote healing. Much nursing care can be rescheduled.
Provide opportunities for the client to see and hold her baby. Provide photos and encourage phone calls if infant is restricted to nursery.	The mother and baby need opportunities to engage in the attachment process.
Role model infant care and appropriate parenting behaviors when infant is in room. Point out positive features and infant responses to sensory stimulation.	Client may not have experienced appropriate mothering behaviors. Noting infant's features and responses facilitates attachment.
Provide nonsedating pain relief before client holds or attempts to feed infant.	Pain or sedation may distract or decrease attention and interfere with attachment.

INTERVENTIONS	RATIONALES
Assist client to feed her infant if possible or to pump breasts to maintain milk supply if unable to nurse (e.g., drug therapy).	Feeding the infant is a primary parental task that facilitates attachment and self-esteem. Many drugs cross into the breast milk.
Encourage father or family to feed and care for the infant, in the client's room if possible, when the client is unable to do so.	Providing care and feeding promotes parenting skills. The client may observe care and offer parenting advice.
Offer praise and positive feedback for effective parenting behaviors.	Praise promotes self-esteem. Feedback provides information about effective behaviors.
Perform infant assessments at client's bedside while providing information about the infant (e.g., reflexes, fontanels, behaviors, etc.).	Assessment at the bedside provides the client with the opportunity to get to know her baby as an individual.
Make referrals as needed (specify: e.g., social services, counseling, parenting groups).	Client may need additional help to parent effectively.

NIC: *Attachment Promotion*

Evaluation

(Date/time of evaluation of goal)

(Has goal been met? not met? partially met?)

(Does client make eye contact with infant? Does she touch and talk to her baby? Does client report the desire to care for her infant?)

(Revisions to care plan? D/C care plan? Continue care plan?)

PUERPERAL INFECTION

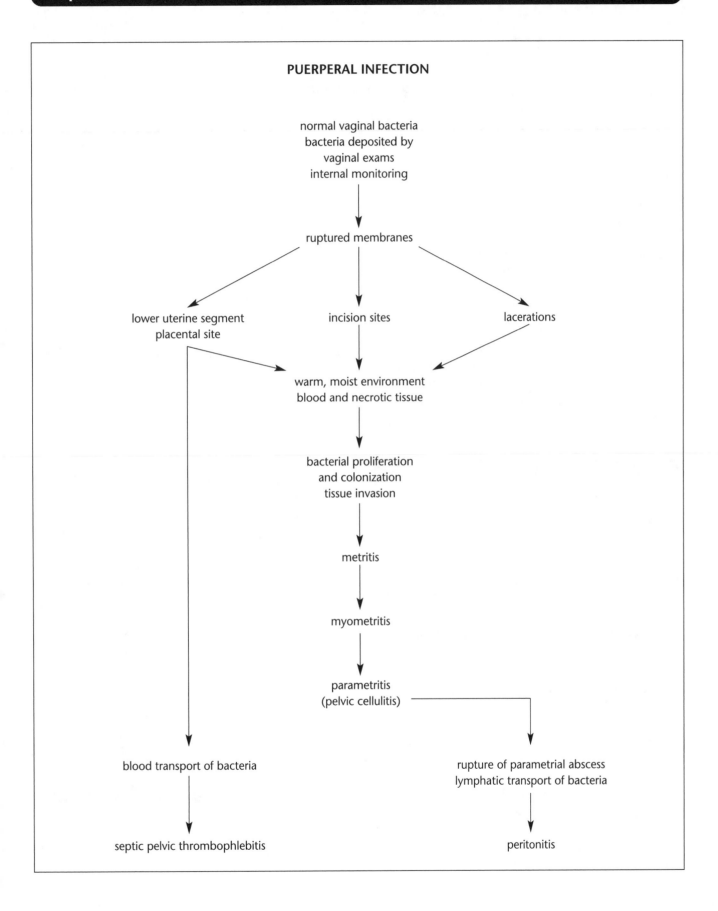

CHAPTER 3.9

THROMBOPHLEBITIS

The formation of blood clots in either superficial (SVT) or deep veins (DVT) is a potential complication of childbirth. The term thrombophlebitis refers to thrombus (clot) formation caused by inflammation of the veins, as in septic pelvic thrombophlebitis. Emboli are clots that have detached from the vein wall and travel through the bloodstream. Pulmonary embolism describes the situation when a clot lodges in the pulmonary artery. Complete occlusion of the artery results in severe respiratory distress and death.

Puerperal physiology that predisposes to thrombus formation includes increased clotting factors and platelets, decreased fibrinolysis, and release of thromboplastin from the placenta, membranes, and decidua.

RISK FACTORS

- Venous stasis: immobility
- History of thrombus formation
- Varicose veins, heart disease, hemorrhage, anemia
- Traumatic birth
- Puerperal infection
- Maternal obesity, advanced age, grand multiparity

SIGNS AND SYMPTOMS

Pulmonary Embolism

- sudden onset respiratory distress: dyspnea, tachypnea, cough, rales, hemoptysis, chest pain, tachycardia, diaphoresis, pallor, cyanosis, feelings of impending doom

SVT	DVT
more common with history of varicosities	more common with history of thrombosis
saphenous vein most common	femoral vein, pelvic veins; symptoms begin around 10 days postpartum
symptoms begin 3–4 days postpartum	

SVT	DVT
local heat, and redness along vein	fever, chills, pale, cool, edematous leg: "milk leg"
tenderness, firmness or bumps along vein	positive Homan's sign; pain: foot, leg, inguinal, pelvic

MEDICAL CARE

Pulmonary Embolism

- respiratory support: oxygen
- medications: IV heparin, streptokinase, and others
- surgical embolectomy

SVT	DVT
bedrest with elevation of leg above heart	strict bedrest with elevation of legs above heart
support hose	application of moist heat
heat application	Medications: IV heparin gradually converted to warfarin, analgesics, antibiotics if pyrexic
analgesics prn	Serial clotting studies: PT, PTT
	gradual return to ambulation with support hose
	Discharged on warfarin (Coumadin)

COMMON NURSING DIAGNOSES

See PAIN

Related to: Inflammation and ischemia secondary to phlebitis.

Defining Characteristics: Client reports pain in affected extremity (specify using quotes and a pain scale). Positive Homan's sign (specify extremity).

See ANXIETY

Related to: Perceived threat to biologic integrity secondary to risk for pulmonary embolism.

Defining Characteristics: Client expresses feelings of apprehension (specify). Client is (specify: e.g., restless, tense, crying, etc.).

See RISK FOR IMPAIRED PARENTING

Related to: Interruption of bonding process secondary to maternal illness.

> ### ADDITIONAL NURSING DIAGNOSES

RISK FOR INJURY

Related to: Venous obstruction, anticoagulant medications, risks for embolism.

Defining Characteristics: None, as this is a potential diagnosis.

Goal: Client will not experience any injury by (date/time to evaluate).

Outcome Criteria

✔ Client's leg doesn't exhibit pain, pallor, redness, or edema.

✔ Bilateral pedal pulses are equal.

✔ No signs of respiratory distress: dyspnea, tachypnea.

✔ Client doesn't experience abnormal bleeding: bleeding gums, bruising, petechiae, or hematuria.

NOC: *Risk Control*

INTERVENTIONS	RATIONALES
Assess client's VS and lower extremities for color, temperature, edema, and tenderness (Homan's sign) q 8h.	Assessment provides information about the development of superficial or deep vein thrombosis.
Instruct client to maintain bedrest with legs elevated as ordered (specify). Avoid massaging affected leg.	Elevation of legs facilitates venous return. Rest and avoiding massage ↓ activities that might lead to embolism.

INTERVENTIONS	RATIONALES
Maintain warm, moist heat to affected leg as ordered.	Heat causes vasodilatation and ↑ circulation to area to resolve thrombus faster.
Observe client for signs of pulmonary embolism. Notify physician and provide respiratory support.	Observation helps identify pulmonary embolism early. Respiratory support may help if the embolus is not occluding the pulmonary artery.
Administer anticoagulant medications as ordered (specify: e.g., drug, dose, route, and times).	Specify action of individual drug. Anticoagulants prevent further thrombus formation while the body naturally dissolves the clot.
Monitor lab values. Inform physician before giving heparin if APTT is outside of range (specify).	Usual range for APTT during heparin therapy is 1.5 to 2.5 times normal. Longer times may indicate risk of hemorrhage.
Keep antidotes to anticoagulant drugs available: protamine sulfate for heparin, vitamin K for warfarin.	Antidotes reverse the effects of anticoagulant medications and decrease the risk of hemorrhage.
Closely monitor client for signs of abnormal bleeding: bleeding gums, easy bruising, epistaxis, or hematuria. Assess stools for occult blood as indicated.	Abnormal bleeding may indicate excessive anticoagulant therapy.
Administer antibiotics as ordered (specify drug, dose, route, times).	Specify action of drug.
Measure client's leg and apply antiembolism stockings (TED hose) as ordered.	Antiembolism stockings promote venous return and ↓ venous stasis.
Assist client with ambulation when ordered.	Assistance avoids injury and allows early identification of complications.
Explain all interventions and rationales to client and family.	Understanding promotes compliance and decreases anxiety.

NIC: *Risk Identification*

Evaluation

(Date/time of evaluation of goal)

(Has goal been met? not met? partially met?)

(Does client's leg exhibit pain, pallor, redness, or edema? Are bilateral pedal pulses equal? Does client exhibit any signs of respiratory distress? Did client experience abnormal bleeding?)

(Revisions to care plan? D/C care plan? Continue care plan?)

 INEFFECTIVE THERAPEUTIC REGIMEN MANAGEMENT

Related to: Insufficient understanding of condition and therapeutic regimen.

Defining Characteristics: Client verbalizes desire to learn about conditions and manage own care (specify).

Goal: Client will manage therapeutic regimen effectively by (date/time for evaluation).

Outcome Criteria

✔ Client describes factors contributing to and actions she can take to avoid venous thrombosis.

✔ Client relates intent to comply with therapeutic regimen.

NOC: *Knowledge: Treatment Regimen*

INTERVENTIONS	RATIONALES
Assess client's previous knowledge about venous thrombosis.	Assessment provides information about client's knowledge base.
Encourage questions at any time and family participation in learning.	Encouragement assures comfort when asking questions. Family support promotes compliance.
Discuss the impact of venous stasis on thrombus formation.	Discussion provides information about physiologic cause and effect.
Assist client to identify ways to avoid venous stasis: avoid prolonged standing or sitting, change positions at least every 2 hours, avoid crossing legs or using knee Gatch on bed.	Assisting client to identify risk factors empowers her to gain control over her risk.
Assist client to identify ways to increase venous return: need to wear support hose correctly, planned rest periods with legs elevated.	Assistance empowers the client and enhances self-esteem. Incorrectly applied hose may cause constriction.

INTERVENTIONS	RATIONALES
Teach client about her medications: (specify: e.g., warfarin, heparin, antibiotics), dose, route, time, drug interactions, need for follow-up lab tests, excretion in breast milk, and so forth.	Anticoagulant drugs may have serious adverse effects if taken improperly. Client should not take other drugs including OTC without checking with caregiver.
Inform client about risks of bleeding with anticoagulants and signs and symptoms to report immediately.	Early identification of abnormal bleeding allows prompt administration of the antidote.
If client is taking warfarin, teach about dietary sources of vitamin K (green, leafy vegetables) and possible effects on drug therapy.	Ingestion of large amounts of vitamin K may ↓ the effectiveness of warfarin.
Ask client to review teaching and repeat important concepts. Provide with written information as well as verbal feedback.	Interventions reinforce learning of new material. Written information may be reviewed at home.
Praise client for demonstrated learning of new material. Provide with phone number to call for further questions.	Praise reinforces self-esteem. Provision of phone number ensures access to additional information.

NIC: *Behavior Modification*

Evaluation

(Date/time of evaluation of goal)

(Has goal been met? not met? partially met?)

(Does client describe factors contributing to and actions she can take to avoid venous thrombosis? Does client relate intent to comply with therapeutic regimen?)

(Revisions to care plan? D/C care plan? Continue care plan?)

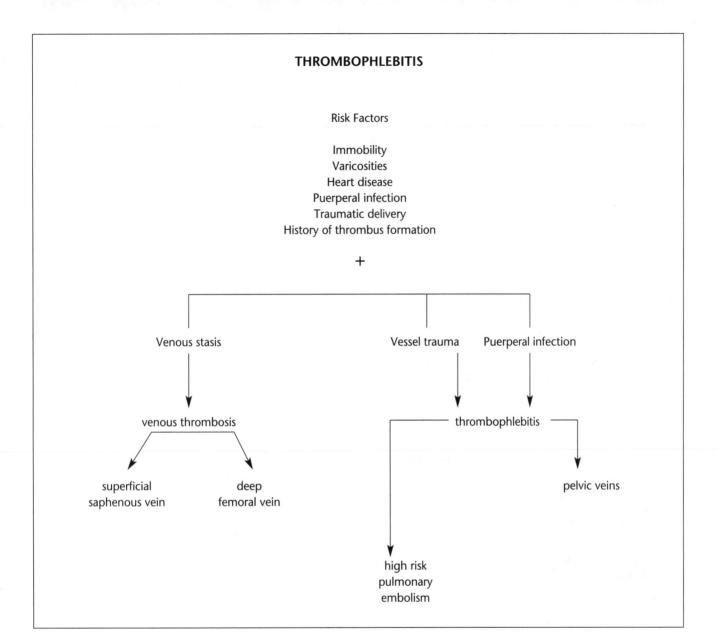

THROMBOPHLEBITIS

Risk Factors

Immobility
Varicosities
Heart disease
Puerperal infection
Traumatic delivery
History of thrombus formation

+

Venous stasis   Vessel trauma   Puerperal infection

venous thrombosis   thrombophlebitis

superficial   deep   pelvic veins
saphenous vein   femoral vein

high risk
pulmonary
embolism

CHAPTER 3.10

ADOLESCENT PARENTS

The adolescent mother may feel overwhelmed by the reality of her infant and the physical discomforts of the puerperium. In addition, she and her baby may have experienced a complicated pregnancy or birth. These factors may lead to a prolonged "Taking-In" phase characterized by withdrawal and preoccupation with physical needs.

Teaching methods should take into account the client's age and maturity level. The baby's father should be included when possible. Adolescents may focus on the concrete physical tasks of infant care and neglect sensory stimulation. They may feel shy about asking questions. A supportive atmosphere fosters learning. Contraceptive counseling and sex education are important topics, as many adolescent mothers will experience a repeat pregnancy. Social support, financial ability, and educational goals need to be assessed and appropriate referrals made.

In addition to the basic care plans for vaginal or cesarean birth, the following nursing diagnoses may apply to the adolescent mother.

COMMON NURSING DIAGNOSES

See IMPAIRED PARENTING

Related to: Conflict between meeting own needs and those of infant secondary to parental immaturity.

Defining Characteristics: Specify behaviors: for example, inappropriate or nonnurturing behavior towards infant, lack of attachment behaviors (give examples). Client verbalizes dissatisfaction with infant or own parenting skills. Father of infant expresses dissatisfaction with level of involvement with infant.

See INEFFECTIVE COPING

Related to: Inadequate psychological/maturational resources to adapt to adolescent parenting.

Defining Characteristics: Specify: for example, parents verbalize inability to cope or meet expectations of parental roles (quotes). Clients exhibit/report use of inappropriate coping mechanisms (specify: e.g., substance abuse).

ADDITIONAL NURSING DIAGNOSES

DISTURBED BODY IMAGE

Related to: Effects of pregnancy and birth, surgery (specify).

Defining Characteristics: Client verbalizes negative response to body after childbirth (specify: e.g., "Look how ugly I am!"). Client exhibits negative nonverbal response to body changes (specify: grimacing, crying, etc.).

Goal: Client will demonstrate acceptance of body changes by (date/time to evaluate).

Outcome Criteria

✔ Client will verbalize acceptance of body changes associated with pregnancy and birth.

✔ Client plans health-promoting postpartum diet and exercise program.

NOC: *Body Image*

INTERVENTIONS	RATIONALES
Establish a trusting relationship with client. Provide for privacy and time for discussion. Sit down.	Discussion of body image requires a trusting safe relationship. Sitting down shows the client that the nurse is available and willing to talk.
Encourage client to express her feelings about body changes, how she views her body now, and fears about the permanency of changes.	Client may need encouragement to express negative feelings and fears about her body changes. Expression increases self-awareness.

INTERVENTIONS	RATIONALES
Assist client to list her concerns and provide accurate information about each concern.	Identification of specific concerns allows development of a plan to address each concern.
Reassure client that abdominal muscle tone will return and may be improved with postpartum exercises as approved by her caregiver.	The flabby abdominal appearance after childbirth may be the most apparent, unusual, and distressing change for new mothers.
Inform client that she may not be able to wear her prepregnancy clothes for a while if they have a fitted waist. Suggest clothing with loose or elastic waistbands (e.g., sweat pants).	Client may assume that she will return to her usual shape as soon as the baby is born. Clothing may be an important indication of social status for client.
If client has an abdominal incision, prepare her for its appearance before removing the dressing (specify: e.g., size, location, staples, or stitches).	Preparation helps decrease anxiety when viewing an incision for the first time.
Describe how the incision may look when healed and the importance of incision care to avoid infection and abnormal scarring.	Description provides anticipatory guidance and reinforces teaching about care of the incision.
Discuss the appearance and cause of stretch marks on hips, abdomen, and breasts.	Stretch marks are common during pregnancy and may be very distressing to the client.
Reassure client that stretch marks will fade with time and may become hardly noticeable. Inform her that creams and lotions will not fade the marks but may make her feel more comfortable.	Reassurance and information help the client cope with permanent changes and incorporate them into her new body image.
Provide information about weight loss during the puerperium. Assist client to plan an individualized diet and exercise program.	Information empowers the client to develop strategies to improve body image after childbirth. Optimum diet and exercise will assist the client to look and feel her best.
Teach client about breast changes during the puerperium. Reassure her that breast size doesn't indicate ability to nurse her baby. Inform her that breastfeeding will not make her breasts sag but will help her lose weight.	Teaching corrects common misconceptions about breastfeeding and its effects on body image.
Encourage client to discuss concerns about body image and sexuality (e.g., she is unattractive to men now, her vagina is	Discussion of concerns allows correction of misconceptions that may be fostered by society and some care providers.

INTERVENTIONS	RATIONALES
stretched out, and she will be sexually unappealing, etc.). Correct misconceptions.	Promotes positive sexual identify.
Provide information about self-care related to postpartum diaphoresis and lochia flow (e.g., frequent showers, pad changes, use of peri bottle, sitz baths).	Information assists the client with personal grooming and care of her body.
Encourage family and friends to be supportive to client; correct any misconceptions they may express.	Social support increases the adolescent client's self-esteem.
Provide positive reinforcement for indications of positive body image: grooming, posture, and so forth.	Positive responses reinforce client's attempts to reconcile her new body image and make the most of it.
Arrange consults as indicated (specify: e.g., psychiatric, dietary, etc.).	Anorexia nervosa and bulimia are psychiatric disorders related to a distorted body image.
Refer client to community agencies as indicated after discharge (specify: e.g., teen parent program, support groups, etc.).	Support groups provide the client with additional information and self-help skills.

NIC: *Body Image Enhancement*

Evaluation

(Date/time of evaluation of goal)

(Has goal been met? not met? partially met?)

(Does client verbalize acceptance of body changes associated with pregnancy and birth? Does client plan health-promoting postpartum diet and exercise program?)

(Revisions to care plan? D/C care plan? Continue care plan?)

 INTERRUPTED FAMILY PROCESSES

Related to: Specify (e.g., role confusion secondary to adolescent parenthood, illness of a family member, birth of a high-risk newborn, etc.).

Defining Characteristics: Specify (e.g., family doesn't communicate openly and effectively among members [Grandmother tells client "You're doing it all wrong, let me do it"]. Family is not adapting effectively with crisis of birth [specify: e.g., family express anger and disapproval towards client or infant. Family or father of the baby refuses to visit client, won't talk about or hold the baby, etc.]).

Goal: Family will adapt to birth and resume effective functioning by (date/time to evaluate).

Outcome Criteria

✔ Family shows signs of acceptance of infant and new mother.

✔ Family identifies external agencies and support resources.

NOC: *Family Coping*

INTERVENTIONS	RATIONALES
Observe family interactions and reactions to the mother and infant.	Observation provides information about family dynamics and reactions to birth.
Demonstrate respect and concern for family in a caring and nonjudgmental manner.	Disrespect or judgmental behavior will close lines of communication between the family and the nurse.
Provide the family with feedback about perceptions (specify: e.g., "This must be difficult for your family. It's hard to adjust to being a grandmother when you're so young," etc.).	Feedback helps the family to verify or correct perceptions, and acknowledge feelings and conflicts.
Encourage verbalization of individual feelings without attacking family members (e.g., guilt, anger, blame, etc.).	Expression of negative feelings allows the family to acknowledge the problems they need to work on.
Provide accurate information to family members about client's/infant's condition and prognosis.	Information assists the family to adapt to a changing situation and helps allay unrealistic fears.
Encourage family members to identify primary concerns. Assist them to note similarities and areas of conflict.	Encouragement facilitates open communication about concerns.
Assist the family to list priorities, identify choices, and plan ways to adjust to the situation.	Assisting the family to prioritize and problem-solve builds on family strengths.
Encourage family to maintain open communication and support of each other.	Open communication and support help the family adapt to change.
Provide feedback about observed family strengths.	Feedback helps the family evaluate effectiveness of family adaptation during and after discussion.

INTERVENTIONS	RATIONALES
Assist family to identify additional social supports they can call on (specify: e.g., extended family, friends, religious groups).	Additional support may be needed to foster family adaptation. Family may not recognize that help is available from sources other than themselves.
Provide referrals as indicated (specify: support groups, counseling, etc.).	Referrals provide the family with additional information and help.

NIC: *Family Integrity Promotion*

Evaluation

(Date/time of evaluation of goal)

(Has goal been met? not met? partially met?)

(Does family verbalize acceptance of infant and new mother? Specify using an example. Did family identify external agencies and support resources to contact? Which ones?)

(Revisions to care plan? D/C care plan? Continue care plan?)

 INEFFECTIVE HEALTH MAINTENANCE

Related to: Substance abuse (specify: tobacco, alcohol, marijuana, etc.). Poor dietary habits (specify: high fat diet, inadequate nutrients, etc.). Lack of understanding about (specify: sexuality/reproductive health care needs).

Defining Characteristics: Clients report smoking cigarettes (specify number of cigarettes or packs/day), drinking, or using other drugs (specify type and amount). Clients report poor dietary habits (specify: e.g., ↑ fat diet, skip meals, drink soda instead of milk, etc.). Clients state inaccurate information about sexuality/reproductive needs (specify: e.g., "We don't need contraception because we're never having sex again").

Goal: Clients will change behaviors to maintain health by (date/time to evaluate).

Outcome Criteria

✔ Clients will identify unhealthy behaviors.

✔ Clients will verbalize plan to engage in healthy behaviors (specify: stop smoking, avoid alcohol and other drugs, eat a balanced diet, use contraception to avoid repeat pregnancy, etc.).

NOC: *Knowledge: Health Promotion*

INTERVENTIONS	RATIONALES
Assess client's reasons for unhealthy behaviors (may lack knowledge, poverty, addiction, peer pressure, cultural norms, etc.).	Assessment provides information about motivation for unhealthy behaviors.
Discuss the possible consequences associated with the behaviors (specify).	Clients will be informed of the risks of unhealthy behaviors.
Assist clients to plan healthy behaviors (specify: quit smoking, change dietary habits, use contraception, etc.).	Clients will identify the problems and decide on a plan for change.
Offer praise and positive reinforcement for plans to change behaviors.	Praise and reinforcement increase clients' motivation for change.
Relate healthy behaviors to good parenting of the clients' new baby.	Maternal health and role modeling affects the child's health and behavior as he grows up.
Provide information as needed about healthy behaviors (specify: e.g., nutrition, sexuality teaching).	The clients may lack necessary knowledge about nutrition, sexuality, and so forth.
Assist clients to obtain additional resources if indicated (specify: WIC, AFDC, social services, etc.).	Poverty may be a factor in poor dietary habits. Lack of transportation may affect ability to obtain health care.
Refer clients to supportive services (specify: smoking cessation program, substance abuse programs, peer support groups, resource mothers programs, home tutors, etc.).	Referral provides resources that have been successful in helping clients to overcome addiction and maintain healthy lifestyles. Peer groups and resource mothers programs are especially effective with adolescents.

NIC: *Health System Guidance*

Evaluation

(Date/time of evaluation of goal)

(Has goal been met? not met? partially met?)

(Does client identify unhealthy behaviors? Did client make plans to engage in healthy behaviors? Specify.)

(Revisions to care plan? D/C care plan? Continue care plan?)

DELAYED GROWTH AND DEVELOPMENT

Related to: Physical changes of pregnancy and birth. Interruption of the normal psychosocial development of adolescence.

Defining Characteristics: Specify clients' ages and maturity levels. Mother is underweight/overweight (specify ht, wt, and percentile). Clients report difficulty with peers, or parent(s) related to the pregnancy and baby. Clients verbalize confusion about plans for the future (specify).

Goal: Clients will demonstrate adequate growth and age-appropriate psychosocial development while accomplishing the developmental tasks of parenting.

Outcome Criteria

✔ Mother will obtain needed nutrition for recovery, lactation, and normal physical growth. Clients will make plans to complete at least a high school education. Clients report satisfactory relationship with each other, parent(s), significant others, and peers.

NOC: *Child Development: Adolescence*

INTERVENTIONS	RATIONALES
Assess mother's physical growth compared to norms for age.	Assessment provides information about physical growth.
Assess teen parent's maturity of thinking and ability to plan for the future. Tailor discussion to developmental level (specify: e.g., concrete thinking, formal operations, etc.).	Assessment guides planning. Young adolescents may have difficulty relating current behaviors to future consequences.
Reinforce nutrition teaching relating it to the mother's growth needs as well as recovery and lactation if indicated.	Reinforcement promotes compliance. Young adolescents may need more nutrients and calories than adult mothers do.
Assess the impact of parenthood on clients' education and future plans for a vocation or career.	Teen parenting may adversely affect education and skill attainment and the development of a mature identity.
Discuss body image issues and correct misconceptions (e.g., "I'll never wear a bikini again").	The adolescent may fear mutilation or permanent disfigurement from birth.
Encourage clients to finish basic schooling and make realistic	Encouragement assists the clients to plan for the future. Inadequate

(continues)

(continued)

INTERVENTIONS	RATIONALES
plans for the future including childcare.	education and low income become a vicious circle for many teen parents.
Assist clients to assess relationships with parent(s), each other, and peers (plan ways to improve these if needed).	Parenthood may affect relationships. Teens need social interaction in order to develop identity and independence.
Teach clients about the developmental tasks of adolescence (Erikson).	Teaching may decrease some confusion from conflicting feelings and desires.
Refer clients as needed (specify: e.g., special schooling/vocational programs, etc.).	Referrals may assist the clients to plan a future for themselves and the infant.

NIC: *Self-Responsibility Facilitation*

Evaluation

(Date/time of evaluation of goal)

(Has goal been met? not met? partially met?)

(Does client choose appropriate nutrition? Does client have plans to finish high school? Does client report satisfaction with relationships?)

(Revisions to care plan? D/C care plan? Continue care plan?)

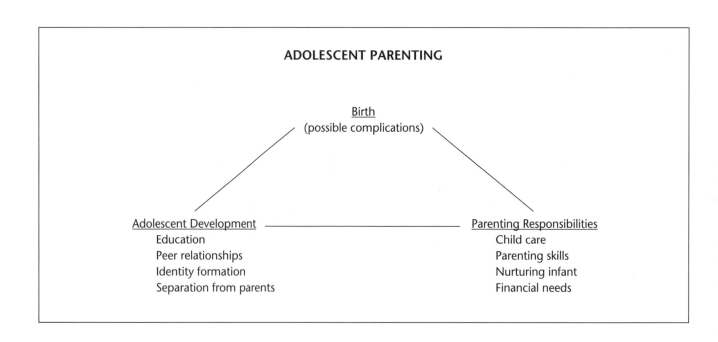

ADOLESCENT PARENTING

Birth
(possible complications)

Adolescent Development
Education
Peer relationships
Identity formation
Separation from parents

Parenting Responsibilities
Child care
Parenting skills
Nurturing infant
Financial needs

CHAPTER 3.11

POSTPARTUM DEPRESSION

Fifty to eighty percent of new mothers experience an "adjustment disorder with depressed mood" (DSM-IV, 4th ed.), commonly known as the "baby blues" in the first few days after giving birth. This is a self-limiting condition related to hormonal changes and periods of increased sensitivity and unexplained crying. "Postpartum major mood disorder," also known as postpartum depression, is a more serious condition that affects fewer women. The third recognized postpartum psychiatric condition is "postpartum psychosis" which is more common in women with a history of previous psychiatric disorders. Clients experiencing postpartum depression or psychosis must be evaluated and protected from harming either themselves or their infants.

RISK FACTORS

- History of psychiatric illness or postpartum depression
- Unwanted pregnancy
- Lack of stable relationships
- Lack of financial and emotional support
- Multiple babies
- Low self-esteem, dissatisfaction with self

The client who exhibits signs of depression, and her family, need information and assessment to differentiate the "blues" from major depression.

SIGNS AND SYMPTOMS

"Blues"	*Depression*
Early onset: first few days	Late onset: 4th week up to 1 year
Short-lived: 2–3 days	Continue for more than 2 weeks
Mild depression	

"Blues"	*Depression*
Anxiety, irritability, crying episodes	Hopelessness, helplessness
Appropriate fatigue	Agitation or exaggerated slowness of movement
	Insomnia or excessive sleeping
	↓ interest ↓ energy Unable to concentrate
	Appetite changes
	Feelings of guilt or worthlessness
	Thoughts of death or suicide

MEDICAL CARE

- "Blues": anticipation, recognition, reassurance
- Major depression or psychosis: psychotropic medications including antidepressants, antipsychotics, lithium, tranquilizers. Psychotherapy, counseling or day-treatment programs. Possible hospitalization and/or electroconvulsive therapy (ECT).

COMMON NURSING DIAGNOSES

See ANXIETY

Related to: Actual or perceived threat to self-concept secondary to difficulty adapting to birth and parenting.

Defining Characteristics: Client reports feelings of (specify: e.g., nervousness, helplessness, and loss of control). Client exhibits (specify: e.g., irritability, lability, crying, withdrawal, etc.).

See RISK FOR IMPAIRED PARENTING

Related to: Ineffective adaptation to stressors associated with parenting a new infant.

Defining Characteristics: Client exhibits a lack of or inappropriate parenting behaviors (specify). Client verbalizes (specify: e.g., frustration with baby, self, or ability to care for infant).

 ### See INTERRUPTED FAMILY PROCESSES

Related to: Gain of new family member.

Defining Characteristics: Family system is not supportive (specify). Family doesn't (specify: e.g., communicate openly, meet the physical or emotional needs of its members, etc.).

ADDITIONAL NURSING DIAGNOSES

 ## INEFFECTIVE COPING

Related to: Inadequate psychological resources to adapt to motherhood; unsatisfactory support systems; altered affect secondary to imbalance of neurotransmitters.

Defining Characteristics: Client verbalizes that she is unable to cope (specify). Client is unable to care for self or infant (specify: e.g., poor hygiene, doesn't respond to infant's cues, etc.). Client uses inappropriate coping mechanisms (specify: e.g., denial, substance abuse, etc.). Client exhibits destructive behavior (specify).

Goal: Client will engage in more effective coping behaviors by (date/time to evaluate).

Outcome Criteria

✔ Client will identify current stresses leading to ineffective coping.
✔ Client will explore personal strengths and plan new ways to cope with stresses.

NOC: *Coping*

INTERVENTIONS	RATIONALES
Assess client's affect, personal hygiene, and interaction with a support system (e.g., visitors, phone calls).	Assessment provides information about client's ability to cope.

INTERVENTIONS	RATIONALES
Assess client's attachment behavior towards her infant: eye contact, holding, touch, talking to the baby, and so forth. Evaluate cultural variation if indicated.	Poor attachment behavior may signal a risk for neglect or abuse of the infant. In some cultures the new mother is not expected to provide infant care in the early puerperium.
Notify caregiver if client avoids looking at or touching infant or makes negative comments about infant.	Negative comments and avoidance of infant may signal that the infant needs protection.
Establish trusting relationship with client. Spend time with client, provide for privacy, and remain nonjudgmental.	Establishment of trust promotes a sense of safety and support for the client.
Encourage client to explore how she is feeling using therapeutic communication skills (e.g., use of open-ended questions: "Can you tell me how you're feeling now?" or reflection: "You seem to be sad today").	Therapeutic communication assists the client to identify and explore her emotions.
Assess client for severe depression or thoughts about death or suicide. Notify caregiver immediately about any indication of suicidal ideation.	Clients who are severely depressed or talking about death/suicide need immediate psychiatric help.
Evaluate client's ability to relate information in a coherent and generally organized manner.	Evaluation provides information about organization of client's thought processes.
Note any bizarre behaviors: inappropriate laughter, talking to someone who isn't present, evidence of delusional thinking or hallucinations. Inform caregiver of client's behavior.	Bizarre behavior may indicate mania or psychosis.
Assist client to identify, and rank in intensity, all current stressors in her life.	Identification and ranking of stressors helps the client organize her thinking.
Observe client's nonverbal behaviors as she describes feelings and stressors.	Observation provides additional information about the client and what she is saying.
Ask client how she usually copes with similar stressors in her life and if this is an effective method.	Asking the client to identify and evaluate usual coping mechanisms increases client's self-awareness.
Explore alternative coping mechanisms with client. Help client identify ways to avoid the stressor, change the situation, or cope with what can't be changed.	Exploration assists the client to identify the potential to alter a stressor and alternatives to usual coping methods.

INTERVENTIONS	RATIONALES
Help client identify personal strengths that have helped her in the past. Explore how these can help in the present.	Identification of strengths promotes self-esteem and decreases feelings of helplessness.
Provide positive reinforcement for description of positive coping mechanisms.	Positive reinforcement enhances client's self-esteem and encourages effective coping.
Assist client to identify healthy behaviors she can use to reduce unavoidable stresses (e.g., exercise, meditation, relaxation techniques, etc.).	Exercise, meditation, and relaxation techniques help to relieve stress and improve health.
Assist client in formulating a plan to cope more effectively with stressors in her life.	Assistance encourages the client to commit to positive changes.
Encourage client to seek and accept social support during the puerperium.	Client may have unrealistically high expectations for herself or may need "permission" to ask for help.
Teach client and significant other the signs and symptoms of postpartum "baby blues": transient feelings of sadness, crying, common emotional lability, and feelings of milk depression in the first few days after childbirth.	Information provides anticipatory guidance for recognition of emotional fragility that occurs in the first few weeks after birth.
Encourage significant other to be supportive to client during this time and reassure them that this only lasts 2 or 3 days.	Encouragement of support promotes effective family coping.

INTERVENTIONS	RATIONALES
Provide information about signs and symptoms of developing major depression to report to client's caregiver: severe depression with late onset, lasts more than 2 weeks, and interferes with normal activities of daily living.	Information allows client and significant other to differentiate between the "blues" and major depression after childbirth.
Encourage client and significant other to plan ways to cope with stress of having a new baby when they go home.	Planning helps family cope with stresses related to caring for a newborn.
Provide information about community support services (specify: e.g., support groups, mental health agencies, etc.).	Information helps client and family to obtain additional help after discharge.
Provide for follow-up phone call or arrange a home visit with client at 2 to 3 weeks postpartum.	Follow-up helps reinforce effective coping and identify additional problems that may develop after discharge.

NIC: *Coping Enhancement*

Evaluation

(Date/time of evaluation of goal)

(Has goal been met? not met? partially met?)

(Did client identify current stresses leading to ineffective coping? Did client explore personal strengths and plan new ways to cope with stresses?)

(Revisions to care plan? D/C care plan? Continue care plan?)

POSTPARTUM DEPRESSION

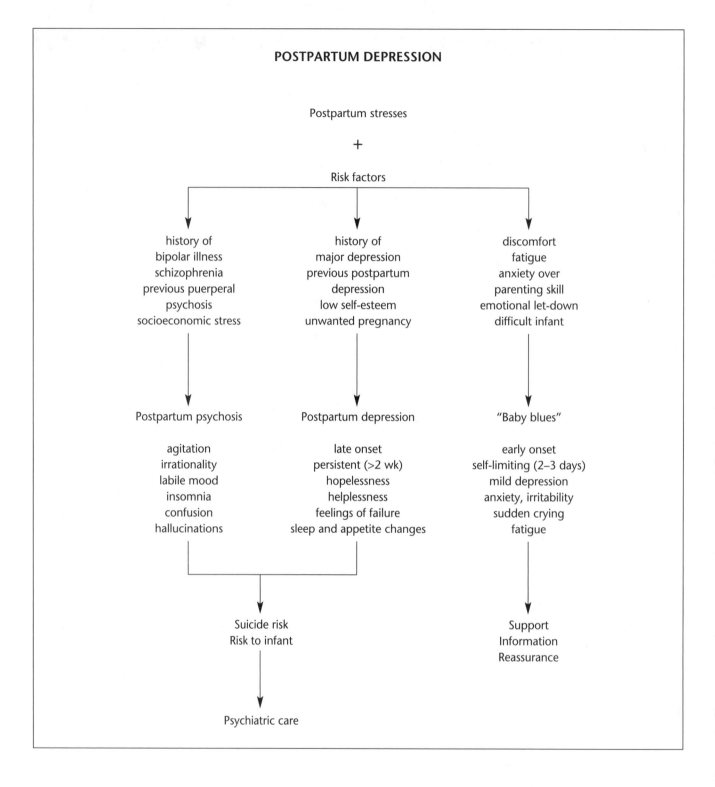

Postpartum stresses

+

Risk factors

| history of bipolar illness schizophrenia previous puerperal psychosis socioeconomic stress | history of major depression previous postpartum depression low self-esteem unwanted pregnancy | discomfort fatigue anxiety over parenting skill emotional let-down difficult infant |

Postpartum psychosis

agitation
irrationality
labile mood
insomnia
confusion
hallucinations

Postpartum depression

late onset
persistent (>2 wk)
hopelessness
helplessness
feelings of failure
sleep and appetite changes

"Baby blues"

early onset
self-limiting (2–3 days)
mild depression
anxiety, irritability
sudden crying
fatigue

Suicide risk
Risk to infant

Support
Information
Reassurance

Psychiatric care

CHAPTER 3.12

PARENTS OF THE AT-RISK NEWBORN

The birth of a preterm infant, an infant with a congenital anomaly, or a compromised newborn requiring intensive care disrupts the normal parent–infant attachment process. In the case of preterm birth, the client may not have completed the developmental tasks of pregnancy. Congenital anomalies may be life-threatening or disfiguring. An otherwise normal term newborn may experience distress during labor and require resuscitation at birth, or the baby's condition may deteriorate in the first few hours of life.

All parents must relinquish their "fantasy" baby in order to form an attachment with their real baby. For parents of an at-risk newborn, shock, disbelief, grief, guilt, and a sense of failure may complicate this process.

COMMON NURSING DIAGNOSES

 ### SEE FEAR

Related to: Life-threatening condition of the newborn (specify).

Defining Characteristics: Parents express great apprehension about condition and prognosis of newborn (specify using quotes). Parents exhibit physiologic indications of sympathetic response (specify: e.g., pallor, tremor, etc.).

 ### SEE INTERRUPTED FAMILY PROCESSES

Related to: Disruption of family routines and expectations secondary to birth of high-risk newborn.

Defining Characteristics: Family is not adapting constructively to crisis (specify: e.g., lack of communication between family members, lack of emotional support for each other, etc.).

ADDITIONAL NURSING DIAGNOSES

 ### RISK FOR IMPAIRED PARENT– INFANT ATTACHMENT

Related to: Unexpected outcome to pregnancy (specify: preterm birth, infant with congenital anomalies, compromised neonate). Barriers to attachment secondary to intensive care environment.

Defining Characteristics: None, as this is a potential diagnosis.

Goal: Parents will engage in the attachment process with their infant by (date/time to evaluate).

Outcome Criteria

✔ Parents will see, touch, and talk to their baby.

✔ Parents will verbalize positive feelings towards their baby.

NOC: *Parent–Infant Attachment*

INTERVENTIONS	RATIONALES
Provide parents with information about their infant at birth (specify: e.g., breathing, need for resuscitation, visible anomalies).	Information helps the parents to cope with reality rather than fears of the unknown. Parents pick up on nonverbal cues from staff when there is a problem at birth.
Encourage parents to see and touch their baby before transfer to the nursery.	Seeing and touching the baby are important to facilitate attachment even if the baby is ill.
If infant is to be transferred to another facility, take parents to the nursery to see the baby or have the baby brought to them in a warmer before transport. Take pictures of the baby and give to parents with a set of footprints.	The parents need to see their baby to begin the attachment process. When the infant is transported, pictures and footprints provide tangible evidence of the baby's existence.

(continues)

183

(continued)

INTERVENTIONS	RATIONALES
Ask transport team to call when they arrive and provide parents with an update on the baby's condition. Provide parents with phone number of receiving facility and encourage calls to check on baby.	Providing information allays fears the parents may have and establishes a relationship with the new facility.
Assess parents' level of understanding about the baby's condition.	Assessment provides information about parent's learning needs.
Provide accurate information from a consistent source for parents (e.g., neonatologist, primary NICU nurse, etc.).	Accurate information from a trusted source helps the parents resolve their grief and attach to their baby.
Arrange for the parents to visit their baby in the NICU as soon as possible after birth.	Early visitation encourages attachment. There may be a "sensitive period" for optimal parental attachment.
Provide parents with anticipatory guidance before going to the NICU: what they will see and hear in the unit, what they may expect their baby to look like including equipment around him. Use written materials or videos to reinforce teaching.	Anticipatory guidance decreases the anxiety encountered in an unfamiliar environment. The infant may have many monitors attached to him. Pictures in books, or videos help the parents visualize what the NICU is like.
Focus parents' attention on their baby. Point out attractive features or individual attributes. Address variations from the way a normal term newborn looks (e.g., preterm skin may be red, thin; immature genitalia; baby may be pale, retracting, etc.). Show pictures of babies with corrected anomalies if indicated (e.g., cleft lip).	Parents may be distracted by the noise and machinery of the NICU, increasing their feeling of separation from the infant. Drawing their attention to the baby helps them begin the identification process. Parents may be afraid to ask questions about abnormal-looking attributes. Pictures of corrections are reassuring with disfiguring anomalies.
Encourage parents to make eye contact, talk to, and touch their infant. Explain that the infant needs to hear their familiar voices, see them, and feel their touch too.	Parents may be afraid they will hurt their baby or interfere with equipment if they touch him. Providing comfort in the form of sound and touch is a parenting task.
Explain each monitor that is attached to the baby: what it monitors, how it's attached, where the readout is, and what is normal range. Explain any alarms that "go off."	Parents may harbor misconceptions about equipment attached to their baby. They may become upset when the numbers on the read-out change or an alarm sounds.

INTERVENTIONS	RATIONALES
Provide parents with the phone number of the unit, the name of their baby's nurses and instruct them to call or visit when they want to.	Intervention promotes trust and a sense of security for parents to know how to get information about their baby.
Assist parents to review their labor, birth, and any resuscitation events. Provide accurate information and correct misconceptions.	Review helps parents incorporate the events surrounding the birth into their present situation.
Encourage parents to express their feelings about their baby's birth. Reassure them that many parents feel guilty, angry, helpless, or depressed.	Encouragement promotes, expression of normal feelings that the parents may think are shameful.
Provide parents with information about parent–infant attachment. Note the importance even if the baby doesn't survive (if this is indicated).	Resolution of grief is facilitated if the parents have been able to form an attachment to their baby. Knowing that they cared for their baby in some way comforts them.
Encourage parents' assistance with caregiving activities for their baby: changing diapers, helping with skin care, and so forth. Acknowledge ambivalent feelings they may have about the baby's nurses.	Encouraging parents to assist promotes attachment to the infant. Parents may feel grateful and jealous of NICU nurses who care for their baby.
Encourage the mother who planned on breast-feeding her baby to pump her breasts and bring in the milk for her baby when he is allowed to eat. Praise mother's commitment to her baby.	Breast milk is usually the ideal food for the at-risk newborn. The mother will need to make a major commitment to pump, store, and deliver her milk for the baby.
Compliment parents on caregiving activities and interest in their baby.	Compliments provide feedback about parenting skills and attachment.
Teach parents about their baby's individual responses. Plan neonatal behavioral assessments for a time when parents are visiting and show them appropriate ways to stimulate their baby (specify).	Assessments provide parents with important information about their baby's behavior. A preterm or compromised neonate may not respond to parental stimulation as older siblings did.
Promote family support and participation (e.g., grandparents, siblings, etc.).	Intervention facilitates the whole family's attachment to the baby.
Keep a record of parents' or family's visiting patterns and phone calls about their baby.	A record provides information about family attachment or avoidance of the baby.

INTERVENTIONS	RATIONALES
Encourage parents to discuss how they feel towards their baby after several visits.	Encouragement helps parents identify beginnings of emotional attachment.
Notify caregiver and initiate referrals to social services if family avoids contact with their baby.	Infants who are separated from their parents for a long time after birth are at high risk for neglect or abuse.
Provide support to parents whose infant has a genetic defect. Arrange consultation with a genetic counselor.	Genetic defects may engender guilt and blame in the parents. Genetic counselors are experienced in helping parents cope and plan for future pregnancies.
Provide information about additional support systems: e.g., NICU parents groups, parents of children with congenital anomalies.	Support groups can offer information and ideas to enhance parents adaptation.

NIC: *Environmental Management: Attachment Process*

Evaluation

(Date/time of evaluation of goal)

(Has goal been met? not met? partially met?)

(Did parents see, touch, and talk to their baby? Have parents verbalized positive feelings towards their baby?)

(Revisions to care plan? D/C care plan? Continue care plan?)

ANTICIPATORY GRIEVING

Related to: Potential for neonatal loss secondary to prematurity, compromised neonate or infant with congenital anomalies (specify).

Defining Characteristics: Client and significant other report perceived threat of loss (specify quotes: for example, "Our baby is going to die isn't he? Will our baby ever be normal?").

Goal: Client and significant other will begin the grieving process.

Outcome Criteria

✔ Client and significant other identify the meaning of the possible loss to them.

✔ Client and significant other are able to express their grief in culturally appropriate ways (specify).

NOC: *Family Coping*

INTERVENTIONS	RATIONALES
Assess the parents' beliefs about the perceived potential loss.	Assessment provides information and clarification.
Provide accurate information about the baby's condition and prognosis. Provide information updates from a consistent source.	Parents may be overly anxious from being uninformed about current condition. Provision of a consistent source helps prevent conflicting information.
Encourage and assist parents to form an attachment to their baby. (If the baby is nonviable, allow parents to hold the infant until he or she expires.)	Grief-work is facilitated if the parents formed an attachment to the baby and provided some care before death.
Assist parents to describe what the perceived loss means to them. Don't minimize the loss (e.g., "Well at least she isn't brain-damaged").	Identifying the meaning of this loss helps the parents know what they are grieving for and begin the grief process.
Support the family's cultural expressions of loss/grief in a respectful and nonjudgmental manner.	Different cultures express grief in different ways—the nurse needs to allow and facilitate grief-work without being judgmental.
Teach parents about normal grieving and relate it to their loss of a perfect baby. Describe feelings that they may experience. Provide written materials if literate.	Knowing that shock, anger, disbelief, guilt, and depression, and so forth are normal reactions will help the parents to cope with these feelings.
Support parents in the stage they are in and assist with reality-orientation (specify: e.g., "I can see that you are angry, this is a normal way to feel," or "I can see that you are hoping things will turn out OK; I am hoping so too").	Support assists the parents to identify the stage they are in and work through the process without feeling that the nurse is judging them.
Encourage parents to ask for support from family and social support system.	Social support helps ease the burden of grief and may help with future needs.
Offer to contact the parents' clergy or the hospital chaplain if desired.	Religious support may be helpful to parents.

NIC: *Grief-Work Facilitation*

Evaluation

(Date/time of evaluation of goal)

(Has goal been met? not met? partially met?)

(What do client and significant other describe as the meaning of the possible loss? Use quotes. Describe grief reactions the client and significant other express: crying, anger, being stoic, culturally prescribed responses, etc.)

(Revisions to care plan? D/C care plan? Continue care plan?)

INTERRUPTED BREAST-FEEDING

Related to: Specify (e.g., prematurity, NPO status of high-risk neonate, congenital anomalies: cleft lip/palate, etc.).

Defining Characteristics: Mother desires to breast-feed her infant but is unable to do so because of (specify: e.g., infant is on IV fluids only; preterm infant or infant with congenital anomaly is unable to suck/swallow effectively, etc.).

Goal: Client will maintain lactation and provide milk for infant until breast-feeding can be resumed.

Outcome Criteria

✔ Client will identify actions to promote lactation.

✔ Client will verbalize understanding of pumping, storing, and delivering breast milk for her baby.

NOC: *Knowledge: Breast-Feeding*

INTERVENTIONS	RATIONALES
Discuss client's original intent and desire to provide breast milk for her infant.	Client may be unaware that she can still provide milk for her baby if nursing is contraindicated.
Assess beliefs, previous experience, knowledge, and role models for breast-feeding.	Lack of knowledge or support for breast-feeding may interfere with client's ability to succeed with pumping until nursing can be resumed.
Provide information (written and verbal) about the benefits of breast milk for her baby. Teach client that breast milk is easily digestible, provides antibody protection, reduces development of allergies.	Teaching provides reinforcement for providing breast milk for the high-risk neonate.

INTERVENTIONS	RATIONALES
Provide information (written and verbal) about pumping the breasts, storing milk (plastic bottles only), and bringing the milk to the hospital for the baby.	Information helps the client to initiate lactation and store her milk safely.
Provide for privacy and a calm, relaxed atmosphere. Reassure client that lactation is a natural activity in which her body is prepared to engage.	Anxiety and embarrassment interfere with learning, the "let down" reflex, and milk production. Reassurance helps client to believe in the wisdom of her body.
Teach client that relaxation is necessary for effective lactation. Describe how the "let-down" reflex is affected by her emotions.	Teaching promotes effective breast milk production. Maternal tension, emotional upset, or embarrassment may inhibit the "let-down" reflex.
Instruct client to get into comfortable positions for pumping. Suggest she keep a glass of water close by.	Comfort promotes relaxation. Pumping (or breast-feeding) stimulates thirst.
Describe the feedback loop of milk production and breast stimulation.	Understanding the relationship between milk supply and stimulation enhances the client's ability to provide breast milk for her baby.
Teach client to pump at least 8 times in 24 hours. Instruct client to stroke her breast while pumping: the "hind milk" or last milk in the breast contains high fat content to promote growth.	Frequent pumping stimulates milk production. Understanding the physiology of lactation promotes self-confidence.
Instruct client in breast care: wash hands before pumping; wash nipples with warm water and no soap; allow to air dry.	Instruction promotes self-care. Handwashing prevents the spread of pathogens; soap may dry the nipples causing cracks.
Praise client for commitment, skill development, and nurturing behaviors.	Praise increases self-worth and promotes confidence in abilities.
Describe what client will feel when her milk "comes in" (breast engorgement) and what she can do to ease discomfort: suggest warm showers, application of warm, moist cabbage leaves, ↑ frequency of expression of milk, mild analgesics (acetaminophen) as ordered by caregiver.	Anticipatory guidance decreases anxiety and promotes effective self-care. Moist heat causes vasodilatation and decreases venous and lymphatic congestion. Cabbage leaves are anecdotally reported to be effective in relieving discomfort. Emptying the breast ↓ the sensation of fullness.
Encourage client to explore her feelings about pumping. Discuss client concerns about working, etc.	Client may have concerns that increase anxiety and interfere with successful lactation.

INTERVENTIONS	RATIONALES
Praise client's attempts and successes. Reinforce the benefits of breast milk, if only for the first few weeks or months.	Praise helps build self-confidence and intent to continue supplying breast milk.
Assist client to obtain a breast pump after discharge from the hospital.	The client may be able to purchase, rent, or borrow a pump from different agencies.
Refer client as indicated (specify: e.g., to a lactation specialist, other mothers, or La Leche League, etc.).	A lactation specialist is prepared to assist mothers with special needs. La Leche League provides information and support for breast-feeding mothers.

NIC: *Lactation Counseling*

Evaluation

(Date/time of evaluation of goal)

(Has goal been met? not met? partially met?)

(Did client identify actions to promote lactation? Does client verbalize understanding of pumping, storing, and delivering breast milk for her baby?)

(Revisions to care plan? D/C care plan? Continue care plan?)

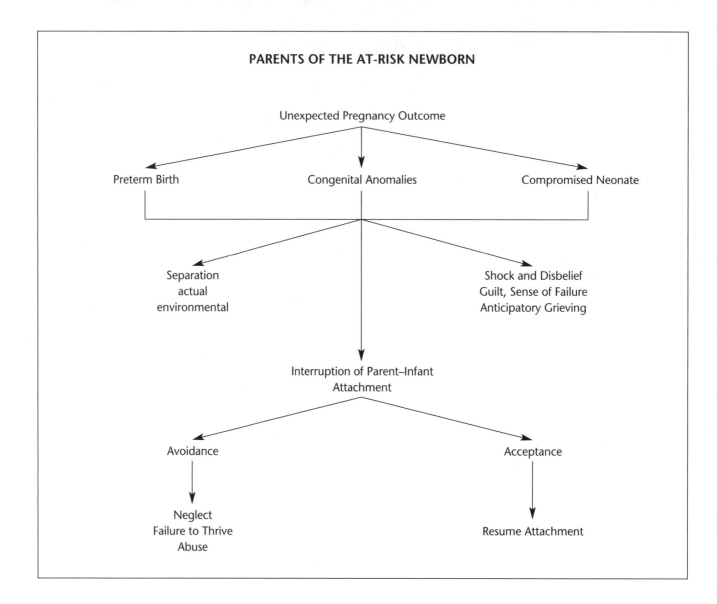

PARENTS OF THE AT-RISK NEWBORN

Unexpected Pregnancy Outcome

Preterm Birth   Congenital Anomalies   Compromised Neonate

Separation
actual
environmental

Shock and Disbelief
Guilt, Sense of Failure
Anticipatory Grieving

Interruption of Parent–Infant
Attachment

Avoidance   Acceptance

Neglect
Failure to Thrive
Abuse

Resume Attachment

UNIT 4

NEWBORN

CHAPTER 4.0

HEALTHY NEWBORN

The healthy term infant is prepared for the dramatic transition to extrauterine life by the events of normal labor and vaginal birth. Contractions result in gradually decreased fetal oxygen and pH and increased carbon dioxide during labor. Descent through the birth canal squeezes the chest, removing excess lung fluid. Changes in blood chemistry combine with thermal stimulation of birth into a cooler environment and a suddenly expanded chest to stimulate the first breath. Respiration causes pressure changes in the cardiopulmonary system that result in gradual closure of the foramen ovale, ductus arteriosus and ductus venosus thus initiating adult-type circulation. The infant is born awake, alert, and with the necessary reflexes to begin breast-feeding and bonding with his parents.

The goals of nursing care for the newborn are to provide warmth and safety, identify any life-threatening problems, and facilitate postnatal adaptation and parent-infant attachment.

WARMTH AND SAFETY

- The infant is dried immediately and placed in a warm environment: skin-to-skin with the mother or on a prewarmed dry blanket under a radiant warmer with controlled temperature

- Medications: vitamin K 0.5 to 1 mg, IM to prevent hemorrhagic disease of the newborn; eye prophylaxis to prevent ophthalmia neonatorum (1% silver nitrate, 0.5% erythromycin, or 1% tetracycline ophthalmic preparations) following birth; hepatitis B vaccination, genetic, and hearing screening before discharge

- Identification includes matching leg and armbands with the mother and possibly footprints and fingerprints before the mother and infant are separated

- Infant security systems to prevent abduction vary by agency

- Bathing is delayed until temperature stabilizes (gloves are worn until the initial bath is completed)

- Cord care and circumcision care to prevent infection or hemorrhage

- Use of a car seat for discharge

ASSESSMENTS

- Immediate assessment of respiratory effort, heart rate, and color followed by appropriate resuscitation measures

- Apgar scoring at 1 and 5 minutes: heart rate, respiratory effort, color, muscle tone, and reflex irritability; continued at 5 minute intervals until a score of 7 or better is obtained

- Physical assessment and measurements

- Gestational age assessment correlated with newborn weight and length

- Neonatal behavioral assessment

- Parent–infant attachment assessments

- Hearing screening

ATTACHMENT AND BONDING

- Encouragement of breast-feeding and interaction during the periods of infant reactivity: first period during the first 30 minutes after birth is followed by sleep; the second period begins around 4 to 6 hours after birth and lasts 2 to 4 hours

- Encouragement and support for rooming-in

- Parent teaching: normal newborn appearance and behavior; infant care and feeding

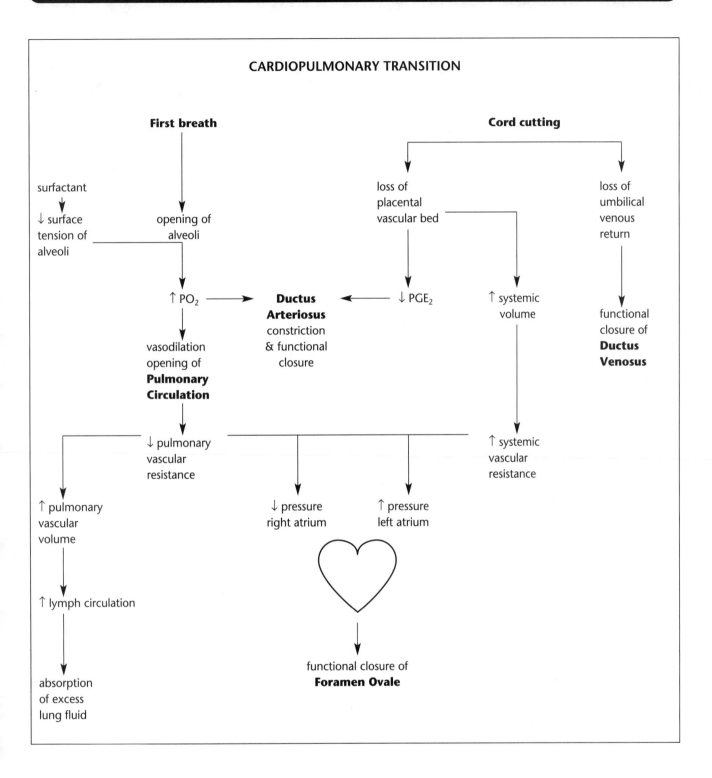

CARDIOPULMONARY TRANSITION

TABLE 4.1   Newborn Care path

BIRTH	ASSESSMENT	MEDS/TX	NUTRITION ELIMINATION	TEACHING/ OTHER

1st hour	Apgar
	
	TPR (hourly × 4)
	# cord vessels
	
	cord blood to lab
	(Rh neg. mom)
	
	weight, length
	OFC, chest circ.
	
	breast-feeding technique,
	nipple soreness at each
	feeding
		neonatal resuscitation prn
		
		vit. K 0.5 mg IM
		triple dye or alcohol swab
		to cord if ordered
		
		skin-to-skin or warmer
		(37°C) w/probe in place
			breast-feeding
			
			√ suck/swallow
			
			                     √ stool
			                     √ urine
				promote attachment
				
				ID bands
				footprints/thumbprint
				Infant security
				
				instruction: breast-feeding
				burping, holds, bulb
				syringe, newborn
				characteristics

2nd hour	BP × 1 heel-stick Hct physical assessment gestational-age assessment attachment	erythromycin 0.5% ophthalmic, O.U. XT √ blood glucose all SGA, LGA, & prn	first water (bottle baby)	hepatitis B information
4 hours	TPR q 8 hr if stable √ maternal HBsAg	hepatitis B vaccine per protocol first bath if temp stable Kangaroo care or return to warmer until stable then open crib cord care as ordered	first formula breast feeding q 2–4	ongoing teaching at bedside
8 hours			formula q 3–4 breast q 2–4 assess feeding q 8 hr	lactation specialist prn
1st day	weight (MD exam w/in 24 hr) assess voiding after circ.	circumcision circ care		photos hearing screen teaching circ care
Discharge	weight & % loss MD exam metabolic screen hearing screen			√ ID bands & remove remove cord clamp provide PKU info appointment for √ up infant-care information sheets gift pack car seat

CHAPTER 4.1

BASIC CARE PLAN: TERM NEWBORN

The care plan is based on a review of the prenatal record, labor and delivery summary, gestational-age assessment and a thorough physical assessment. Specific infant data should be inserted wherever possible.

COMMON NURSING DIAGNOSES

 ### INEFFECTIVE AIRWAY CLEARANCE

Related to: Excessive secretions (specify if cause is identified: e.g., secondary to cesarean birth).

Defining Characteristics: Infant experiences choking or gagging on excessive secretions; tachypnea; abnormal breath sounds (specify).

Goal: Infant will experience a clear airway by (date/time to evaluate).

Outcome Criteria

✔ Infant's respiratory rate will be between 30–60 bpm.
✔ Bilateral breath sounds will be clear to auscultation.

NOC: *Aspiration Control*

INTERVENTIONS	RATIONALES
Suction infant's mouth, then nares with bulb syringe after birth of the head.	Suctioning before birth of the shoulders clears the upper airway before the first breath. Neonates are obligate nose-breathers; suctioning the nares may cause gasping and aspiration of oral contents if mouth has not been cleared first.
Position infant with head slightly down and on a side. Stimulate crying if needed.	Positioning facilitates drainage of fluid by gravity. Crying opens the airway and improves lymph drainage and absorption of excess lung fluid.

INTERVENTIONS	RATIONALES
Assess respiratory rate and effort, note nasal flaring, retractions, or grunting (specify frequency of assessment).	Assessment provides information about effectiveness of suctioning and stimulation to clear the airway. Tachypnea, flaring, grunting, and retracting are signs of respiratory distress.
Repeat suctioning with bulb syringe or wall suction only as needed to remove excessive secretions.	Excessive suctioning may stimulate a vagal response, causing bracycardia and further compromise.
Auscultate bilateral breath sounds and apical pulse (specify frequency).	Auscultation provides information about fluid in the lungs and heart rate, rhythm, and regularity.
When stable, place infant skin-to-skin with mother covered by a warm blanket with bulb syringe readily available.	Skin-to-skin promotes warmth and attachment. Bulb syringe allows immediate clearance of secretions.
Monitor infant for episodes of increased secretions (choking and gagging) during periods of reactivity. Clear airway with bulb syringe as needed.	Infant may experience additional secretions and need for suctioning during the first and second periods of reactivity.
Teach mother to use bulb syringe: Depress bulb first then insert syringe into side of infant's mouth and release bulb compression. Remove from mouth and depress bulb to discharge contents. Clear mouth before suctioning nose.	Teaching parents promotes timely airway clearance. Depressing bulb first avoids blowing secretions into infant's lungs. Inserting syringe into side of mouth avoids vagal stimulation from touching back of pharynx.
Notify caregiver if secretions continue to be excessive.	Copious secretions are a sign of tracheoesophageal malformations.

NIC: *Airway Management*

Evaluation

(Date/time of evaluation of goal)
(Has goal been met? not met? partially met?)

(What is respiratory rate? Are breath sounds clear bilaterally?)

(Revisions to care plan? D/C care plan? Continue care plan?)

 ## INEFFECTIVE THERMOREGULATION

Related to: Limited neonatal compensatory metabolic temperature regulation.

Defining Characteristics: Temperature fluctuations in response to environmental factors (e.g., birth into cool environment, wet body, etc.).

Goal: Infant will be maintained in a neutral thermal environment by (date/time to evaluate).

Outcome Criteria

✔ Infant's axillary temperature will remain between 36.5 and 37° C (97.7–98.6° F).

NOC: *Thermoregulation: Neonate*

INTERVENTIONS	RATIONALES
Dry newborn thoroughly and quickly and discard the wet blanket. Place infant on a warm blanket under a pre-warmed radiant warmer for initial assessment.	Drying quickly and placing on a warm, dry surface prevents heat loss by evaporation.
Assess axillary temperature at birth and when indicated (specify frequency).	Axillary temperature is preferred to avoid risk of rectal perforation. Assessment provides information about the neonate's temperature regulation.
Wrap infant in warm blanket and carry to mother. May place infant skin-to-skin with mother and place blanket over mother and baby.	Kangaroo care provides for warmth and bonding.
Teach family about the infant's need for warmth and to keep the infant's head covered.	Teaching provides information the family needs to care for their baby. The infant's head provides a large surface area for heat loss.
Return infant to warmer as needed. Unwrap infant (except diaper) while under warmer.	The radiant warmer heats surfaces exposed to it. Covering the infant decreases the amount of warmth reaching his skin.

INTERVENTIONS	RATIONALES
Position the warmer's temperature probe over nonbony area on infant's abdomen and secure with foil patch. Set controls to maintain skin temperature of 36.5 and 37° C. Check that alarms are turned on.	Placing the probe over a bony area will give a false-high skin temp. reading causing the warmer to shut off prematurely. The warmer should be set to a physiologic range and alarms turned on to prevent overheating the infant.
When temperature is 37° C, infant may be quickly bathed while remaining under radiant warmer. Wash and dry the head first, then expose and wash one area of body at a time and dry thoroughly before moving on to another area.	Bathing quickly in a warm environment avoids heat loss from evaporation and convection.
Avoid placing infant on cool surfaces or using cold instruments in assessment (e.g., scale, stethoscope).	Placing the infant on a cool surface or using cool instruments increases heat loss by conduction.
When temperature has stabilized after bath, dress infant in a shirt, diaper and hat, wrap in 2 blankets and transfer to open crib. Monitor temp per protocol and return to warmer if needed.	Interventions promote warmth while assessing the infant's ability to regulate his temperature in an open crib.
Place cribs away from windows, avoid drafts or air conditioning blowing on the sides of the crib or on the infant.	Heat may be lost directly from the infant's body to cooler air (convection) and to cooler surfaces close to the infant's body by radiation.
Maintain room temperature at 72° F. Teach family to adjust infant's coverings after discharge to the room temperature based on how they are feeling (e.g., if it is very warm, the baby doesn't need to be dressed in sweaters).	Teaching assists parents to care for their infant. The infant may suffer from hyperthermia if overdressed.

NIC: *Temperature Regulation*

Evaluation

(Date/time of evaluation of goal)

(Has goal been met? not met? partially met?)

(What is infant's temperature? Has it been stable? Specify.)

(Revisions to care plan? D/C care plan? Continue care plan?)

RISK FOR INFECTION

Related to: Exposure to pathogens, invasive procedures (specify: e.g., cord cutting, injections, heel sticks, circumcision), breaks in skin integrity (specify: e.g., abrasions, spiral electrode site, etc.), immature immune system.

Defining Characteristics: None, as this is a potential diagnosis.

Goal: Infant will not experience infection by (date/time to evaluate).

Outcome Criteria

✔ Infant receives prophylactic eye ointment (specify).

✔ Sites of invasive procedures or broken skin (specify) show no signs of infection (specify for each: e.g., no redness, edema, purulent discharge, etc.).

NOC: *Risk Control*

INTERVENTIONS	RATIONALES
Perform a 3-minute hand scrub prior to caring for mothers and infants. Wash hands before and after touching infant. Wear gloves until after the infant's first bath and when changing wet or soiled diapers.	A 3-minute scrub removes most pathogens. Washing hands before and after touching infant prevents the transmission of microorganisms between babies. Gloves protect the caregiver from blood-borne pathogens.
Do not place shared-items in infant's bed (e.g., thermometers, stethoscopes, etc.).	Sharing equipment may transfer microorganisms from one infant to the next.
Assess maternal records for: history of infections and their treatment, HBsAg, time of membrane rupture, maternal fever, application of internal fetal monitoring, operative delivery.	Assessment of maternal records provides information about the risk of infection for this neonate.
Assess newborn's axillary temperature at birth and report hyperthermia to caregiver.	An infant born with a fever may have experienced intrauterine infection.
Assess newborn for compromised skin integrity: punctures from scalp electrodes, abrasions, and so forth. Document findings and include areas in future assessments for development of redness, edema, or purulent drainage.	Assessment provides information about potential sites for invasion by pathogens. Monitoring ensures early identification of infection.

INTERVENTIONS	RATIONALES
Assess cord for number of vessels without touching the cut surface. Provide cord care if ordered (specify: e.g., triple dye, bacitracin, alcohol, etc.). Assess cord for foul odor or purulent drainage at each diaper change. Fold diapers down to expose the cord.	The cut surface of the umbilical cord presents a site for proliferation of microorganisms. Keeping the cord exposed facilitates drying and inhibits bacterial growth.
Wipe excess secretions from infant's eyes. Administer eye prophylaxis as ordered (specify: e.g., erythromycin 0.5% ophthalmic ointment O.U.) within 2 hours of birth.	Neonatal eye prophylaxis prevents ophthalmia neonatorum caused by exposure to gonorrhea and/or Chlamydia in the vagina. Waiting for a short time promotes attachment during the first period of reactivity.
Provide mother with information about hepatitis B vaccination; obtain consent. Administer 1st dose of vaccine to infant per protocol (specify drug, dose, and route).	Infants of mothers who are positive for HBsAg should receive the vaccine at birth. It is recommended for all newborns to prevent hepatitis B infection.
Administer injections and perform heel sticks using aseptic technique. Document sites and add to future assessments.	Aseptic technique prevents introduction of pathogens during injections and heel sticks.
Assess circumcision for signs of infection during each diaper change. Rinse penis with water only and place a gauze pad with petroleum jelly over penis (unless a Plastibell has been used) at least 4–5 time per day.	Assessment provides information about developing infection. Gauze protects the surgical site; petroleum jelly prevents gauze sticking to the site.
Assess infant for signs of infection: temperature instability beyond the first few hours, feeding problems, lethargy, pallor, apnea, or diarrhea. Notify caregiver.	Neonates may exhibit subtle signs of infection compared to older infants. The infant may merely not "look right" or behave "normally."
Teach parents to care for circumcision and not to remove yellowish exudate.	Yellowish exudate is granulation tissue. Removal may cause hemorrhage and increase the risk of infection.
Teach family to avoid exposing the infant to people with infections. Instruct family to wash their hands before handling the infant.	Teaching helps the family to care for their baby and prevent infection.
Teach parents to use a thermometer before discharge. Instruct them to take the infant's temperature only if he appears ill (hot, lethargic, refusal to eat,	Parents may not know how to use and read a thermometer. Guidelines are provided to ensure prompt treatment if the infant becomes ill.

(continues)

(continued)

INTERVENTIONS	RATIONALES
diarrhea, dehydrated, etc.) and to call the doctor for fever >101° F rectally or 100.4° F axillary.	

NIC: *Infection Protection*

Evaluation

(Date/time of evaluation of goal)

(Has goal been met? not met? partially met?)

(Did infant receive eye prophylaxis? Specify time, drug, etc. Provide an assessment of cord, circumcision, injection sites, and any areas of broken skin.)

(Revisions to care plan? D/C care plan? Continue care plan?)

IMBALANCED NUTRITION: LESS THAN BODY REQUIREMENTS

Related to: Limited intake during the first few days of life.

Defining Characteristics: Weight loss (specify birth weight compared to current wt.). Mother's milk has not come in. Insufficient intake of calories (specify caloric needs for individual infant and compare with caloric intake. A term newborn needs 120 calories/kg/day: mature breast milk and regular formula usually contain about 20 cal/oz).

Goal: Infant will establish feeding pattern to obtain needed nutrients by (date/time to evaluate).

Outcome Criteria

✔ Newborn demonstrates effective suck and swallow reflexes.

✔ Breast-fed baby nurses well during first 4 hours after birth.

✔ Bottle-fed baby retains first water and formula feeding.

✔ Infant produces at least six wet diapers per day. Total weight loss is <10% of birth weight.

NOC: *Nutritional Status: Nutrient Intake*

INTERVENTIONS	RATIONALES
Weigh infant at birth and each day without diaper or clothing. Cover scale with blanket and zero before weighing. Protect from	Monitoring infant's weight losses/gains provides information about nutritional status.

INTERVENTIONS	RATIONALES
falls without touching infant. Compare to previous weights.	
Assess infant's suck reflex during initial assessment. Check swallowing during first feeding.	Infant needs to be able to suck and swallow effectively to obtain nourishment from breast or bottle.
Observe infant for first stool and urine. Monitor all intake and output.	Passage of first stool indicates a patent anus, first urine indicates renal function. Monitoring I&O provides information about nutrition and fluid balance.
Assess airway clearance and bowel sounds during the periods of reactivity. Encourage breast-feeding after birth, during second period of reactivity and every 2–3 hours.	Infants may have ↑ secretions during reactive periods that should be cleared to prevent aspiration or choking during feeding. Usually bowel sounds are ↑ during reactive periods indicating readiness to feed.
Assist breast-feeding mother as needed. Instruct her to burp infant when changing breasts and when finished and to place infant on right side after eating.	Assistance helps mother to feed her infant. Burping ↓ discomfort and spitting-up. Placing on right side facilitates stomach emptying.
Refer to lactation specialist as needed.	Lactation specialist can assist the breast-feeding mother who is having difficulty.
Inform parents that the infant is getting enough milk if he gains weight and produces six or more wet diapers per day.	Parents, especially breast-feeding, may worry about whether their baby is getting enough to eat. Information provides reassurance.
Provide culturally sensitive care to clients who wish to wait until their milk comes in to breast-feed their babies. Provide water and formula as ordered (specify).	Some cultures believe that colostrum is not good for the baby. Culturally sensitive care promotes maternal role-attainment.
Provide sterile water to infants whose mothers choose not to breast-feed within 4 hours. Assess for excessive gagging, choking, or vomiting and notify caregiver.	Sterile water (like colostrum) is nonirritating if aspirated. Assessment provides information about patency of esophagus.
If infant tolerated water feeding, assist mother to provide first formula feeding (specify formula and amount) as ordered.	Formula feeding may begin after assessment of the infant's ability to ingest water.
Monitor infant for signs of feeding intolerance: excessive spitting up, abdominal distention, abnormal stools. Notify caregiver.	Feeding intolerance may indicate congenital anomalies or complications.

INTERVENTIONS	RATIONALES
Provide teaching to bottle-feeding family as needed: hold infant close with head higher than stomach (do not prop the bottle); ensure nipple is full of formula; burp infant after each ounce or more frequently, and when finished; place infant on right side after eating.	Teaching promotes parent–infant attachment; prevents aspiration; ↓ middle ear infections; ↓ gas, discomfort, and spitting up; facilitates stomach emptying.
Teach parents that a small amount of regurgitated formula is normal after eating but to notify caregiver if infant vomits the whole feeding.	Feeding may need to be repeated if large amount was vomited. Increasing force and frequency of vomiting may indicate pyloric stenosis.
Inform bottle-feeding mothers of the schedule suggested by her caregiver (specify) and ensure that sterile formula is available for feedings.	Formula takes longer to digest than breast milk so the infant can usually go longer between feedings. Formula should be thrown away after 1 hour to prevent contamination.
Praise parents for successful feeding of their new baby. Inform mothers that newborns may be sleepy while they recover from birth but will wake up and be hungry by the time the milk normally comes in.	Praise enhances self-esteem and promotes parental role-attainment. Mothers may feel like failures if the infant is sleepy and won't nurse "on time." Reassurance promotes confidence.
Teach parents about the normal newborn's stools; meconium, transitional, and milk stools: color, consistency, smell, and frequency (specify for bottle- or breast-fed babies).	Teaching helps parents to identify normal variations in infant stools.
Teach parents that weight loss of up to 10% is normal after birth but then their baby should gain about an ounce per day after that for the first 6 months.	Teaching provides information the parents need to assess their infant's growth.
Provide written and verbal instructions on infant feeding (and formula preparation) at discharge per infant's caregiver. Provide phone number of nursery and information about community resources (specify: e.g., WIC, La Leche League).	Instruction and resources help parents care for their baby after discharge.

NIC: *Nutrition Management*

Evaluation

(Date/time of evaluation of goal)

(Has goal been met? not met? partially met?)

(Did newborn demonstrate effective suck and swallow reflexes? Did breast baby nurse well during 1st 4 hours? Did bottle baby retain 1st water and formula? How many wet diapers in last 24 hours? What % of birth-weight has infant lost?)

(Revisions to care plan? D/C care plan? Continue care plan?)

RISK FOR INJURY

Related to: Immaturity and dependency on others for care.

Defining Characteristics: None, as this is a potential diagnosis.

Goal: Infant will not experience injury by (date/time to evaluate).

Outcome Criteria

✔ Newborn receives vitamin K injection.

✔ Mother demonstrates safety when handling, positioning and caring for infant.

✔ Metabolic screening is begun before discharge.

NOC: *Risk Control*

INTERVENTIONS	RATIONALES
Administer vitamin K, per order (specify time, dose) IM into the middle third of the vastus lateralis.	Vitamin K is synthesized by intestinal bacteria and used in production of prothrombin. Injection is provided to prevent neonatal hemorrhage. The vastus lateralis is a safe site for neonatal injections.
Place matching identification bands on infant's arm and leg and mother's arm before separating mother and baby. Check numbers before giving infant to mother.	Matching identification prevents mix-up of mothers and babies.
Obtain footprints and mother's fingerprint per protocol before separation.	Prints may be used for identification if well done. Also given as souvenirs.
Inform parents about hospital's infant security system (specify).	Infant security system prevents abduction.

(continues)

(continued)

INTERVENTIONS	RATIONALES
Promote attachment and bonding at every opportunity. Perform most infant care at bedside and teach parents to provide care. Praise parents' skill and point out infant's individuality and response to them.	Interventions enhance parents' motivation and caregiving skills to promote infant safety.
Perform physical assessment and gestational age assessment of newborn. Obtain BP and heel-stick Hct per order (specify). Notify caregiver of abnormal findings.	Assessments provide information about abnormalities and risk factors. ↓ BP may indicate hypovolemia, ↑ Hct >65% indicates polycythemia.
Assess blood glucose level per protocol (specify). Initiate feeding per orders (specify) if blood sugar is <40 mg/dL, and re-check blood glucose level.	Hypoglycemia may result in brain damage.
Monitor infant for development of jaundice. Notify caregiver.	Neonatal jaundice indicates hyperbilirubinemia that, if severe, may cause kernicterus and brain damage.
Teach family to pick up and always hold infant by supporting neck and spine. Demonstrate various positions (e.g., football hold, cradling, and upright). Assist family to return-demonstrate. Instruct family to never shake the baby.	Teaching family to support infant's neck and spine helps prevent injury to the spinal cord.
Teach family to position infant on right side, supported by a rolled blanket, after feeding. Inform family that infant should not sleep on his stomach or with a pillow.	Infants sleeping on their stomach have an increased incidence of SIDS. Placing infant on right side after eating facilitates stomach emptying.
Show family how to use the bulb syringe to clear excess secretions and stimulate the infant to cry should he become pale or apneic. Reassure family that a nurse will respond quickly to their concerns during hospitalization.	Information assists family to clear infant's airway.

INTERVENTIONS	RATIONALES
Teach parents how to bathe their baby, preventing chilling or burning. Instruct them to give sponge baths only until the cord falls off.	Teaching helps family prevent cold stress or hyperthermia. Sponge bathing helps keep the cord dry to prevent infection.
Teach family to never leave infant alone on an unprotected surface.	Teaching prevents falls. Infant may roll or turn over before parents expect.
Provide information on normal infant behavior and care. Teach ways to comfort a crying infant: burping, feeding, changing, motion, use of a pacifier, and so forth.	Anticipatory guidance helps parents to provide safe care for their baby.
Obtain specimens for metabolic screening before discharge. Inform parents of the need for repeat testing (specify where and when).	Metabolic screening provides information about conditions that can cause mental retardation or handicaps unless treated.
Provide appointment for newborn check up. Inform parents about the need for immunizations for their baby.	Newborn exams and immunizations help identify abnormalities and prevent serious illness.
Reinforce teaching and provide the nursery phone number and written information on infant care at discharge. Ensure that infant is properly placed in a car seat at discharge.	Reinforcement helps parent assimilate information. Phone number provides additional help after discharge. A properly used car seat protects the infant riding in an automobile.

NIC: *Risk Identification*

Evaluation

(Date/time of evaluation of goal)

(Has goal been met? not met? partially met?)

(Date, time, dose, route and site of vitamin K injection? Was metabolic screening begun? Did mother demonstrate safe care and handling of her baby?)

(Revisions to care plan? D/C care plan? Continue care plan?)

CHAPTER 4.2

BASIC CARE PLAN: NEWBORN HOME VISIT

The newborn home visit allows assessment of the home environment and family adaptation to having a new baby. The family benefits from an opportunity to have their questions answered in the comfort of their own home. Anticipatory guidance is provided to promote optimal growth and development of the infant. The care plan is based on a review of prenatal and hospital records and assessments made during the visit.

COMMON NURSING DIAGNOSES

 See READINESS FOR ENHANCED FAMILY COPING

Related to: Effective family adaptation to birth and care of newborn.

Defining Characteristics: Family members are able to describe the impact of the new baby. Family members are moving in the direction of providing a healthy and growth-promoting environment and lifestyle.

ADDITIONAL NURSING DIAGNOSES

 HEALTH-SEEKING BEHAVIORS

Related to: Limited knowledge and experience caring for a newborn.

Defining Characteristics: Infant's mother and family seek information to promote the infant's health (specify: e.g., "When should I feed him cereal? Does he need to eat more?", etc.).

Goal: Family will obtain information about promoting infant health by (date/time to evaluate).

Outcome Criteria

✔ Family participates actively in home visit by asking questions about their baby.

✔ Family states intentions to keep all well-baby appointments and obtain immunizations on schedule.

NOC: *Health-Seeking Behavior*

INTERVENTIONS	RATIONALES
Invite family to participate in assessments of their baby. Provide continual information as obtained and praise positive parenting evidence.	Participation enhances family's knowledge about their baby and promotes feeling comfortable when asking questions.
Note general appearance, hygiene, warmth, and color of infant.	Assessment provides information about family's need for more information related to hygiene, appropriate coverings, or neonatal jaundice.
Evaluate anterior fontanel, infant's head and eye movement. Evaluate baby's response to noise.	Provides information about hydration and neurosensory status.
Auscultate infant's heart rate and rhythm, and breath sounds. Note respiratory rate and effort.	Cardiorespiratory assessment provides information about infant's physiologic health.
Inspect umbilicus for redness or drainage. Note whether cord has fallen off. Ask family about bathing and skin care practices. Teach not to use powders on baby.	Assessment provides information about family's understanding of bathing and skin care for their baby. Powders may be aspirated and cause irritation.
Evaluate diaper area for rashes. Suggest frequent diaper changes, exposing the area to air several times a day and use of a barrier ointment (e.g., A & D) for diaper rash.	Diaper rash is a common parental concern. Exposure to air facilitates healing; ointments protect the skin from urine and feces.
Ask family about infant's elimination patterns: frequency, color, and consistency of stools; # of wet diapers per day.	Information about elimination indicates adequate nutrition and function of the gastrointestinal system.

(continues)

(continued)

INTERVENTIONS	RATIONALES
Ask family about infant's sleeping pattern during the day and night. Provide reassurance and suggest sleeping when the baby does for the first few weeks.	Many babies seem to have their days and nights confused during the early weeks. Parents often seek information about how to cope with fatigue.
Weigh the infant and compare to birth weight. Ask family about infant feeding behavior: (If breast-feeding, is milk in? How often, and for how long does baby nurse? For formula babies, how often and how many ounces does he take?)	Successful feeding with weight gain indicates adequate infant nutrition.
Provide information and support for feeding as needed (specify).	Mothers may have many questions and concerns about feeding their baby.
Assess attachment and bonding: (Does family touch and comfort infant? Do they talk to him making eye contact? Do they say nice things about the baby? Does baby respond?)	A lack of bonding behavior may indicate ineffective parenting. Lack of infant attachment behavior may indicate sensory deficits.
Assess sibling's response to the new baby. Provide information about safety related to siblings.	Focusing on siblings promotes self-esteem. Sibling rivalry depends on the older child's age and dependency needs.
Assess infant's sleeping area for safety concerns: screens on windows, firm crib mattress without pillows. Crib: not painted with lead-based paint; slats not greater than 2⅜ inches apart; side rails kept up and locked. Provide information as needed.	Assessment provides information about family's knowledge, or need for information about safety.
Encourage family to ask questions. Reinforce need for follow-up immunizations, metabolic screening, and well-baby check-ups.	Family should feel comfortable seeking information about healthy behaviors for their baby. Reinforcement of important preventive-care needs improves compliance.
Refer family as indicated (specify: e.g., additional home visit for specific need, social services, WIC, AFDC, support groups, etc.).	Family may need additional assistance to provide optimum care for their new baby.

NIC: *Health Education*

Evaluation

(Date/time of evaluation of goal)

(Has goal been met? not met? partially met?)

(Did family participate in home visit? Does family state intent to provide preventive health care for their baby?)

(Revisions to care plan? D/C care plan? Continue care plan?)

READINESS FOR ENHANCED ORGANIZED INFANT BEHAVIOR

Related to: Normal infant behavior.

Defining Characteristics: Infant is able to regulate heart rate and respiration (specify rates). Infant exhibits normal reflexes (specify). Infant's movements are smooth without tremors. Infant exhibits appropriate state behaviors (specify: e.g., sleeps soundly, is alert upon waking, follows object with eyes, responds to sound, etc.). Infant is consoled easily (describe).

Goal: Infant will continue appropriate growth and development.

Outcome Criteria

✔ Parents verbalize understanding of normal infant behavior.

✔ Parents verbalize intent to stimulate infant development appropriately (specify: e.g., provision of visual, auditory, and tactile sensory input).

✔ Parents demonstrate ways to decrease excessive stimulation.

NOC: *Child Development: Infant*

INTERVENTIONS	RATIONALES
Discuss infant's needs for sleep and stimulation with parents. Identify different infant states: deep sleep, active REM sleep, drowsy, awake, quiet alert, overstimulated, and crying.	Discussion facilitates parents' understanding of their baby's behaviors and needs.
Provide parents with a list of possible infant behavioral cues.	A list helps parents identify infant behaviors they may have overlooked.
Assist parents to identify their baby's behavioral cues indicating stability and organization (quiet, alert, consolable or self-consoling)	Assistance enables parents to explore their infant's behavioral cues and what they mean.

INTERVENTIONS	RATIONALES
compared with periods of disorganization and distress (crying, arching, looking away, yawning).	
Instruct parents to respond appropriately to infant's cues by providing interaction and stimulation during periods of organization and comfort with decreased stimulation when disorganized.	Instruction provides information about ways to enhance infant's development.
Suggest ways to provide visual stimulation: changing mobiles with medium-range, high-contrast colors and geometric shapes or human faces; changing facial expressions and mimic infant's expressions.	The newborn prefers distinct shapes, colors, and the human face. Infant responds by fixed staring, bright, wide eyes to new visual stimuli.
Suggest ways to provide auditory stimulation: classical music, vary speech tone and patterns, reciting poetry, using the infant's name frequently.	Infants respond to sound by becoming alert and searching for the source.
Suggest ways to provide tactile stimulation: skin-to-skin contact, gentle touch, stroking, infant massage, and toys with varied textures.	Touch may help the newborn return to organized state when upset (e.g., swaddling, patting).
Suggest rocking, infant swing, placing infant in a front-carrier and going to a walk.	Movement is often soothing to the infant and provides vestibular stimulation.
Discuss hand-to-mouth behaviors as self-consoling. Provide information about the infant's need for nonnutritive sucking.	Infants have an innate need to engage in sucking which eating alone may not satisfy. Allowing hand-to-mouth or use of a pacifier may meet the infant's needs.
Help parents identify ways to decrease excess stimulation: providing a quiet place to sleep, decreasing excess noise, and so forth.	Infants need periods of calm and decreased stimulation in order to reorganize behaviors.
Praise parents for promotion of their infant's development.	Praise promotes parental self-esteem and enhances developmentally appropriate infant care.
Provide anticipatory guidance about infant growth and developmental changes. Provide referral to parent groups or community agencies as indicated.	Anticipatory guidance and support groups assist parents to provide appropriate stimulation to meet their baby's changing developmental needs.

NIC: *Environmental Management: Attachment Process*

Evaluation

(Date/time of evaluation of goal)

(Has goal been met? not met? partially met?)

(Did parents verbalize understanding of normal infant behavior? Did parents verbalize intent to stimulate their baby appropriately? Did parents demonstrate comforting and ways to ↓ stimulation of their infant?)

(Revisions to care plan? D/C care plan? Continue care plan?)

IMBALANCED NUTRITION: RISK FOR MORE THAN BODY REQUIREMENTS

Related to: Parents' lack of knowledge about infant nutrition needs, familial obesity.

Defining Characteristics: Parents and/or siblings of infant are obese. Infant is gaining excessive weight for age (specify). Parent reports feeding infant solid food before 4–5 months of age (specify).

Goal: Infant will receive nutrition appropriate for age by (date/time to evaluate).

Outcome Criteria

✔ Infant will gain appropriate weight for age (specify: e.g., 1 ounce per week).

✔ Infant is fed a diet appropriate for age (specify: e.g., breast milk, iron-fortified infant formula).

NOC: *Knowledge: Diet*

INTERVENTIONS	RATIONALES
Assess infant's weight gain compared to expected gain. Assess daily intake.	Assessment provides information about excessive weight gain and feeding.
Assess parents' beliefs about infant feeding and weight gain (e.g., does cereal help the baby sleep through the night? A fat baby is a healthy baby?).	Parental beliefs may need to be challenged to promote proper infant feeding.
Provide information about the infant's nonnutritive sucking needs.	Parents may be feeding the infant too much just because he appears to enjoy sucking.

(continues)

(continued)

INTERVENTIONS	RATIONALES
Provide accurate information to parents about their baby's daily calorie needs (specify) and how many ounces of formula he needs daily (specify) or approximation with nursing mothers.	Accurate information helps parents develop an appropriate feeding plan for their baby.
Provide information about infant's iron needs. Teach parents to use iron-fortified formula as instructed by their caregiver. Instruct breast-feeding mothers to continue to take prenatal vitamins and iron and eat a healthy diet while nursing their babies.	Term newborns have stored enough iron in their liver for approximately 4–6 months. Milk has little iron content.
Explain to parents that solid food remains mostly undigested in the newborn's stomach, providing him with little nourishment. Teach parents to delay introduction of solid food until 4–6 months.	Feeding the infant doesn't result in appreciably longer sleep periods and is not beneficial to the infant.
Assist family to evaluate their eating habits. Reinforce positive eating habits and discuss the consequences of obesity.	If the family has poor eating habits with obesity, the infant will grow up learning poor habits. Obesity is implicated in heart disease, diabetes, and early death.

INTERVENTIONS	RATIONALES
Help family plan a nutritious diet based on the food guide pyramid and excluding excess fat and calories. Provide written (or picture) resources.	Parents may be unfamiliar with nutritional needs and meal-planning using the food guide pyramid. Written or picture resources will help in the future.
Refer family members to a dietitian or community resources as indicated (specify: e.g., weight-loss groups).	Referral helps the family gain additional information and support for dietary changes.

NIC: *Nutrition Management*

Evaluation

(Date/time of evaluation of goal)

(Has goal been met? not met? partially met?)

(Is infant's weight gain appropriate? Specify. Is infant being fed an appropriate diet? Specify.)

(Revisions to care plan? D/C care plan? Continue care plan?)

CHAPTER 4.3

CIRCUMCISION

Male circumcision is the surgical removal of the foreskin (prepuce) covering the glans penis. This is usually done for religious, cultural, or social reasons. There have been conflicting medical recommendations for and against circumcision in recent years. The American Academy of Pediatrics (AAP) issued a policy statement in 1999 recommending against routine newborn circumcision. If parents choose to circumcise their sons for religious or cultural reasons, the AAP recommends that pain relief measures be used.

Religious circumcision rites are usually performed after the infant is discharged. When circumcision is to be performed in the hospital, the parents need to give informed consent and the procedure is usually done on the day before discharge. The procedure is delayed if the infant is preterm, unstable, has urethral anomalies, or evidence of a bleeding disorder.

RISKS

- Pain
- Hemorrhage
- Infection
- Tissue damage

MEDICAL CARE

- The infant should have received his vitamin K injection at birth; the procedure is done several hours after a feeding to prevent vomiting and aspiration
- The infant is restrained on a circumcision board with arms and legs secured to prevent movement
- Anesthesia: anesthetic cream applied topically, or dorsal penile nerve block with 1% lidocaine without epinephrine
- Circumcision is performed using a clamp (Gomco, Mogen) or Plastibell; the clamp is removed after circumcision, the rim of the Plastibell remains in place until it falls off after a week

COMMON NURSING DIAGNOSES

See RISK FOR INFECTION

Related to: Incision site for microorganism invasion and colonization.

ADDITIONAL NURSING DIAGNOSES

PAIN

Related to: Tissue trauma secondary to surgery.

Defining Characteristics: Infant is crying, irritable, and restless with interrupted sleep patterns (describe for individual infant).

Goal: Infant will demonstrate decreased pain by (date/time to evaluate).

Outcome Criteria

- ✔ Infant sleeps without disturbance.
- ✔ Infant is not grimacing or crying.

NOC: *Pain Control*

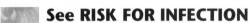

INTERVENTIONS	RATIONALES
Assess infant for signs of pain during and after procedure: grimacing, crying, restlessness and interruption in normal sleep patterns.	Assessment provides information about physiologic responses to pain.
Apply sterile 4×4 gauze pad with petroleum jelly or A&D ointment to circumcised penis (except if Plastibell was used). Cover with a loose diaper.	Sterile lubricated gauze prevents the wound sticking to the gauze and protects the wound from pathogens. Loose diapers decrease pressure on the wound.

(continues)

(continued)

INTERVENTIONS	RATIONALES
Dress and wrap infant in a blanket and take him to his mother to be fed and comforted immediately after circumcision.	The infant has not eaten for several hours before circumcision and may have become chilled during the procedure.
Instruct mother to cuddle and talk to her baby while feeding him and to avoid putting pressure on the penis until healed.	Instruction helps the mother comfort her baby and avoid discomfort.
Position infant on his side after circumcision. Provide access to his hands or a pacifier if mother agrees, for nonnutritive sucking.	Lying on the side decreases pressure on the penis. Sucking provides comfort for the infant.
Observe infant for voiding after circumcision. Note amount and adequacy of stream. Instruct parents to monitor voiding and notify caregiver if infant has problems voiding.	Edema after surgical procedure may interfere with infant's ability to void.
Change and teach parents to change diapers frequently after circumcision.	Teaching prepares parents to care for their baby. Urine is irritating to the open wound.
Cleanse and teach parents to clean the penis by squeezing water over it and apply the lubricated gauze (except Plastibell circumcision) and loose diaper for 2 to 3 days after circumcision.	Cleaning removes urine and promotes healing. Water only is squeezed over penis to avoid chemical or mechanical injury.
Administer mild analgesics if ordered (specify drug, dose, route, times).	Specify action and side effects of drug if ordered.
Teach parents whose infant was circumcised with a Plastibell that the rim should fall off within 8 days and to notify caregiver if it doesn't.	Parents need information to prevent complications after discharge.

NIC: *Analgesic Administration*

Evaluation

(Date/time of evaluation of goal)

(Has goal been met? not met? partially met?)

(Is infant crying? grimacing? Sleeping uninterrupted?)

(Revisions to care plan? D/C care plan? Continue care plan?)

 RISK FOR DEFICIENT FLUID VOLUME

Related to: Active losses secondary to surgical complication. Increased vulnerability secondary to immaturity.

Defining Characteristics: None, as this is a potential diagnosis.

Goal: Infant will exhibit adequate fluid volume by (date/time to evaluate).

Outcome Criteria

✔ Infant will exhibit no bleeding from circumcision site after procedure.

✔ Infant's intake will be similar to output.

✔ Infant's mucous membranes will be moist, fontanels flat, and skin turgor elastic.

NOC: *Fluid Balance*

INTERVENTIONS	RATIONALES
Ensure that vitamin K was given at birth. Assess family history for bleeding disorders. Notify caregiver before surgical procedures are done.	Vitamin K is needed for prothrombin synthesis. Infant may have an inherited clotting disorder.
Assess surgical site for bleeding after procedure. Apply gentle pressure to the area with sterile gauze and notify the physician.	Pressure is used to obtain hemostasis. The physician may order application of gel foam or need to ligate the blood vessel.
Teach parents not to wipe off the yellow-white exudate that forms on the penis after circumcision.	The exudate is granulation tissue. Removal may cause bleeding.
Assess infant's heart rate and respiration after procedure.	Tachycardia and tachypnea may be signs of excessive fluid loss.
Observe and instruct parents to check circumcision site for signs of bleeding during each diaper change.	Frequent observation prevents hemorrhage.
Weigh infant daily and compare to previous weight.	Weight loss should not be more than 1% to 2% per day. Excess may indicate dehydration.
Monitor all intake and output (specify: e.g., weigh or count diapers), check fontanels and skin turgor q 8 hours.	Intake and output provides information about fluid balance. Dry mucous membranes and poor skin turgor indicate tissue dehydration.

INTERVENTIONS	RATIONALES
If infant is receiving IV fluids, monitor hourly I&O, urine specific gravity and glucose, and lab values for Hgb, Hct, and electrolytes as obtained.	IV fluids put the infant at risk for FVD or FVE. Urine sp. gravity >1.013 indicates dehydration, glycosuria may cause osmotic diuresis, lab values indicate hydration and electrolyte balance.
Maintain a neutral thermal environment. Humidify any oxygen the infant receives.	Excessive heat from radiant warmers or phototherapy ↑ fluid losses. Humidified oxygen prevents drying of mucous membranes.

NIC: *Fluid Management*

Evaluation

(Date/time of evaluation of goal)

(Has goal been met? not met? partially met?)

(Did infant have any bleeding after circumcision? What is infant's I&O? Describe infant's skin turgor, mucous membranes, and fontanels.)

(Revisions to care plan? D/C care plan? Continue care plan?)

NEWBORN CIRCUMCISION

■ Circumcision is uncommon in Europe, South America, and Asia (AAP, 1999)

■ Circumcision is generally performed as a religious custom or for health promotion

■ Jewish males are circumcised on the 8th day

■ Muslim males are circumcised between ages 4 and 13 years

■ In the United States, circumcision is often performed to conform to the cultural norm: because the baby's father or brothers were circumcised

■ Circumcision is practiced among African and Aboriginal tribes, Native Americans, and was performed by the ancient Aztecs and Mayans

■ Some cultures practice male (and female) circumcision as a rite of passage performed at puberty

■ Hinduism and Bikhism are religiously against circumcision

CHAPTER 4.4

SMALL FOR GESTATIONAL AGE (SGA, IUGR) NEONATE

The infant who is at or below the tenth percentile for weight compared to gestational age is designated as SGA or small for gestational age. Benign factors that can affect size include heredity, sex, and altitude, with high altitudes producing smaller infants. Chromosomal defects (e.g., trisomies) and dwarf syndromes also result in SGA neonates. Intrauterine growth retardation (IUGR) results in an SGA newborn that has not received optimum intrauterine oxygen and nutrients for appropriate growth.

IUGR infants who have been chronically deprived, exhibit symmetric growth retardation. All organs and body systems are proportional but small. Causes include drug and alcohol abuse, maternal smoking, chronic maternal anemia (e.g., sickle cell), vascular disease (heart, renal), multiple gestation, chromosomal anomalies, and congenital infections (TORCH, syphilis).

The infant who experiences deprivation later in pregnancy, may reveal asymmetric growth retardation. The newborn exhibits normal head circumference and length, but appears wasted with a small chest and abdomen. Hypertensive disorders (PIH), placental infarcts, and advanced diabetes mellitus may result in vascular damage with decreased uteroplacental perfusion.

COMPLICATIONS

- Decreased fetal reserves
- Oligohydramnios
- Labor intolerance: fetal distress
- Meconium aspiration
- Cold stress
- Hypoglycemia
- Hypocalcemia
- Polycythemia
- Hyperbilirubinemia

MEDICAL CARE

- Identification of the infant at risk for IUGR: fundal height, serial ultrasound growth measurements; ultrasound to rule out congenital anomalies
- Delivery if close to term or deteriorating condition
- Suctioning of meconium and neonatal resuscitation at birth
- Thermoregulation, early feeding
- CBC, TORCH titer, urine CMV and drug screening, chromosome studies, total bilirubin

COMMON NURSING DIAGNOSES

See INEFFECTIVE THERMOREGULATION

Related to: Limited metabolic compensatory regulation secondary to age and inadequate subcutaneous fat.

Defining Characteristics: Temperature fluctuations (specify age/wt, temperature changes and use of warmers).

See IMPAIRED GAS EXCHANGE

Related to: Specify (e.g., decreased reserves, ineffective respiratory effort, meconium aspiration).

Defining Characteristics: Specify (e.g., pale color or central cyanosis, blood gas results, etc.).

See IMPAIRED PARENTING

Related to: Specify (e.g., separation secondary to infant illness, maternal substance abuse during pregnancy, unwanted pregnancy, etc.).

Defining Characteristics: Specify (e.g., infant is in NICU because of meconium aspiration, mother used drugs or alcohol during pregnancy, etc.).

ADDITIONAL NURSING DIAGNOSES

RISK FOR INJURY

Related to: Insufficient glucose for CNS secondary to IUGR and ↓ glycogen stores, ↓ enzymes needed for gluconeogenesis, and ↑ metabolism.

Defining Characteristics: None, as this is a potential diagnosis.

Goal: Infant will not experience injury from hypoglycemia by (date/time to evaluate).

Outcome Criteria

✔ Infant's blood glucose levels remain above 40 g/dL for the first 24 hours, then above 45 g/dL.

✔ Infant does not exhibit signs of CNS injury: tremors, jitteriness, lethargy, seizures. and coma.

NOC: *Risk Detection*

INTERVENTIONS	RATIONALES
Provide a neutral thermal environment for infant.	Cold stress causes ↑ metabolism and further depletion of glucose.
Assess for and respond quickly to signs of respiratory distress.	Respiratory distress results in ↑ energy expenditures and depletion of glucose.
Feed infant as soon as possible after birth: breast-feeding or formula followed by feedings q 2–3 hours.	Early feeding promotes normal blood glucose levels after the stress of labor and birth. Frequent feeding helps maintain a steady blood glucose level until the infant is able to replenish stores.
Assess heel stick blood glucose level within first hour and per protocol (specify: e.g., q 1–2 hours × 6, then q 6h). Notify caregiver if <40 mg/dL.	SGA infants are at high risk for hypoglycemia because of decreased glycogen reserves and increased metabolism.
Supplement breast- or bottle feedings with OG feeding as ordered (specify).	The SGA infant may have a weak suck and need supplements in order to maintain blood glucose and to receive adequate calories: 120–130 cal/kg/day.

INTERVENTIONS	RATIONALES
Administer IV fluids as ordered (specify solution, rate) via pump.	IV fluids with 10–15% glucose solution may be needed. Excessive rate of infusion can lead to hyperglycemia and cellular dehydration.
Assess IV site, fluid, and rate hourly. Do not increase rate to "catch up" nor stop infusion abruptly.	Extravasation of fluids can cause tissue necrosis. Increasing the rate causes hyperglycemia, abrupt discontinuation causes hypoglycemia. The infusion needs to be tapered off for infant to adapt.
Monitor hourly intake and output.	Intake and output and daily weights provide information about adequate intake and weight gain or loss.
Observe infant for signs of hypoglycemia: tremors, jitteriness, lethargy, muscle tone, sweating, apnea, seizure activity, LOC. Assess blood glucose level.	Signs of cerebral hypoglycemia are similar to signs of other complications. Blood glucose level is tested to verify behavioral clues.
Monitor lab results for hypocalcemia or sepsis.	Hypocalcemia is frequently associated with hypoglycemia. The symptoms of hypocalcemia and sepsis are similar to those of hypoglycemia.
Explain all procedures and rationales to parents. Provide time for questions and offer reassurance as needed.	Explanations and reassurance help parents to cope with unexpected and unfamiliar procedures.

NIC: *Hypoglycemia Management*

Evaluation

(Date/time of evaluation of goal)

(Has goal been met? not met? partially met?)

(What is infant's blood glucose level? Describe infant's behavior: Are there any tremors, jitteriness, lethargy, signs of seizures or ↓ LOC?)

(Revisions to care plan? D/C care plan? Continue care plan?)

INEFFECTIVE TISSUE PERFUSION

Related to: Increased viscosity of blood.

Defining Characteristics: Infant exhibits (specify: Hct >65%, plethora, persistent peripheral cyanosis, ↓ peripheral pulses, respiratory distress, jitteriness, hypoglycemia, seizures, hyperbilirubinemia).

Goal: Infant will experience adequate tissue perfusion by (date/time to evaluate).

Outcome Criteria

✔ Infant's Hct will be <65%.

✔ Infant will be pink without cyanosis.

NOC: *Tissue Perfusion*

INTERVENTIONS	RATIONALES
Monitor infant's Hct levels as obtained.	Hct levels above 65% indicate polycythemia, which causes sluggish blood flow and poor tissue perfusion.
Observe continuously for signs of respiratory distress (tachypnea, flaring, grunting, retractions, and apnea). Provide respiratory support as needed.	Respiratory distress is related to poor pulmonary tissue perfusion with resultant ↑ PVR and persistent fetal circulation.
Assess heart rate, peripheral pulses, color and color changes q 1 hour.	Hypoxemia results in tachycardia and possibly heart failure. Peripheral pulses may be ↓, with peripheral cyanosis while the rest of the infant appears ruddy.
Assess intake and output (specify frequency).	Poor renal perfusion may result in kidney damage.
Monitor blood glucose levels (specify frequency).	Hypoglycemia results from ↓ stores and ↑ consumption of glucose related to ↑ metabolic demands.
Observe infant for signs of CNS perfusion: behavior changes, seizure activity.	Observation provides information about signs of ↓ central nervous system perfusion.
Provide IV fluids as ordered (specify).	Fluids may be ordered to decrease blood viscosity.
Assist with exchange transfusions as indicated.	Partial plasma exchange transfusion may be indicated to lower blood viscosity.
Monitor bilirubin levels as obtained.	Excessive RBCs become damaged in the capillaries and break down releasing bilirubin. The infant is at high risk for hyperbilirubinemia.
Explain all procedures and assessments to parents.	Explanations help the parents to cope with unfamiliar procedures.

NIC: *Tissue Perfusion—Peripheral*

Evaluation

(Date/time of evaluation of goal)

(Has goal been met? not met? partially met?)

(What is infant's Hct? Describe infant's color.)

(Revisions to care plan? D/C care plan? Continue care plan?)

DELAYED GROWTH AND DEVELOPMENT

Related to: Insufficient nutrients and oxygen for optimal intrauterine growth and development; preterm birth.

Defining Characteristics: Size/gestational age discrepancy (specify: e.g., SGA, IUGR, LGA). Preterm birth (specify gestational age). NICU environment instead of with parents.

Goal: Infant will experience improved growth and development by (date/time to evaluate).

Outcome Criteria

✔ Infant gains 20–30g. per day after stabilization.

✔ Infant is able to maintain a quiet–alert state with varying facial expressions indicating interest.

✔ Infant exhibits hand-to-mouth movements and sucking.

NOC: *Growth*

INTERVENTIONS	RATIONALES
Assess infant's weight daily without diaper.	Daily weights provide information about continuing patterns of loss or gain.
Promote optimum nutrition by assisting parents with feedings as needed (specify: e.g., referral to a lactation consultant, offering formula q 2h, etc.).	Adequate nutrients are needed for growth.
Discuss infant development with parents and solicit ideas for appropriate stimulation.	Parents need information in order to promote optimal development of their baby.
Observe infant's behavioral cues and provide stimulation only as tolerated (specify signs of stress for this infant: e.g., tachycardia, tachypnea, yawning, withdrawal, crying, etc.).	Observation provides information about the individual infant's need for rest or appropriate stimulation.

INTERVENTIONS	RATIONALES
Promote rest by clustering care, decreasing unnecessary noise and stimulation, and covering the isolette during sleep.	Promoting periods of rest allows the infant to reorganize and decrease oxygen and glucose use.
Describe and promote kangaroo care with parents.	Skin-to-skin contact between parent and infant promotes infant development and parental bonding.
Suggest ways to stimulate the infant (specify: e.g., mobiles, photos, talking to the baby, tapes of music, womb sounds, rocking, stroking, etc.).	Provision of infant stimulation to promote development is a parenting role. Parents may benefit from suggestions.
Assist parents to provide short periods of infant stimulation and note infant's responses.	Short periods of stimulation help the parents assess how their baby is responding without offering too much stimulation at once.
Encourage sibling visits with preparation for what they will see and hear in the NICU environment.	Sibling visits promote family bonding, stimulate the infant, and reassure the siblings that their baby is real. Preparation decreases anxiety.

INTERVENTIONS	RATIONALES
Provide additional information about infant development and referrals to support groups as indicated (specify).	Additional information promotes engagement and effective parenting. Books, videos, and other parents are potential resources.

NIC: *Developmental Enhancement*

Evaluation

(Date/time of evaluation of goal)

(Has goal been met? not met? partially met?)

(What is infant's weight gain pattern? Describe infant's behaviors and responses to stimulation.)

(Revisions to care plan? D/C care plan? Continue care plan?)

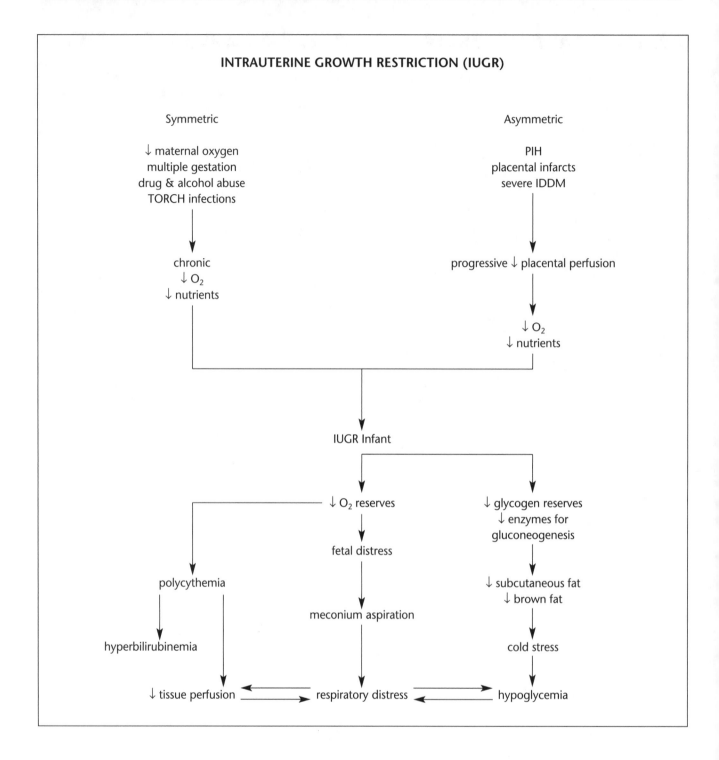

INTRAUTERINE GROWTH RESTRICTION (IUGR)

Symmetric

↓ maternal oxygen
multiple gestation
drug & alcohol abuse
TORCH infections

chronic
↓ O_2
↓ nutrients

Asymmetric

PIH
placental infarcts
severe IDDM

progressive ↓ placental perfusion

↓ O_2
↓ nutrients

IUGR Infant

↓ O_2 reserves

fetal distress

meconium aspiration

↓ glycogen reserves
↓ enzymes for
gluconeogenesis

↓ subcutaneous fat
↓ brown fat

cold stress

polycythemia

hyperbilirubinemia

↓ tissue perfusion → respiratory distress ← hypoglycemia

CHAPTER 4.5

LARGE FOR GESTATIONAL AGE (LGA, IDM) NEONATE

The infant who is at or above the 90th percentile for weight compared to gestational age is designated as LGA or large for gestational age. Benign factors associated with LGA infants include heredity (large parents tend to have large infants) and sex, with males being generally larger than females. Pathologic factors may be hydrops fetalis, transposition of the great vessels, Beckwith–Wiedemann syndrome, and the infant of a diabetic mother (IDM).

The diabetic mother with poor glycemic control and an uncompromised vascular system delivers large amounts of glucose to her fetus. The fetus responds with increased insulin production by the islet cells in the pancreas. Insulin facilitates uptake of glucose and glycogen synthesis, lipogenesis, and protein synthesis. This results in a macrosomic infant with increased fat stores and organomegaly. Birth deprives the infant of the expected glucose supply placing the neonate at high risk for complications of hypoglycemia. Insulin also acts as an antagonist to lecithin synthesis and inhibits production of phosphatidylglycerol (PG), thereby delaying pulmonary maturation.

COMPLICATIONS (IDM)

- CPD, birth trauma: shoulder dystocia, cephalhematoma, fractures, Erb's palsy, facial paralysis
- Oxytocin use, forceps or cesarean delivery
- RDS, slow respiratory development
- Hypoglycemia, hypocalcemia
- Polycythemia, hyperbilirubinemia
- Cardiomegaly, congenital heart defects, caudal regression syndrome

MEDICAL CARE

- Prevention through maternal glycemic control during pregnancy

- Estimation of fetal size and pelvic adequacy—possible planned cesarean birth
- Frequent blood glucose testing after birth
- IV therapy with 10%–15% glucose until stable
- Assessment for injury: X-ray, CT scan

COMMON NURSING DIAGNOSES

 See IMPAIRED GAS EXCHANGE

Related to: Immature respiratory development and insufficient surfactant production secondary to maternal diabetes mellitus.

Defining Characteristics: Specify (e.g., signs of respiratory distress at birth, central cyanosis, blood gases, or oximetry readings).

 See INEFFECTIVE TISSUE PERFUSION

Related to: Obstruction secondary to blood viscosity/polycythemia.

Defining Characteristics: Specify (e.g., color, respiratory effort, hematocrit, etc.).

See DELAYED GROWTH AND DEVELOPMENT

Related to: Excessive glucose use secondary to maternal diabetes mellitus.

Defining Characteristics: Specify infant's age, weight, and percentile compared to gestation.

ADDITIONAL NURSING DIAGNOSES

 RISK FOR INJURY

Related to: Birth trauma secondary to large size; insufficient glucose secondary to transient hyperinsulinism.

Defining Characteristics: None, as this is a potential diagnosis.

Goal: Infant will not experience injury from macrosomia or hypoglycemia by (date/time to evaluate).

Outcome Criteria

✔ Infant does not exhibit signs of birth trauma: fractures, cephalhematoma, Erb's palsy, or facial paralysis.

✔ Infant's blood glucose levels remain above 40 g/dL in the first 24 hours.

NOC: *Risk Control*

INTERVENTIONS	RATIONALES
Review labor progress and birth records for indications of prolonged labor or difficult delivery (e.g., forceps, shoulder dystocia, etc.).	Review provides information about potential injuries and guides a thorough assessment.
Provide warmth and assess for cardiorespiratory stability at birth.	Cold stress and respiratory distress deplete the infant's blood glucose supply.
Assess for signs of congenital anomalies: heart defects, caudal regression syndrome.	Infants of diabetic mothers are at increased risk for congenital defects: transposition of the great arteries, VSD, PDA, femoral hypoplasia, and caudal regression syndrome.
Assess infant for bruising, decreased movement of arms or facial asymmetry. Palpate clavicles for fractures: note crepitus. Assess head for molding and injury. Differentiate between caput succedaneum and cephalhematoma by noting position of swelling relative to cranial sutures.	Macrosomia or forceps intervention may result in bruising or injury. Nerve injury to the brachial plexus or facial nerve results in decreased movement.
Report findings of injury to caregiver. Arrange further testing as ordered (specify: e.g., X-ray, CT scan, etc.).	Additional testing may be indicated to confirm clinical findings.
Discuss birth injuries and treatment plan with parents. Allow time for questions and refer to caregiver as needed.	Parents may become angry about birth injuries. Discussion and referral helps increase understanding.
Feed stable infant within the first hour after birth: breast-feeding or formula followed by feedings q 2–3 hours.	The infant with hyperinsulinism will quickly deplete his blood glucose after birth.

INTERVENTIONS	RATIONALES
Assess heel-stick blood glucose level within first hour and per protocol (specify: e.g., q 1–2 hours × 6, then q 6h). Notify caregiver if <40 mg/dL.	Frequent blood glucose assessments provide information about effectiveness of feedings or IVF in maintaining blood glucose.
Monitor lab results for glucose, calcium, hematocrit, and bilirubin levels.	The infant of a diabetic mother is also at risk for hypocalcemia, polycythemia, and hyperbilirubinemia.
Administer IV fluids via pump as ordered (specify solution, rate). Assess IV site and rate hourly. Monitor hourly intake and output.	IV glucose may be indicated to maintain blood sugars. Frequent assessment prevents complications of IV therapy. Hourly I&O provides information about fluid balance.
Titrate feedings and IVF as ordered to maintain adequate blood glucose levels.	The infant will gradually decrease insulin production as glucose supply is decreased. Titration ensures adequate blood sugar levels during this transition.
Observe infant for signs of hypoglycemia: tremors, jitteriness, lethargy, ↓ muscle tone, sweating, apnea, seizure activity, ↓ LOC. Assess blood glucose level.	Observation provides early recognition of complications.
Explain condition to parents. Reassure them that the infant's insulin production will probably adapt within a few days.	Parents may have high anxiety if their infant requires IV fluids.
Refer parents to additional resources as indicated (specify: e.g., infants with congenital heart defects may be referred to American Heart Association for more information).	Referrals provide additional resources to parents with special needs.

NIC: *Risk Identification*

Evaluation

(Date/time of evaluation of goal)

(Has goal been met? not met? partially met?)

(Does infant have any birth injuries? What is infant's blood glucose level?)

(Revisions to care plan? D/C care plan? Continue care plan?)

INFANT OF A DIABETIC MOTHER (IDM)

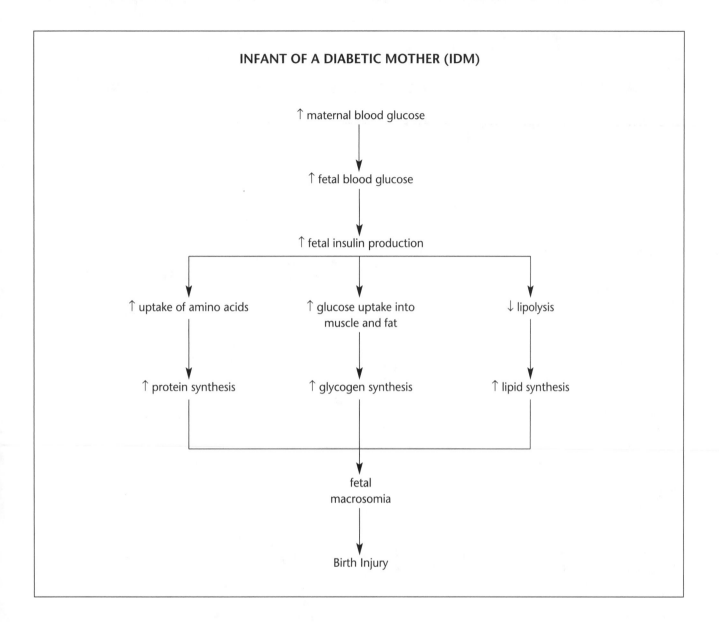

CHAPTER 4.6

POSTTERM INFANT

The infant born after 42 weeks of gestation is defined as postterm. Primiparity, grand multiparity, and history of prolonged pregnancy are factors associated with postterm gestation. In some pregnancies thought to be postterm, an error has been made in calculating gestational age because of variations in menstrual cycles and ovulation. Rare fetal conditions associated with prolonged pregnancy are anencephaly and fetal adrenal hypoplasia.

Complications of postmaturity are thought to be associated with oligohydramnios and placental degeneration. The fetus receives inadequate nourishment and oxygen and suffers distress related to cord compression. Meconium is passed and remains thick because of decreased amniotic fluid. The postmature infant has a characteristic appearance. The infant is alert with eyes wide open. The body appears long and thin with almost no subcutaneous fat. The infant's skin is stained with meconium, loose, dry, and cracked, without vernix or lanugo. Fingernails are long and may also be stained.

COMPLICATIONS

- Meconium aspiration syndrome
- Perinatal hypoxia
- Cold stress
- Hypoglycemia
- Polycythemia
- Hyperbilirubinemia
- Neonatal seizures

MEDICAL CARE

- Ultrasound for gestational age and fetal anomalies
- NST, CST, delivery before 43 weeks
- Suctioning on the perineum with visualization and suction of meconium below the vocal cords before initiation of respiration
- Respiratory support, blood gas analysis, X-ray
- Labs: blood glucose, Hct, bilirubin

COMMON NURSING DIAGNOSES

See INEFFECTIVE THERMOREGULATION

Related to: Immature regulatory mechanisms. Insufficient subcutaneous fat and brown fat secondary to postmaturity.

Defining Characteristics: Specify infant's gestational age. Describe temperature fluctuations and warming devices used.

See RISK FOR INJURY

Related to: Insufficient glucose levels for metabolism secondary to postmaturity.

See RISK FOR IMPAIRED PARENT–INFANT ATTACHMENT

Related to: Abnormal infant appearance secondary to postterm birth. Separation of infant and parents secondary to need for intensive care.

ADDITIONAL NURSING DIAGNOSES

IMPAIRED GAS EXCHANGE

Related to: Meconium obstruction of airway. Pulmonary immaturity resulting in deficient surfactant production. Persistence of fetal circulation.

Defining Characteristics: Progressive signs of respiratory distress (specify: nasal flaring, grunting, retractions, tachypnea, tachycardia, pallor, cyanosis). Acidosis (specify ABGs). (Specify X-ray results: e.g., "ground glass appearance"). Specify thick meconium visualized below the vocal cords.

Goal: Infant will experience adequate gas exchange by (date/time to evaluate).

Outcome Criteria

✔ Infant will have a PaO_2 >50–80 torr, $PaCO_2$ of 45–55 torr, pH 7.25–7.45, SaO_2 >94%.

NOC: *Respiratory Status: Ventilation*

INTERVENTIONS	RATIONALES
Assist caregiver to suction the infant's mouth and nose when head is born but before trunk delivers.	Suctioning the oropharynx clears meconium before the chest is expanded at birth.
At birth, gently place infant under a radiant warmer. Dry quickly, remove wet blankets, and place on a dry, warm blanket.	Interventions prevent cold stress, which also depletes oxygen reserves.
Suction or assist with suctioning the neonate at risk for meconium aspiration before stimulating respiration.	Clearing the airway before initiation of breathing prevents meconium aspiration.
When airway is clear, stimulate respiration and resuscitate per Neonatal Resuscitation Protocol.	The Neonatal Resuscitation Protocol provides for optimal oxygenation of a distressed neonate.
Assess respiratory rate. Observe for signs of distress: flaring, grunting, retracting, tachypnea, apnea.	Tachypnea (rate over 60) indicates respiratory distress. Observations promote early recognition and treatment for the compromised neonate.
Assess infant's color and muscle tone.	Assessment provides information about the infant's tissue oxygenation and energy reserves.
Auscultate apical heart rate and breath sounds, assess BP (specify frequency).	Tachycardia may indicate distress, bradycardia may indicate severe distress. Rales may indicate meconium aspiration. Blood pressure needs to be maintained for adequate pulmonary perfusion.
Provide oxygen as needed (specify: blow-by, oxyhood, PPV with ambu bag and mask or endotracheal tube).	Oxygen needs to be provided based on infant's condition and respiratory ability.
Assist with exogenous surfactant administration as indicated (specify preventive or rescue).	Exogenous surfactant may be administered to infants with RDS or meconium aspiration to replace deficient surfactant and decrease surface tension of alveoli.

INTERVENTIONS	RATIONALES
Assist with initiation of mechanical ventilation as indicated (specify: e.g., CPAP, IMV, IPPB with PEEP, HFV, ECMO)	(Specify rationale for type of mechanical ventilation prescribed.)
Monitor blood gas status as obtained (specify: e.g., $TcPaCO_2$, $TcPaO_2$, SaO_2, and ABGs).	Mechanical ventilation and high oxygen levels are associated with air leaks, pneumothorax, retinopathy, and bronchopulmonary dysplasia. The goal is to decrease settings and wean the infant as soon as tolerated.
Monitor ventilator settings and FiO_2. Assist with assessments and weaning infant from ventilator when stable.	Monitoring blood gases provides information about infant's response to oxygen administration and ventilation.
Administer IV fluids via infusion pump as ordered (specify fluid, site, rate). Assess IV hourly.	IV fluids are initiated to maintain circulating volume and replenish glucose. Hourly assessments prevent fluid overload or injury from infiltration.
Monitor hourly intake and output. Weigh diapers.	Monitoring I&O provides information about fluid balance. Urine output should be 1–3 cc/kg/hr.
Administer medications (e.g., antibiotics, aminophylline, calcium gluconate, Priscoline, dopamine) as ordered; (specify: drug dose, route, times).	(Specify action of prescribed drugs in facilitating gas exchange).
Monitor infant for therapeutic and adverse effects of medications.	(Specify therapeutic effects expected related to gas exchange. Provide rationale for adverse effects.)
Assist respiratory therapist with chest physiotherapy as ordered (specify).	Chest physiotherapy (CPT) may be ordered to facilitate removal of meconium and thick secretions from the lungs.
Monitor X-ray results as obtained.	Serial X-rays may indicate worsening or improvement of condition.
Provide nutrition by TPN or OG until infant is stable and able to suck.	TPN or OG feedings provide glucose and nutrients without excess energy expenditure for the neonate with respiratory distress.
Suction infant only as necessary. Preoxygenate and postoxygenate infant when suctioning.	Pre- and postoxygenation replaces gases lost during suctioning.
Provide stimulation if infant becomes apneic.	Stimulation increases sympathetic nervous system activity and stimulates respiration.

(continues)

(continued)

INTERVENTIONS	RATIONALES
Explain all equipment and procedures to infant's parents.	Information reduces parent's anxiety about unfamiliar procedures and equipment.

NIC: *Airway Management*

Evaluation

(Date/time of evaluation of goal)

(Has goal been met? not met? partially met?)

(What are infant's blood gases? Is the PaO_2 >50–80 torr? $PaCO_2$ between 45–55 torr? pH 7.25–7.45? SaO_2 >94%?)

(Revisions to care plan? D/C care plan? Continue care plan?)

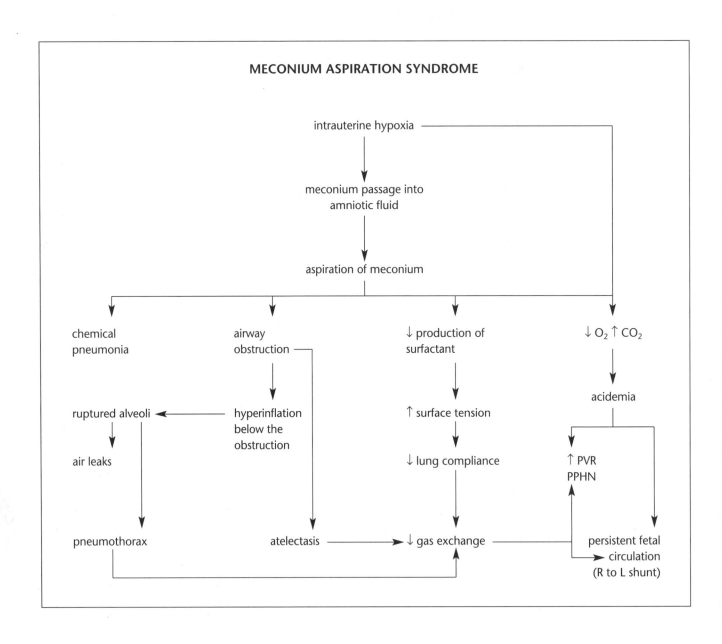

MECONIUM ASPIRATION SYNDROME

CHAPTER 4.7

BIRTH INJURY

Infants at high risk for birth injury include breech presentations, macrosomic infants, those experiencing a prolonged second stage of labor, or operative obstetrics (forceps, vacuum extraction, and cesarean delivery). Injuries may be minor such as bruises, petechiae, abrasions, subconjunctival hemorrhages, or small lacerations. Cephalhematoma, fractures, and peripheral nerve damage are more serious injuries that usually resolve without further complication. Life-threatening injuries include abdominal or spinal cord injury, subdural or intracranial hemorrhage, and perinatal asphyxia with hypoxic-ischemic encephalopathy (HIE). Hypoxic–ischemic injury may result in seizure disorder, cerebral palsy, or mental retardation.

The goals of nursing care are to identify the infant at risk and promote safe birth practices. All infants should be assessed for potential injury soon after birth. Prompt identification promotes early treatment and may prevent further complications.

MEDICAL CARE

- Neonatal resuscitation
- Diagnostic studies: X-ray, ultrasound, CT scan, EEG
- Laboratory: Hgb, Hct, blood glucose, bilirubin, electrolytes, spinal fluid
- Prevention or treatment of metabolic and respiratory acidosis
- Fluid and electrolyte administration
- Medication to control seizures
- Surgical repair

COMMON NURSING DIAGNOSES

See IMPAIRED GAS EXCHANGE

Related to: Insufficient oxygen supply secondary to intrauterine hypoxia, difficult delivery, birth trauma.

Defining Characteristics: Progressive signs of respiratory distress (specify: nasal flaring, grunting, retractions, tachypnea, tachycardia, pallor, cyanosis). Acidosis (specify ABGs).

See RISK FOR INFECTION

Related to: Impaired defenses secondary to birth trauma.

ADDITIONAL NURSING DIAGNOSES

RISK FOR INJURY

Related to: Tissue trauma secondary to difficult or precipitous birth process (specify: e.g., malpresentation: breech, face; nuchal cord; shoulder dystocia; forceps/vacuum assisted birth; prolonged second stage, unattended precipitous birth, etc.).

Defining Characteristics: None, as this is a potential diagnosis.

Goal: Infant will not experience further injury by (date/time to evaluate).

Outcome Criteria

✔ Identified birth injuries are resolved without complication.

NOC: *Symptom Control*

INTERVENTIONS	RATIONALES
Review labor and delivery summary before assessment.	Review of the labor and birth record guides focused assessment for potential birth trauma.
Examine the infant under a warmer with an adequate light source.	Examining the infant under a radiant warmer allows complete visualization without causing cold stress. A good light source is needed to examine skin discoloration.

(continues)

(continued)

INTERVENTIONS	RATIONALES
Observe infant's resting posture for flexion, symmetry, and spontaneous movement.	Before disturbing the infant, observation provides information about possible fractures or neurologic damage. Infant should have all 4 extremities flexed (except frank breech infants whose legs may be extended because of uterine positioning).
Assess skin for erythema, ecchymosis, petechiae, abrasions, or lacerations.	Skin assessment provides information about soft tissue trauma incurred during birth. Facial petechiae may result from a tight nuchal cord, shoulder dystocia, or facial presentation. Forceps injuries are usually the shape of the forceps.
Assess head for shape, position, and neck movement. Palpate for appropriate molding, caput succedaneum, cephalhematoma, or signs of skull fracture. Palpate fontanels.	Holding the head at an angle implies neck injury, inability to move indicates damage. Caput is edema of the presenting part that usually crosses sutures. Cephalhematoma is bleeding into the periosteum and usually does not cross sutures. Fractures may be palpated as depressions.
Observe face for symmetry of muscle tone. Assess blink, pupil, and such reflexes.	Abnormal reflexes indicate cranial nerve injury.
Assess eyes for subconjunctival hemorrhage.	Subconjunctival hemorrhages are usually benign, resulting from pressures on the head during birth.
Assess nares for patency.	Deviated septum may result from compression during birth. Infants are obligate nasal breathers.
Assess extremities for symmetry of movement and intact long bones. Palpate clavicles noting any bumps or crepitus.	Asymmetry of movement or tone in extremities may indicate nerve injury or fractures. Palpation of the clavicles provides information about fractures, which are common with large infants.
Evaluate equality of palmer and plantar grasp.	Inequality of plantar or palmer grasps may indicate neurologic injury.
Assess abdomen for size, shape, and distention or discoloration. Auscultate bowel sounds.	Abdominal trauma may result in internal bleeding and shock.

INTERVENTIONS	RATIONALES
Evaluate infant reflexes; Moro, Babinski, and trunk incurvation.	Abnormal or lack of reflex response to appropriate stimulation may indicate neurologic injury.
Document and report abnormal findings from physical exam to infant's caregiver.	Accurate documentation facilitates evaluation of subsequent changes in condition. Infant's caregiver should verify abnormal findings.
Assist with diagnostic studies as ordered (e.g., X-ray, CT scan).	Diagnostic studies provide information about the suspected injury.
Explain injury to parents. Provide reassurance that the condition should resolve spontaneously (if appropriate).	Explanation and reassurance promote parent understanding and bonding with their baby. Frequently the injury will resolve spontaneously without disfigurement.
Monitor identified injuries every shift for resolution and healing or development of complications.	Continued assessment provides information about resolution or need for additional interventions.

NIC: *Neurologic Monitoring*

Evaluation

(Date/time of evaluation of goal)

(Has goal been met? not met? partially met?)

(Describe injuries identified. Is there evidence of resolution without complications? Describe.)

(Revisions to care plan? D/C care plan? Continue care plan?)

IMPAIRED PHYSICAL MOBILITY

Related to: Neuromuscular injury; musculoskeletal injury secondary to difficult birth.

Defining Characteristics: Inability to move body part, ↓ muscle strength (specify for infant: e.g., signs of Erb's palsy, facial paralysis, fractures, neck or spinal cord injuries, etc.).

Goal: Infant will regain physical mobility by (date/time to evaluate).

Outcome Criteria

✔ Infant is able to move affected body part normally.

✔ Infant doesn't experience complications from impaired mobility (specify: e.g., aspiration, displaced fractures, contractures, etc.).

NOC: *Mobility Level*

INTERVENTIONS	RATIONALES
Review labor and delivery summary and physical and neurologic assessment findings.	Review of birth events and assessment findings provides information about identified injuries affecting physical mobility.
Assess for spontaneous movement of affected area, muscle tone, preferred position, range of motion or indications of pain, (specify frequency).	Assessment provides information about the degree of immobility and signs of improvement.
Maintain anatomic alignment with use of blanket rolls. Position infant on unaffected side.	Anatomical alignment prevents abnormal stress on joints and tissues when the infant is unable to move area spontaneously.
Dress and handle infant carefully to avoid putting additional strain on affected area.	Careful handling prevents further injury and complications.
Immobilize fractures as indicated (specify: e.g., with a fractured clavicle, the long sleeve of the infant's shirt may be pinned across chest to immobilize the arm on the affected side).	Immobilization promotes comfort and healing of fractures.
Teach family to care for the infant without putting stress on the injured arm or shoulder.	Teaching empowers family to care for their infant safely.
Evaluate the infant with facial paralysis for ability to suck and swallow. Assist with feeding by use of a soft nipple and holding the infant's mouth as needed. Provide artificial tears or lubrication for the affected eye if it remains open.	Evaluation and assistance prevents aspiration and promotes adequate nutrition. Lubrication prevents drying of the eye in facial paralysis.
Perform passive range of motion exercises q 2–4 hours on the affected side for infants with Erb's palsy as ordered.	Passive range of motion exercises help to prevent contractures, physical deformities, and promote joint function during periods of paralysis.
Maintain splinting of arm affected with Erb's paralysis as ordered. Assess for circulation and skin integrity q 2 hours.	Splinting may be indicated to maintain correct placement of the humerus. Assessments provide information to prevent complications from splint (obstructed circulation, skin break down)
Teach family to perform range of motion exercises or maintain splinting as indicated.	Teaching family correct techniques for range of motion and splint care ensures that infant will receive needed interventions after discharge.

INTERVENTIONS	RATIONALES
Encourage family to hold and stimulate infant.	Family may be afraid of hurting the infant. Encouragement assists the family to handle the infant safely while meeting emotional and developmental needs.
Provide information about the injury, expected duration of symptoms, and referrals as indicated for.	Information helps the family to cope with the newborn's injury. Referrals provide continuing care after discharge.

NIC: *Positioning*

Evaluation

(Date/time of evaluation of goal)

(Has goal been met? not met? partially met?)

(Is infant able to move affected body part normally? Has infant experienced any complications from impaired mobility? [Specify potential complications for particular injury.])

(Revisions to care plan? D/C care plan? Continue care plan?)

IMPAIRED TISSUE PERFUSION (CEREBRAL)

Related to: Decreased cerebral blood flow and oxygenation secondary to perinatal asphyxia (hypoxia and ischemia). Increased ICP secondary to birth trauma or intracranial bleeding.

Defining Characteristics: Specify for infant (e.g., Apgar scores <7; inadequate resuscitation efforts; acidosis [specify cord blood gases or ABG]. Decreased muscle tone; LOC [lethargy, coma]; seizures; abnormal posturing. Signs of ↑ ICP: apnea, bradycardia, bulging fontanel, wide cranial sutures, etc.).

Goal: Infant will experience adequate cerebral tissue perfusion by (date/time to evaluate).

Outcome Criteria

✔ Infant is well-oxygenated (specify: e.g., SaO_2 >94%) with arterial pH 7.25–7.45.

✔ BP appropriate for age and weight (specify range).

✔ Anterior fontanel is soft and flat.

NOC: *Tissue Perfusion: Cerebral*

INTERVENTIONS	RATIONALES
Identify the at-risk fetus and prepare for birth with adequate personnel and functioning equipment for neonatal resuscitation (specify: e.g., call NICU staff, pediatrician, etc.).	Identification of the at-risk fetus and preparation for birth promotes effective resuscitation of the distressed neonate.
Assess respiratory effort, heart rate, and color at birth. Provide vigorous resuscitation to distressed newborn per Neonatal Resuscitation Protocol.	Timely and correct neonatal resuscitation promotes cerebral oxygenation and prevents or corrects acidosis.
Document immediate assessments (including Apgar and cord blood gases), interventions and infant response.	Documentation assists in identifying infants who experienced intrauterine hypoxia, provides information about appropriate resuscitation efforts and infant's response.
Provide warm humidified supplemental oxygen therapy as ordered (specify: e.g., oxyhood, ventilator: type, FiO_2, rate, etc.).	Interventions promote cerebral oxygenation.
Monitor SaO_2, TcO_2, and ABGs as obtained.	Monitoring oxygen levels provides information about effectiveness of respiratory interventions and guides treatment.
Suction only as needed providing oxygen before and after intervention.	Suctioning may ↓ oxygen levels and ↑ ICP.
Position infant with head midline and HOB elevated. Decrease environmental stimulation. Promote rest by clustering care.	Interventions promote ↓ ICP.
Assess anterior fontanel (specify frequency). Observe infant for behavioral changes, decreasing LOC, or shrill cry.	Assessments provide information about ↑ ICP and CNS irritation or depression.
Maintain a neutral thermal environment and normoglycemia by early feedings or IV fluids (or TPN) as ordered (specify). Monitor blood glucose levels per protocol (specify).	Thermal and glucose regulation promote optimum cerebral oxygenation.
Assess BP, apical and peripheral pulses, skin color, and capillary refill (specify frequency). Monitor Hct as obtained.	Assessments provide information about tissue perfusion.

INTERVENTIONS	RATIONALES
Assess hourly intake and output.	Intake and output provides information about infant's fluid balance and tissue perfusion.
Observe infant for signs of seizure activity (e.g., rhythmic jittery movements that persist when the extremity is flexed or are accompanied by rhythmic eye movements).	Observation provides early identification of subtle signs of cerebral injury.
Assist with diagnostic testing: blood glucose, calcium, and electrolyte levels; spinal tap; EEG, CT scan.	Diagnostic testing helps rule out hypoglycemia, hypocalcemia, or altered electrolyte balance as a cause for jitteriness. CSF is obtained for signs of bleeding or infection. CT scan may identify brain injury. EEG may identify seizure activity.
Administer medications as ordered (specify drug, dose, route, time: e.g., phenobarbital).	(Specify action of drugs ordered: e.g., anticonvulsant, antibiotic.)
Provide support and information for the infant's family. Encourage family participation in care of infant.	Support, information, and encouragement assist the family to cope with their infant's condition and possible poor prognosis. Providing care by the family enhances bonding and attachment.
Provide referrals as indicated after discharge (specify: e.g., pediatric neurologist, social services, programs for children with special needs, early intervention programs, etc.).	Referral is indicated for the family of an infant likely to experience long-term disability (e.g., cerebral palsy, mental retardation, etc.).

NIC: *Cerebral Perfusion Promotion*

Evaluation

(Date/time of evaluation of goal)

(Has goal been met? not met? partially met?)

(What is SaO_2? Is arterial pH 7.25–7.45?)

(Is BP within specified range? Is anterior fontanel soft and flat?)

(Revisions to care plan? D/C care plan? Continue care plan?)

BIRTH INJURY

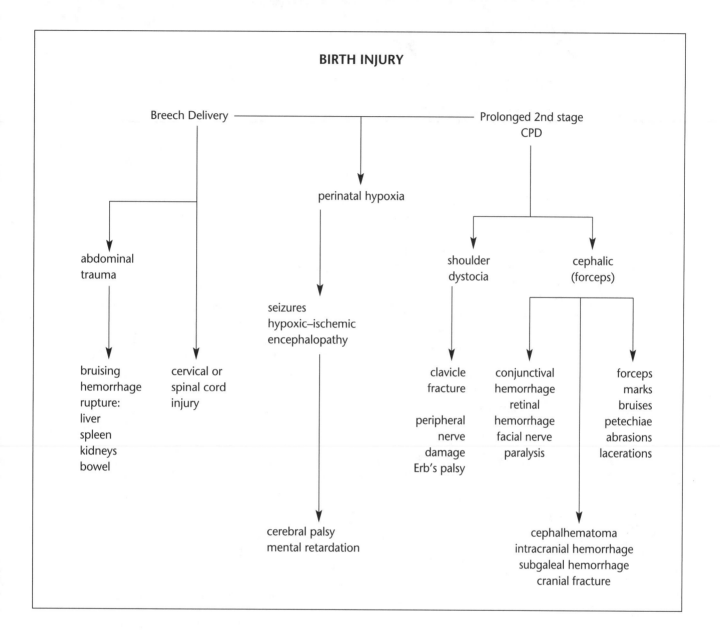

CHAPTER 4.8

PRETERM INFANT

An infant born before 37 weeks of gestational age is described as preterm. The preterm infant may have difficulty adapting to extrauterine existence because of the premature function of body systems. The younger the infant, the more problems are likely to arise. Thus, infants born after 30 weeks gestation have a better prognosis than those born earlier.

Size is not a good indication of gestation as some infants are small for their gestational age (SGA), or large for gestational age (LGA). The term low birth-weight (LBW) is assigned to an infant weighing less than 2500 g., very low birth-weight (VLBW) for those less than 1500 g. and extremely low birth-weight (ELBW) infants weigh less than 1000 g.

COMPLICATIONS

- Respiratory distress syndrome (RDS)
- Ineffective temperature regulation
- Persistence of fetal circulation: patent ductus arteriosus (PDA)
- Intraventricular hemorrhage (IVH)
- Infection
- Necrotizing enterocolitis (NEC)
- Feeding problems
- Fluid and electrolyte imbalances
- Hyperbilirubinemia
- Complications related to intensive care
- Interrupted attachment

MEDICAL CARE

- Respiratory assessment and support; surfactant replacement; oxygen; artificial or mechanical ventilation
- Maintenance of a neutral thermal environment

- Careful management of fluid and electrolytes: insertion of an umbilical artery catheter (UAC) or IV
- Lab tests, X-rays, CT scans, sensory and developmental testing
- Medications as indicated: for example, surfactant, antibiotics, indomethacin for PDA, and so forth
- Nutritional assessment and support: blood glucose monitoring, TPN, breast milk, or 24-calorie formula via gavage if unable to suck and swallow
- Treatment of complications as they arise

COMMON NURSING DIAGNOSES

 ### See INEFFECTIVE THERMOREGULATION

Related to: Immaturity and lack of subcutaneous and brown fat.

Defining Characteristics: Specify infant's gestational age and birth weight. Specify temperature variations and use of warming devices.

See IMPAIRED GAS EXCHANGE

Related to: Insufficient surfactant production. Immature pulmonary and neurologic development.

Defining Characteristics: Specify gestational age, Apgar, blood gases, color, respiratory effort, and so forth.

See RISK FOR DEFICIENT FLUID VOLUME

Related to: Inadequate intake and excessive losses secondary to preterm birth.

 ### See RISK FOR INFECTION

Related to: Sites for invasion of microorganisms. Immature immunologic defenses secondary to preterm birth.

See RISK FOR IMPAIRED PARENT–INFANT ATTACHMENT

Related to: Barriers to attachment secondary to neonatal intensive care of preterm infant.

See DISORGANIZED INFANT BEHAVIOR

Related to: Immature CNS secondary to preterm birth.

Defining Characteristics: Specify for infant (e.g., periods of apnea, bradycardia, muscle twitching/tremors, difficult to console, weak cry, etc.).

ADDITIONAL NURSING DIAGNOSES

INEFFECTIVE BREATHING PATTERN

Related to: Immature neurologic and pulmonary development and fatigue.

Defining Characteristics: Preterm birth (specify gestational age), changes in respiratory rate and patterns: tachypnea, apnea, nasal flaring, grunting, retractions (specify for infant).

Goal: Infant will experience an effective breathing pattern by (date/time to evaluate).

Outcome Criteria

✔ Infant's respiratory rate is between 40 and 60 breaths per minute.

✔ Infant experiences no apnea.

NOC: *Respiratory Status: Ventilation*

INTERVENTIONS	RATIONALES
Assess respiratory rate and pattern. Note nasal flaring, grunting, retractions, cyanosis, and apnea.	Assessment provides information about neonate's ability to initiate and sustain an effective breathing pattern.
Provide respiratory assistance as needed: suction, oxygen, PPV.	Assistance helps the newborn by clearing the airway and promoting oxygenation.
Assist with intubation and surfactant administration if needed.	The infant may need mechanical assistance with breathing. Surfactant is needed to keep the alveoli open.

INTERVENTIONS	R
Collaborate with the physician and respiratory therapist to maintain effective mechanical ventilation for infant as indicated (specify: e.g., IPPB, intermittent positive-pressure breathing).	C__ inf__ Mechan___. required to maintain resp... and oxygenation.
Position infant on side with a rolled blanket behind his back.	Lying on the side position facilitates breathing.
Administer medications as ordered (specify drug, dose, route, times: e.g., calcium gluconate, aminophylline, caffeine).	Specify action of drugs ordered.
Provide tactile stimulation during periods of apnea.	Stimulation of the sympathetic nervous system increases respiration.

NIC: *Respiratory Management*

Evaluation

(Date/time of evaluation of goal)

(Has goal been met? not met? partially met?)

(What is infant's respiratory rate? Is infant experiencing periods of apnea?)

(Revisions to care plan? D/C care plan? Continue care plan?)

IMBALANCED NUTRITION: LESS THAN BODY REQUIREMENTS

Related to: High metabolic rate, inability to ingest adequate nutrients.

Defining Characteristics: Preterm (specify gestational age), respiratory distress, unable to suck or swallow (specify: e.g., gags, drools, tires quickly); (specify current caloric intake compared to calculated needs).

Goal: Infant will obtain adequate nutrition by (date/time to evaluate).

Outcome Criteria

✔ Infant receives adequate calories to meet metabolic needs (specify).

✔ Infant gains 20–30 gm per day after stabilization.

NOC: *Nutritional Status: Nutrient Intake*

INTERVENTIONS	RATIONALES
Weigh infant daily without diaper. Maintain strict hourly intake and output.	Daily weights indicate growth. After stabilization the infant should gain 20–30 g/day. Strict intake and output provides information about FVD or FVE.
Encourage mothers who want to breast-feed their babies. Provide information on pumping, freezing, and delivery of milk to the hospital.	The mother may need to pump her breasts to ensure milk supply for when the infant is able to breast-feed.
Decrease metabolic needs of infant: maintain neutral thermal environment, support oxygenation, decrease stimulation.	Increased metabolism requires ↑ calories and ↓ those available for growth.
Administer parenteral fluids and TPN as ordered (specify). Assess site and rate hourly.	Total parenteral nutrition (glucose, protein, electrolytes, vitamins and minerals) may be needed for extremely preterm infants or those who can't tolerate oral feeding. Complications include infiltration, FVE, and sepsis.
Monitor for complications of TPN (frequent blood glucose checks [specify frequency]; urine glucose, protein, and specific gravity q 8h).	TPN may result in complications such as hyperglycemia, osmotic diuresis and dehydration.
Observe for complications of intralipids (infiltration, ↑ temperature, vomiting, and dyspnea).	Intralipids (fatty acids) are also needed for nutrition and growth.
Assess infant's suck, swallow, and gag reflexes, and bowel sounds.	The infant needs a coordinated suck and swallow reflex, and an effective gag reflex in order to begin oral feeding. Bowel sounds indicate peristalsis.
Administer NG feedings if infant has a weak suck, swallow, and gag reflex, as ordered (specify: e.g., breast milk or ½ strength formula—Pregestimyl). Provide for nonnutritive sucking with a pacifier or hands.	Orogastric feeding provides adequate calories. Nonnutritive sucking may gain weight.
Initiate oral feedings as ordered (specify) if infant has a coordinated suck and swallow reflex. May need to use a nipple for preterm babies if bottle feeding.	When the infant is mature enough, oral feedings are begun. A preterm nipple has a larger hole and is easier to suck on.
Monitor for respiratory distress and fatigue with feeding. Combine oral and OG feedings as indicated by infant's response.	Monitoring provides information about infant's tolerance of feeding. Combined OG and oral nippling ensures adequate calories are obtained.

INTERVENTIONS	RATIONALES
Advance formula strength as tolerated per orders (specify).	Advancing the formula slowly ensures tolerance.
Monitor for complications of oral feeding: assess bowel sounds, measure gastric residual, observe for diarrhea, abdominal distention, occult blood in stools.	Monitoring for complications allows early identification and treatment. The preterm infant is at risk for NEC.
Refer mother to lactation specialist if needed. Praise the quality of the mother's milk and reinforce desirability to breast milk for the baby.	Referral assists the mother to initiate and maintain lactation. Providing milk is an important mothering activity and should be praised.

NIC: *Weight-Gain Assistance*

Evaluation

(Date/time of evaluation of goal)

(Has goal been met? not met? partially met?)

(How many calories is infant receiving? What is infant's weight gain (or loss) pattern?)

(Revisions to care plan? D/C care plan? Continue care plan?)

RISK FOR INJURY

Related to: Immature central nervous system: ↑ ICP, hypoxia, ↑ bilirubin, and stress.

Defining Characteristics: None, as this is a potential diagnosis.

Goal: Infant will not experience CNS injury by (date/ time to evaluate).

Outcome Criteria

✔ Infant does not exhibit any sign of seizures.

✔ Anterior fontanel is flat and soft.

NOC: *Safety Status: Physical Injury*

INTERVENTIONS	RATIONALES
Assess infant's prenatal and birth history for signs of fetal distress or perinatal hypoxia.	Hypoxic events ↑ blood flow to the CNS possibly causing rupture of fragile cerebral capillaries and hemorrhage (IVH).
Provide a neutral thermal environment.	Cold stress results in ↑ need for oxygen and a physiologic stress response.

INTERVENTIONS	RATIONALES
Maintain adequate oxygenation. Avoid rapid fluid administration.	Interventions prevent ↑ ICP or rapid changes in fluid volume that may rupture capillaries.
Suction infant infrequently and only as needed.	Suctioning increases ↓ ICP.
Position and turn infant with head in alignment with body and slightly elevated (15°–30°).	Elevation of head ↓ ICP, turning head to side ↑ ICP.
Monitor TPR and BP per protocol (specify frequency).	Hypotension, apnea and brady-cardia, temperature instability are signs of IVH.
Assess fontanels and head circum-ference (specify frequency).	Signs of IVH include bulging fontanels and increasing head circumference.
Continuously monitor infant for subtle changes in behavior: lethargy, hypotonia, apnea and bradycardia, signs of seizures.	Subtle behavioral changes may indicate IVH.
Monitor diagnostic studies as obtained (specify: e.g., ultra-sound of head).	Routine ultrasound of the head may be ordered within 48 hours to r/o IVH.
Monitor labs as obtained: Hct, blood glucose, calcium, electrolytes, and bilirubin levels.	Alterations in lab values may indicate that the infant is at ↑ risk for CNS damage. Preterm infants are at ↑ risk for kernicterus and brain damage at lower bilirubin levels than term infants.
Decrease stimulation by cluster-ing care and handling infant as little as possible. Decrease environmental stimuli (specify: e.g., noise, lights, movement, and people talking).	Overstimulation results in a physiologic stress response that ↑ BP, P, and ICP that may result in IVH. NICU environments may be brightly lit, noisy, and too stressful for the VLBW or ELBW infant.
Teach parents rationale for restrict-ing handling of infant. Promote gentle touch and comfort mea-sures. Teach parents to recognize when infant is overstimulated.	Parents may feel that they are being excluded from caring for their infant. Teaching helps parents make decisions about their infant.
Provide pacifier as indicated for comfort to prevent crying.	Crying ↑ ICP; a pacifier may be comforting for infant who can suck.
Provide pain medications as needed for procedures (specify drug, dose, route, and indication).	Pain and crying ↑ ICP and should be controlled to prevent IVH.
Administer other medications as ordered (specify: e.g., phenobar-bital, indomethacin, vitamin E, etc.).	Specify action of medications ordered (e.g., phenobarbital to control seizures, indomethacin to close PDA and facilitate oxygenation).

INTERVENTIONS	RATIONALES
Monitor infants who have had an IVH for development of hydrocephalus.	Infants who have experienced IVH are at ↑ risk for development of hydrocephalus within a month.

NIC: *Surveillance*

Evaluation

(Date/time of evaluation of goal)

(Has goal been met? not met? partially met?)

(Does infant exhibit signs of seizures? Is anterior fontanel soft and flat?)

(Revisions to care plan? D/C care plan? Continue care plan?)

 ## RISK FOR IMPAIRED SKIN INTEGRITY

Related to: Premature skin development: thin, fragile skin, ↓ subcutaneous fat; ↓ movement; substances applied to skin.

Defining Characteristics: None, as this is a potential diagnosis.

Goal: Infant will not experience break in skin integrity by (date/time to evaluate).

Outcome Criteria

✔ Infant's skin is intact without reddened or excori-ated areas.

NOC: *Risk Detection*

INTERVENTIONS	RATIONALES
Handle infant gently; do not pull or twist skin.	Preterm infant's skin is fragile and susceptible to injury.
Assess skin daily for impaired integrity: reddened areas, dry, cracked areas, or excoriation.	Assessment provides information about impaired skin integrity so treatment can begin early.
Position infant on a pressure-reducing mattress (fleece, flotation). Change position as tolerated.	The preterm infant has ↓ fat to pad bony areas. Position changes may be stressful to the VLBW or ELBW infant.

(continues)

(continued)

INTERVENTIONS	RATIONALES
Avoid use of tape on infant's skin. If necessary, use protective hydrocolloid barrier under tape.	Preterm infant's skin is thin and not securely attached to under-layers. Pulling on tape may tear the baby's skin. Barriers provide protection to the skin.
Apply barrier to areas of excori-ation and monitor healing. Allow barrier to peel off by itself, do not pull.	Barriers protect the skin, promote healing, and allow visualization of the area.
Use hydrogel electrodes. Rotate daily and inspect skin.	Standard electrodes may damage the infant's skin. Rotation and visualization decrease the poten-tial for skin impairment.
Provide mouth care and apply lubricant if needed for dry lips.	The infant's mouth may become dry and cracked.
Wash infant only as needed with warm water. Use mild soap on diaper area only if needed to remove feces.	The infant doesn't require daily bathing other than eyes, mouth, and diaper area. Soap is irritating and drying to the skin.
Apply oil or lubricant as ordered for dry skin after bathing.	Preterm infant's skin absorbs more substances than term infant's. Safflower oil may pro-vide the infant with additional fatty acids.

INTERVENTIONS	RATIONALES
Cover central line sites with transparent dressing and assess hourly. Change dressing per agency protocol.	Transparent dressings allow hourly assessment to prevent infection.
Ensure that alarms are turned on for warming devices.	Warming devices can burn the infant's delicate skin.
Evaluate the need before putting anything on the infant's skin (e.g., alcohol, tincture of benzoin, provodone iodine, etc.). Wash off after application.	The preterm infant's skin may absorb harmful substances or suffer a chemical burn from substances that are not harmful to mature skin. If the substance must be used, washing it off ↓ the chance of injury.

NIC: *Skin Surveillance*

Evaluation

(Date/time of evaluation of goal)

(Has goal been met? not met? partially met?)

(Is infant's skin intact without reddened or excoriated areas? Describe.)

(Revisions to care plan? D/C care plan? Continue care plan?)

RESPIRATORY DISTRESS SYNDROME (RDS)

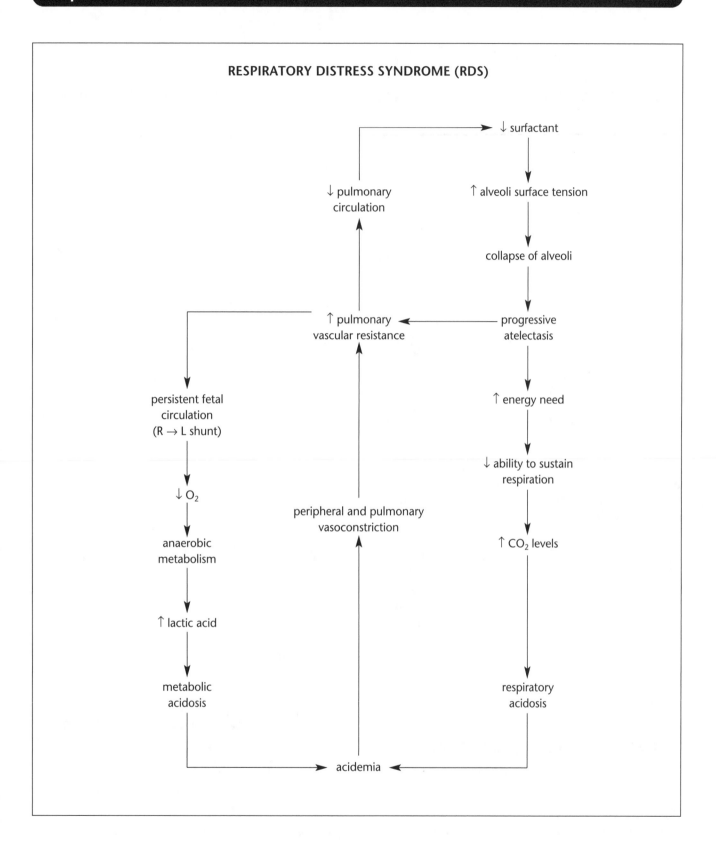

CHAPTER 4.9

HYPERBILIRUBINEMIA

Hyperbilirubinemia is defined as a serum bilirubin level greater than 12 mg/dL for a term neonate or more than 15 mg/dL for a preterm infant. Asian and Native American infants normally have higher bilirubin levels than Caucasian or African-American babies (up to 2 times as high).

Bilirubin is a by-product of red blood cell breakdown. It is normally conjugated in the liver and excreted through the feces and urine, giving them their characteristic color. When blood levels rise above approximately 5 mg/dL, bilirubin moves out of the blood causing jaundice (icterus), a yellow discoloration of the skin or sclera. Higher levels may result in bilirubin deposits in the brain, a condition known as kernicterus. Neurologic consequences of kernicterus may include: seizures, ADHD, cerebral palsy, and mental retardation. Kernicterus may result from bilirubin levels >20 mg/dL in a term infant or as low as 12 mg/dL in a compromised preterm baby. Jaundice is defined as either pathologic or physiologic.

PATHOLOGIC JAUNDICE

- Cause: excessive RBC destruction resulting from Rh or ABO incompatibility (hemolytic disease) infection, polycythemia, cephalhematoma, acidosis, and hypoglycemia
- Jaundice occurs within the first 24 hours of life
- Bilirubin rises more than 5 mg/dL/day
- Bilirubin levels exceed 12 mg/dL

PHYSIOLOGIC JAUNDICE

- Cause: normal RBC breakdown, liver immaturity, and lack of intestinal bacteria
- 50% of term and 80% of preterm neonates
- Jaundice begins after 24 hours (term) or 48 hours (preterm)
- Disappears by 7–10 days

- Bilirubin does not rise more than 5 mg/dL per day
- Bilirubin levels do not exceed 13 mg/dL
- Breast-feeding and/or breast milk jaundice begins 3–5 days after birth and may persist up to 6 weeks

BILIRUBIN AND JAUNDICE

Cephalocaudal progression of jaundice may be used to roughly estimate the level of bilirubinemia.

- 0.2–1.4 mg/dL—normal level, no jaundice
- 3 mg/dL—jaundice of nose only
- 5 mg/dL—jaundice of whole face
- 7 mg/dL—jaundice over chest
- 10 mg/dL—jaundice over abdomen
- 12 mg/dL—jaundice of legs
- 20 mg/dL—jaundice of soles/palms

MEDICAL CARE

- Early feeding, frequent breast-feeding
- Lab work: Hgb, Hct, serum bilirubin, total protein, direct and indirect Coombs, reticulocyte counts
- Transcutaneous bilirubin meter
- Phototherapy
- Exchange transfusion

COMMON NURSING DIAGNOSES

 See INTERRUPTED BREAST-FEEDING

Related to: Excessive bilirubin levels secondary to breast milk jaundice.

Defining Characteristics: Physiologic jaundice beginning at 4–5 days (specify infant's age and bilirubin level). Bilirubin level exceeds 15 mg/dL, mother is instructed to interrupt breast-feeding for 24 hours, pump breasts, and resume nursing as desired when bilirubin levels fall.

ADDITIONAL NURSING DIAGNOSES

RISK FOR INJURY

Related to: Increased blood levels of unconjugated bilirubin; effects of phototherapy; effects of exchange transfusion.

Defining Characteristics: None, as this is a potential diagnosis.

Goal: Infant will not experience injury by (date/time to evaluate).

Outcome Criteria

✔ Infant's bilirubin levels are less than (specify for individual infant).

✔ Infant does not exhibit signs of neurologic injury: irritability, lethargy, rigidity, opisthotonos, or seizures.

✔ Infant's temperature remains between 36.5–37° C (97.7–98.6° F), heart rate between 110–160, respirations between 30–60.

NOC: *Neurologic Status*

INTERVENTIONS	RATIONALES
Review prenatal and labor and delivery summary for infant risk factors for hyperbilirubinemia (e.g., hemolytic disease, preterm, infection, hypoglycemia, etc.).	Review provides information about infants at high risk for pathologic hyperbilirubinemia (e.g., Rh or ABO incompatibility, infection, cephalhematoma, excessive bruising or petechiae, etc.).
Assess infant for jaundice by pressing skin over a bony area and releasing. Assess in natural light moving from head to soles of feet, including mucous membranes and sclera (specify frequency: e.g., q shift). Assess transcutaneous bilirubin levels as indicated.	Jaundice progresses in a cephalo-caudal direction. Artificial light may mask the beginning of jaundice. Transcutaneous monitoring is a noninvasive method of determining bilirubin levels.
Notify caregiver if jaundice is noted within the first 24 hours, or if jaundice extends to the infant's legs, increases by more than 5 mg/dL in one day, or reaches 12 mg/dL.	Pathologic jaundice that may lead to kernicterus begins within the first 24 hours with bilirubin levels rising to >13 mg/dL and increasing ≥5 mg/dL/day. Phototherapy light will degrade sample.

INTERVENTIONS	RATIONALES
Monitor serum bilirubin levels as obtained (specify frequency). If infant is receiving phototherapy, protect blood specimen from light. Monitor other lab work as obtained (e.g., Hgb, Hct, platelets, total protein, serum glucose, etc.).	Monitoring provides information about factors contributing to the hyperbilirubinemia.
Observe infant for subtle signs of neurologic injury: changes in behavior, lethargy, irritability, rigidity, opisthotonos, or seizure activity. Notify caregiver.	Changes may be subtle. There is no specific blood level that signals beginning risk for kernicterus. Preterm or compromised neonates may be affected at lower levels than healthy term infants.
Explain the etiology and significance of hyperbilirubinemia to family. Teach them about the process and goals of therapy (specify: e.g., phototherapy, exchange transfusion).	Explanations assist the family to understand the therapy. Ultraviolet light changes unconjugated bilirubin into a water-soluble form (lumirubin) for easier excretion.
Administer prescribed phototherapy. If infant is to be under bili lights, cover infant's closed eyes with appropriate shield applied to prevent slipping. Place shield over testes per protocol. Place nude infant on diaper under light source (specify type and safety precautions: e.g., distance of light) and turn every 1–2 hours.	Eye shields protect the retina from injury from ultraviolet light. Covering testes may protect them from injury. Turning the nude infant frequently allows greater skin exposure to the light.
Monitor infant's temperature and temperature of isolette (specify frequency).	Exposing the infant may result in hypothermia. Heat from phototherapy lights may cause hyperthermia.
Provide phototherapy with a fiberoptic bilirubin blanket if available.	Bilirubin blankets promote warmth and provide a light source without the need for eye shields. Parents may interact more with their baby.
Provide meticulous skin care to perianal area after each stool. Assess skin q 2 hours. Do not use oil-based products on infant's skin during therapy.	Frequent loose greenish bowel movements are a common effect of phototherapy. Skin care prevents injury. Oil-based products may cause burns.
Remove infant from lights for feedings and parent–infant interaction. Remove patches and assess eyes for injury or drainage.	Isolation during phototherapy may interfere with parent–infant bonding. Frequent eye assessments help detect injury from light or incorrect eye shield application.

(continues)

(continued)

INTERVENTIONS	RATIONALES
For infant who is to receive exchange transfusion, ensure NPO status (specify time frame: e.g., 2–4 hours). Check resuscitation equipment and place at bedside. Place infant under a radiant warmer with temperature probe in place for procedure.	Infants experiencing pathologic hyperbilirubinemia from hemolytic disease may require exchange transfusion. NPO status and emergency equipment at bedside ensure rapid resuscitation if a sensitivity reaction occurs. The infant is under a radiant heat source to prevent complications from cold stress.
Check blood per agency policy (specify). Warm blood as indicated. Monitor vital signs and observe for signs of transfusion reaction before, during, and after exchange transfusion.	Interventions ensure that the correct blood is given to the infant. The blood should be warmed in a blood warmer to protect the RBCs. Close monitoring identifies early signs of transfusion reactions or infant intolerance.
Assist caregiver as needed. Document amounts of blood removed and infused and infant's tolerance of procedure.	Assistance may be needed to perform transfusion smoothly. Documentation details the amounts given and withdrawn and infant's response.
Observe cord for signs of bleeding after procedure and monitor infant for therapeutic or adverse effects.	Observation provides information about hemostasis, improvement of condition, or complications.

NIC: *Surveillance*

Evaluation

(Date/time of evaluation of goal)

(Has goal been met? not met? partially met?)

(What is infant's bilirubin level? Does infant exhibit signs of neurologic injury: irritability, lethargy, rigidity, opisthotonos, or seizures? What is infant's temperature? What are the infant's heart rate and respirations?)

(Revisions to care plan? D/C care plan? Continue care plan?)

 ## RISK FOR DEFICIENT FLUID VOLUME

Related to: Increased losses from evaporation, and frequent loose bowel movements. Decreased intake secondary to the effects of phototherapy.

Defining Characteristics: None, as this is a potential diagnosis.

Goal: Infant will maintain adequate fluid balance during phototherapy (specify date/time to evaluate).

Outcome Criteria

✔ Infant will have at least 6 wet diapers/day.

✔ Infant's skin turgor will be elastic, anterior fontanel soft and flat, and mucous membranes moist.

NOC: *Fluid Balance*

INTERVENTIONS	RATIONALES
Monitor daily weight.	Monitoring weight provides information about excessive fluid losses.
Assess infant's hourly intake and output (weigh diapers, 1 gm = 1 cc).	Assessment of intake and output provides information about fluid balance. Infant should have output of 1–2 cc/kg/hour.
Monitor number, color, and consistency of bowel movements.	Phototherapy may result in fluid loss from frequent loose stools. Monitoring provides information about losses.
Assess urine specific gravity (specify frequency).	Specific gravity provides information about fluid balance. High sp. gravity (>1.030) indicates dehydration, low (>1.010) indicates fluid overload.
Assess skin turgor, mucous membranes, and anterior fontanel q 2 hours.	Assessment provides information about dehydration of tissues: skin turgor, dry mucous membranes, and sunken anterior fontanel.
Notify caregiver of signs of dehydration.	Caregiver may initiate IV fluids if p.o. intake is insufficient to meet fluid needs.
Provide additional fluids during phototherapy (specify: e.g., 25% more formula with more frequent feedings; breast-feed q 2–3 hours; additional water as ordered).	Additional fluids are necessary to balance the losses from therapy. Phototherapy may result in increased fluid losses through the skin, urine, and loose bowel movements.
Show parents how to assess skin turgor, mucous membranes, and fontanel for signs of dehydration. Teach them that the infant should have 6 to 8 wet diapers daily.	Explanations and teaching assist parents to care for their infant after discharge and seek medical treatment for dehydration.
Initiate and maintain IV fluids as ordered (specify: fluid, rate, site).	IV fluids may be required to maintain fluid balance or venous access if infant is to have an exchange transfusion.

INTERVENTIONS	RATIONALES
Assess IV site hourly for rate, color, temperature, and edema.	Assessment provides information about complications of IV therapy: infiltration, infection, or incorrect rate.
Monitor lab values as obtained (specify: e.g., Hct, electrolytes, etc.).	Lab values indicate fluid and electrolyte balance or imbalance.

NIC: *Fluid Management*

Evaluation

(Date/time of evaluation of goal)

(Has goal been met? not met? partially met?)

(How many wet diapers has infant had? Describe skin turgor, mucous membranes, and anterior fontanel.)

(Revisions to care plan? D/C care plan? Continue care plan?)

INTERRUPTED FAMILY PROCESSES

Related to: Disruption of family bonding and attachment with infant caused by treatment restrictions.

Defining Characteristics: Family system cannot interact effectively with infant during phototherapy (specify: e.g., infant under bili-lights except for feeding, mother discharged before infant, etc.). (Specify others: e.g., mother doesn't come to visit infant, parents don't talk to each other, mother is crying, etc.)

Goal: Family will adapt to disruption caused by treatments by (date/time to evaluate).

Outcome Criteria

✔ The family will verbalize feelings associated with disruption of interaction.

✔ Family will maintain a functional process of support for one another.

NOC: *Parent–Infant Attachment*

INTERVENTIONS	RATIONALES
Assess family members' interaction with each other and infant.	Assessment provides information about family processes.

INTERVENTIONS	RATIONALES
Encourage family to talk about their experience regarding infant's treatments. Elicit feelings (e.g., fear, guilt, or isolation). Discuss financial concerns as needed.	Encouragement helps the family to identify and verbalize feelings and concerns. The family may be worried about ability to pay for extra hospital days.
Acknowledge family's feelings and concerns. Assist family to resolve feelings and fears with accurate information.	Acknowledgment indicates respect and validation for family's experience. Providing accurate information decreases fear of the unknown.
Teach family about the usually benign nature of infant's condition as indicated. Explain pathophysiology and treatment rationales on a level they can understand.	Teaching reinforces family's understanding of the condition and treatment. Allays anxiety.
Remove infant from under lights and remove eye shields when family visits. Encourage attachment and bonding activities. Praise parents for interaction and note infant's responses to them.	Interventions promote family-infant attachment and bonding. Eye contact is important for both baby and parents. Praise reinforces positive behaviors.
Promote family cohesiveness by encouraging discussion and problem solving with input from all members.	Encouraging the family to work with each other to solve problems promotes effective family processes.
Help family to identify options and make choices as needed (specify: e.g., who cares for the home and other children, is home therapy an option, etc.).	Assistance helps the family move from feelings to planning solutions to their identified problems.
Refer family as indicated (specify: e.g., social services for financial problems; counseling for dysfunctional communication patterns, etc.).	Referral may be indicated for financial concerns or severely disrupted family processes.

NIC: *Family Integrity Promotion*

Evaluation

(Date/time of evaluation of goal)

(Has goal been met? not met? partially met?)

(Specify feelings family verbalized. Describe how family supports one another and decisions they have made to maintain functionality as a family.)

(Revisions to care plan? D/C care plan? Continue care plan?)

HYPERBILIRUBINEMIA

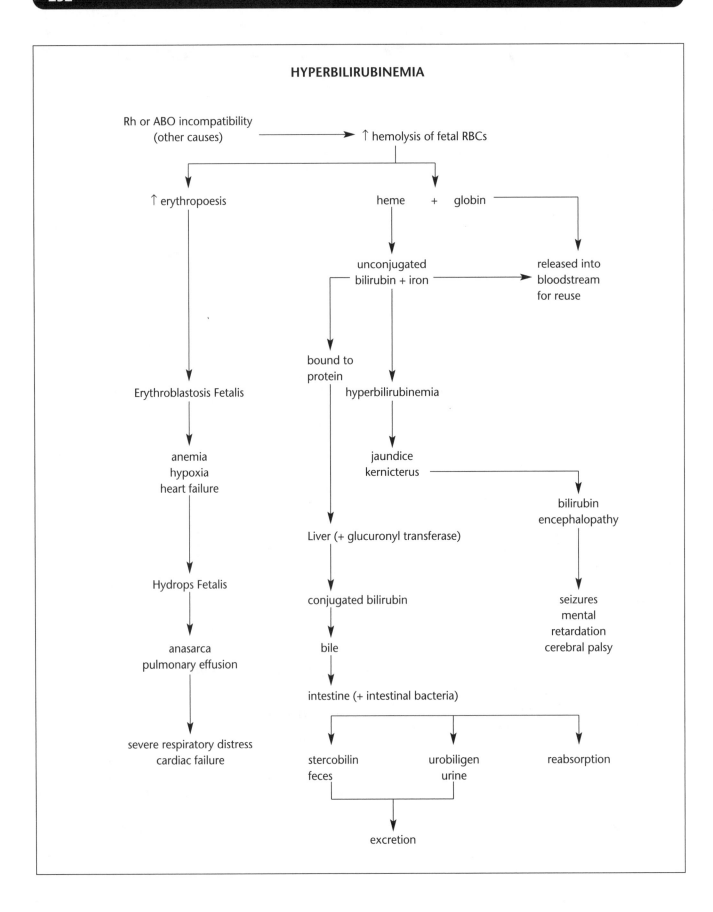

CHAPTER 4.10

HYPOGLYCEMIA

Neonatal hypoglycemia is defined as a blood glucose level below 40 mg/dL in the first 24 hours of life and less than 45–50 mg/dL thereafter. The full-term newborn is supplied with adequate glycogen stores for the first few days of life until oral feeding is well-established. Stressors, such as cold stress or respiratory distress, increase neonatal metabolism and may quickly deplete these stores leaving the infant at risk for hypoglycemia. Infants of diabetic mothers may exhibit hypoglycemia secondary to development of hyperinsulinism in utero. The SGA or preterm AGA infant may not have adequate glycogen stores to prevent transient hypoglycemia after birth.

Signs and symptoms of hypoglycemia are vague and mainly related to CNS glucose deprivation. They include: jitteriness, weak or high-pitched cry, poor tone, apnea, poor feeding, cyanosis, and possible seizure activity. Whenever a newborn's behavior is unusual, a blood glucose level should be obtained as continued hypoglycemia may result in brain damage.

MEDICAL CARE

- Early feeding of all newborns
- Prevention of respiratory distress, cold stress
- Frequent blood glucose monitoring for at-risk newborns: LGA, SGA, preterm, infants of diabetic mothers, and any infant exhibiting signs and symptoms of hypoglycemia
- Laboratory corroboration of bedside glucose monitoring results
- Intravenous glucose (5–10%) based on body weight if necessary

COMMON NURSING DIAGNOSES

See RISK FOR INJURY

Related to: Insufficient CNS glucose level secondary to (specify: e.g., IUGR, IDM, cold stress, etc.).

See ANXIETY (PARENTAL)

Related to: Perceived threat to well-being of newborn.

Defining Characteristics: (Specify for client: e.g., mother states she is "worried," father is pacing at nursery window, etc.).

ADDITIONAL NURSING DIAGNOSES

IMBALANCED NUTRITION: LESS THAN BODY REQUIREMENTS

Related to: (Specify: e.g., increased caloric requirements and inadequate intake, inadequate stores, difficulty obtaining nutrients, etc.).

Defining Characteristics: (Specify blood glucose levels, infant's symptoms such as jitteriness, apnea, etc.).

Goal: Infant will obtain adequate calories for metabolic needs by (date and time to evaluate).

Outcome Criteria

✔ Blood glucose level will be >40 mg/dL in first 24 hours and 45 mg/dL thereafter.
✔ Infant will not exhibit symptoms of hypoglycemia (specify related to what infant had been displaying, e.g., jitters, tremors, etc.)

NOC: *Nutritional Status: Nutrient Intake*

INTERVENTIONS	RATIONALES
Encourage initiation of feeding as soon as possible after birth for all infants. Breast feeding may begin immediately; bottle feed first with water when the infant shows signs of readiness (rooting, suck, swallow reflexes, bowel sounds) followed by formula per protocol.	Early feeding provides nutrients to replace energy stores used during labor and birth. Colostrum contains glucose and is nonirritating if aspirated. First water ensures patency of GI tract before formula is given.

(continues)

(continued)

INTERVENTIONS	RATIONALES
Provide a neutral thermal environment and prevent unnecessary stress for all neonates.	Cold and stress cause the newborn to increase metabolism and rapidly use up energy stores.
Assess blood glucose by heel-stick per protocol and confirm findings with laboratory testing as ordered (specify: e.g., for all LGA, SGA, preterm or symptomatic infants: perform heel-stick glucose at birth and 2 hours, etc.).	Assessment provides information about newborn's glucose levels. Laboratory glucose testing may be more accurate than bedside monitoring.
Feed infants per order if heel-stick glucose is <40 mg/dL. Reevaluate blood glucose level within 30–60 minutes as ordered.	Oral feedings replenish low glucose levels. Testing confirms expected result.
Administer intravenous glucose if ordered (specify strength, amount, rate, etc.) into large peripheral vein via a pump. Do not increase rate to catch up IV.	Glucose may be irritating to small vessels. A pump ensures that the correct amount is given and helps prevent fluid overload or hyperglycemia.
Monitor strict I&O for infants receiving intravenous fluids.	Monitoring helps prevent fluid overload and ensures client receives correct dose.
Discontinue IV glucose slowly and monitor blood glucose levels per protocol.	Tapering glucose slowly prevents hypoglycemia from increased insulin production.
Monitor infants for signs of continued hypoglycemia: jitteriness, apnea, poor feeding, weak cry, poor tone, or cyanosis. Reassess blood glucose levels as needed.	Vague indications of hypoglycemia are confirmed by blood testing.
Teach family about the client's condition, suspected etiology, and treatment (specify for individual client). Allow time for questions and offer support.	Teaching and support encourage the family to participate in the client's care.

NIC: *Nutrition Management*

Evaluation

(Date/time of evaluation of goal)

(Was goal met? Not met? Partially met?)

(What is infant's blood glucose level?)

(Describe infant's behavior relative to previous symptoms of hypoglycemia)

 PAIN

Related to: Frequent heel-sticks.

Defining Characteristics: (Specify for infant: e.g., cries; pulls away; heels are bruised, etc.)

Goal: Infant will experience less pain.

Outcome Criteria

✔ Infant will not cry during procedure.

✔ Infant's heel will not be bruised.

NOC: *Pain Control*

INTERVENTIONS	RATIONALES
Assess infant's heels for signs of injury and avoid additional heel sticks in bruised areas.	Assessment provides information about current injuries.
Apply anesthetic cream to site at least 60 minutes before puncture.	Specify action of drug, time is necessary for topical anesthetic action.
Warm the infant's heel for 5–10 minutes before heel-stick.	Warmth dilates blood vessels so a larger sample may be obtained with less trauma.
Provide a pacifier or other non-pharmacologic method of comfort as needed.	Nonnutritive sucking is comforting to some infants.
Wear gloves. Wipe the area with alcohol and pat it to dry with gauze. Stabilize the infant's foot and puncture the foot on the side of the heel. Obtain blood sample.	Gloves protect the nurse from becoming contaminated with blood. Stabilization prevents movement and allows a careful procedure. Using the side of the heel avoids arteries and nerves in the foot.
Use an automatic heel-stick device rather than a lancet.	Automatic devices are less painful and limit the depth of the puncture.
Apply pressure with gauze over area and a Band-Aid if necessary.	Pressure decreases bleeding. Band-Aids can cause pain when being removed.
Swaddle the infant and take him to his mother if appropriate.	Swaddling and maternal presence promotes comfort for neonates.
Coordinate care and testing to avoid unnecessary heel-sticks.	Obtaining several lab values at once decreases the pain and injury of additional heel-sticks.

NIC: *Pain Management*

Evaluation

(Date/time of evaluation of goal)

(Was goal met? Not met? Partially met?)

(Did infant cry during procedure?)

(Is infant's heel bruised?)

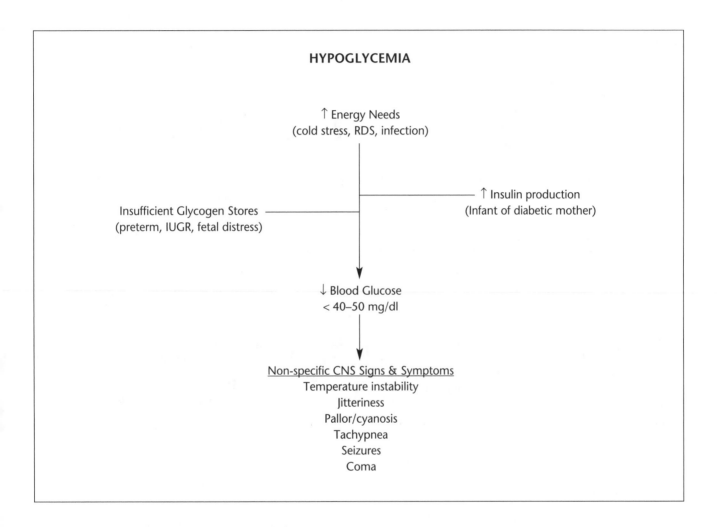

HYPOGLYCEMIA

↑ Energy Needs
(cold stress, RDS, infection)

↑ Insulin production
(Infant of diabetic mother)

Insufficient Glycogen Stores
(preterm, IUGR, fetal distress)

↓ Blood Glucose
< 40–50 mg/dl

Non-specific CNS Signs & Symptoms
Temperature instability
Jitteriness
Pallor/cyanosis
Tachypnea
Seizures
Coma

CHAPTER 4.11

NEONATAL SEPSIS

The newborn is at increased risk for serious infection because of decreased immunity, ineffective leukocytes, and a poorly defined inflammatory response. Maternal immunoglobulin G (IgG) crosses the placenta mainly during the last few weeks of pregnancy and provides protection against some bacteria. Preterm infants do not receive this benefit. Breast-feeding provides immunoglobulin A (IgA) and other substances that protect the newborn from infection.

CAUSES

- Prenatal exposure may be transplacental (rubella, CMV, HIV, syphilis, etc.) or from ascending chorioamnionitis caused by bacteria associated with prolonged SROM.
- During labor and birth, the infant may be exposed to pathogens such as group B ß-hemolytic streptococcus, gonorrhea, herpesvirus, Chlamydia, hepatitis B, and HIV from the mother's reproductive tract.
- External exposure at birth may include staphylococci or enterococci.
- Nosocomial infections most frequently include staphylococcus, enterococci, Klebsiella, or Pseudomonas.

SIGNS AND SYMPTOMS

- Vague, nonspecific changes; infant doesn't "look right"
- Hypothermia, temperature instability
- Poor feeding, abdominal distension
- Hypoglycemia
- Hypotonia, ↓ activity
- Poor perfusion: pallor, mottling, cyanosis

- Signs of respiratory distress (ß-strep)
- Seizure activity

MEDICAL CARE

- Cultures and sensitivity: blood × 2, CSF, urine
- CBC with diff, CRP, blood glucose, ABGs, electrolytes, chest X-ray
- Antibiotics × 2 started before culture results; continue for 1 to 3 weeks if cultures are positive (appropriate drugs), 3 to 5 days if no growth
- Supportive care: IVF, oxygen, ventilation
- Observe for complications: DIC, meningitis

COMMON NURSING DIAGNOSES

 ### See INEFFECTIVE THERMOREGULATION

Related to: Nonspecific effects of infection on neonate.

Defining Characteristics: Specify fluctuations of temperature and use of warming devices.

 ### See RISK FOR DEFICIENT FLUID VOLUME

Related to: Decreased intake secondary to poor feeding.

 ### See RISK FOR IMPAIRED PARENT–INFANT ATTACHMENT

Related to: Separation of mother and infant secondary to need for neonatal intensive care.

ADDITIONAL NURSING DIAGNOSES

RISK FOR INFECTION

Related to: Spread of pathogens secondary to identified sepsis and an immature immune system (specify others: e.g., portal of entry: UAC).

Defining Characteristics: None, as this is a potential diagnosis.

Goal: Infant will not experience spread of infection by (date/time to evaluate).

Outcome Criteria

✔ Infant's heart rate remains <160 (specify range for infant).

✔ Respiratory rate <60 (specify range).

✔ Anterior fontanel is soft and flat.

NOC: *Risk Control*

INTERVENTIONS	RATIONALES
Ensure that all people coming in contact with infant wash their hands well before and after touching the baby.	Hand washing prevents the spread of pathogens from person to person.
Ensure that all equipment used for infant is sterile, scrupulously clean, or disposable. Do not share equipment with other infants.	Interventions prevent the spread of pathogens to the infant from equipment.
Place infant in isolette/isolation room per hospital policy (specify for agency).	Placing the infant in an isolette allows close observation of the ill neonate and protects other infants from infection.
Maintain a neutral thermal environment.	A neutral thermal environment decreases the metabolic needs of the infant. The ill neonate has difficulty maintaining a stable temperature.
Assess TPR and BP, auscultate breath sounds (specify frequency).	Assessments provide information about the spread of infection. ↑ heart rate and respirations, ↓ BP are signs of sepsis. Spread of infection may cause respiratory distress.
Assess anterior fontanel (specify frequency) and continually observe infant for changes in activity or behaviors (e.g.,	Assessment provides information about possible spread of infection to the CNS: signs of meningitis.

INTERVENTIONS	RATIONALES
feeding, sleeping, jitteriness or seizure activity, etc.).	
Provide respiratory support as indicated (specify: e.g., oxyhood, ventilator, etc.).	Respiratory support may be needed during the acute phase of infection to prevent additional physiologic stress.
Feed infant as ordered (specify: e.g., breast, formula, OG feedings, or TPN). Provide for nonnutritive sucking if unable to breast- or bottle feed.	Nutritional needs may increase during infection while the infant may feed poorly. OG feedings or TPN ensure that nutrient needs are met if the infant is too ill to suck effectively.
Administer IV fluids as ordered via an infusion pump (specify: fluids, rate, site). Assess rate and site q hour.	IV fluids help maintain fluid balance. An infusion pump, hourly I&O, and site assessment help prevent complications of therapy: FVE, infiltration, and infection.
Administer antibiotics per order (specify, drugs, doses, routes and method [e.g., syringe pump], and times). Observe for adverse effects (specify for each drug).	(Specify action of each drug. Specify adverse effects.)
Monitor lab results as obtained (culture reports, CBC, differ-, ential CRP, electrolytes, drug peak and trough, etc.). Notify caregiver of abnormal findings.	Lab results provide information about the pathogen and infant's response to illness and treatment.
Assess hourly intake and output and daily weight. Assess urine specific gravity q 8 hours.	Interventions provide information about infant's fluid balance.
Monitor infant for hypoglycemia, jaundice, development of thrush, or signs of bleeding (petechiae, occult blood in stools).	Assessments provide information about development of complications of infection: hypoglycemia, hyperbilirubinemia, opportunistic infections, and coagulation deficits/DIC.
Teach parents effective hand-washing techniques. Encourage participation in caring for their infant.	Teaching parents helps prevent the spread of infection during hospitalization and at home. Participation in care promotes bonding and development of the parenting role.

NIC: *Infection Prevention*

Evaluation

(Date/time of evaluation of goal)

(Has goal been met? not met? partially met?)

(What is infant's heart rate? respiratory rate? Is anterior fontanel flat and soft?)

(Revisions to care plan? D/C care plan? Continue care plan?)

NEONATAL SEPSIS

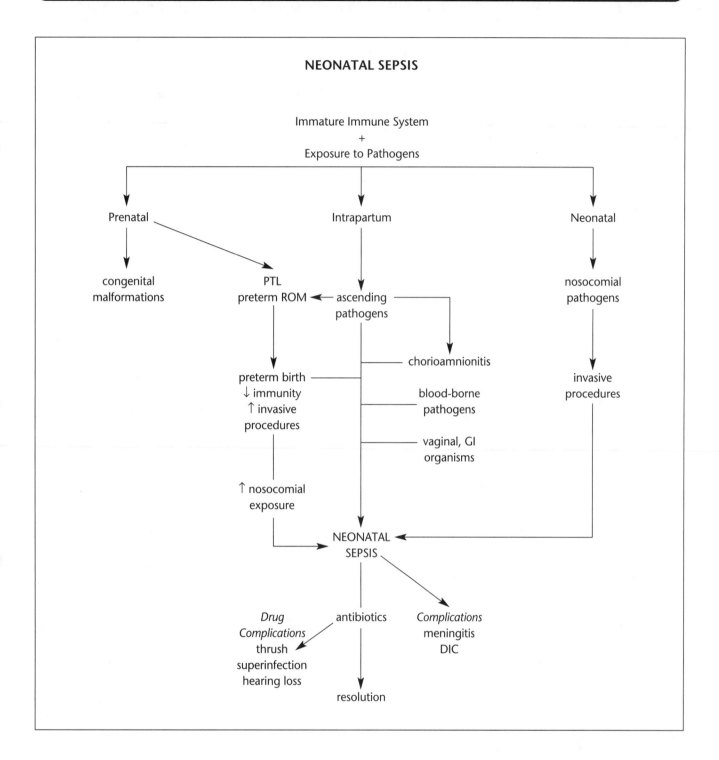

CHAPTER 4.12

NEONATAL HIV/AIDS

Human immunodeficiency virus, type 1 (HIV-1) is the causative organism for AIDS (acquired immunodeficiency syndrome). The HIV retrovirus replicates in the nucleus of T-4 helper lymphocytes (identified by the CD4 surface antigen), causing premature death of those cells. This results in a profound depression of cell-mediated immunity in the host. The body is eventually overwhelmed by opportunistic infections. The virus is transmitted by direct contact with infected blood or body fluids.

There are three perinatal modes of transmission for HIV. The fetus may be infected across the placenta during pregnancy, the neonate may acquire the virus during birth from exposure to maternal blood and body fluids, or HIV virus in the breast milk may infect the infant. The infant infected in utero has a poor prognosis. One goal of nursing care is to prevent the last two modes of transmission.

Newborns of HIV positive mothers will also test positive at birth because of the HIV antibodies received passively from the mother during the last few weeks of pregnancy. Approximately one-third of these infants will actually be infected with the virus. Additional testing is needed to determine which infants have acquired the virus and which have not. The polymerase chain reaction and HIV culture tests may provide a diagnosis as early as 4 to 6 months of age while maternal antibodies are still present for 15 to 18 months (basis of ELISA and Western blot tests). Most infants will be asymptomatic at birth.

SIGNS AND SYMPTOMS

- Possible craniofacial malformations if congenital infection
- Enlargement of liver and spleen
- Swollen lymph glands
- Failure to thrive, poor feeding, diarrhea

- Rash, cough, signs of pneumonia (*Pneumocystis carinii*, interstitial pneumonitis)
- Neurologic or developmental deficits

MEDICAL CARE

- Maternal antiviral drug: zidovudine (ZDT) during the last two trimesters of pregnancy and during labor and delivery
- Avoidance of an episiotomy or other actions creating excess bleeding during birth, careful suctioning of infant at birth, bathing of infant before any injections or invasive procedures, formula feeding
- Laboratory testing: urine screening, baseline immunological tests
- Frequent pediatric follow-up visits; testing for HIV infection
- Prophylactic drugs: infant is started on zidovudine, trimethoprim–sulfamethoxazole (to prevent *Pneumocystis carinii* pneumonia), and monthly doses of gamma globulin IV while diagnostic tests are being done

COMMON NURSING DIAGNOSES

 See RISK FOR DEFICIENT FLUID VOLUME

Related to: Decreased intake secondary to poor feeding. Increased fluid loss secondary to loose stools/diarrhea.

ADDITIONAL NURSING DIAGNOSES

 RISK FOR INFECTION

Related to: Immature immunologic system. Possible exposure to maternal infected blood and body fluids

(HIV, Hepatitis B). Possible immune suppression secondary to transplacental HIV infection.

Defining Characteristics: None, as this is a potential diagnosis.

Goal: Infant will not experience neonatal infection by (date/time to evaluate).

Outcome Criteria

✔ Infant receives prophylaxis (specify: e.g., gamma globulin).

✔ Infant appears free of opportunistic infection: temperature is stable between 36.5 and 37° C (97.7–98.6° F), no respiratory distress, abdomen is soft and nondistended without hepatosplenomegaly.

NOC: *Risk Control*

INTERVENTIONS	RATIONALES
Use Standard Precautions (formerly Universal Precautions) when caring for all clients. Wear gloves, gowns, and eye shields as needed to prevent exposure to blood or body fluids. Dispose of potentially infectious items (diapers, wipes, etc.) per agency policy (specify: e.g., hazardous waste containers, red bags, etc.).	Standard Precautions are implemented to avoid caregiver exposure to blood-borne pathogens such as HIV or hepatitis B viruses.
Identify mothers at risk as well as those with confirmed HIV or hepatitis B infection. Avoid invasive procedures during labor and birth (e.g., fetal scalp electrode, IUPC, episiotomy, or operative delivery).	Risk factors may include IV drug abuse, multiple sexual partners, history of multiple STDs, or blood transfusion before 1985. Invasive procedures during labor may infect the fetus.
Suction infant well at birth with bulb syringe or wall suction device. Do not use mouth suction devices.	Suctioning removes infected maternal secretions. Mouth suction devices create risk of exposure for caregiver.
Provide routine newborn care: dry infant well to remove all blood and body fluids.	The infant requires the same care as any newborn: thermoregulation, and so forth. Drying the infant carefully helps remove maternal blood and body fluid from the infant's skin.
Delay eye prophylaxis, injections or other invasive procedures until after the first bath.	Delay helps avoid transmission of the virus from the infant's skin into the body.

INTERVENTIONS	RATIONALES
Bathe infant thoroughly as soon as possible after initial assessment. Return to warmer until temperature is stabilized.	Early and thorough bathing removes maternal blood and body fluids from infant's skin. Infants bathed soon after birth regain temperature stability as well as those bathed later.
Wash skin with soap and water before injections or heel sticks.	Additional washing helps prevent exposure from skin during invasive procedures.
Label all specimens and notify lab of infant's HIV exposure per protocol. Monitor lab results.	Interventions help prevent exposure of laboratory personnel to potentially infected specimens.
Monitor infant for signs of opportunistic infection: temperature instability, respiratory distress, abdominal distension, hepatosplenomegaly, enlarged lymph glands, activity, seizures, jaundice, petechiae, skin lesions, candidiasis (thrush), or chorioretinitis.	Monitoring provides information about early signs and symptoms of opportunistic infection.
Isolate infant if indicated by presence of infection (specify: e.g., CMV, enteric infection, etc.).	Isolation prevents transmission of infection to other infants in the nursery.
Administer prophylactic medications as ordered (specify: e.g., immune globulin for infants of hepatitis B infected mothers).	(Specify action of prophylactic medication.)
Teach mother to wash her hands before caring for infant and to avoid exposing the infant to visitors with infections.	Washing hands help prevent transmission of the virus from the mother to the infant. The infant may already be HIV infected and immune suppressed at birth.
Teach mother that she will need to bottle feed her baby. Provide assistance as needed.	HIV may be transmitted through breast milk. Instruction helps the mother provide optimum nutrition for her baby.
Teach family about HIV testing and prophylactic medications that will be provided for the infant.	Instruction ensures that family understands the delay in diagnosing whether the infant is infected or not and those medications will be given until then.
Instruct family in Standard Precautions to use when caring for infant (specify: e.g., wash hands before and after care, avoid contact with wet diapers, etc.). Verify understanding.	Standard Precautions help prevent transmission of the virus from the infant to family members. Routine infant care using standard precautions is unlikely to cause infection.

(continues)

(continued)

INTERVENTIONS	RATIONALES
Make appointments for follow-up care before discharge. Instruct family to monitor the infant for signs of infection and to call the caregiver. Provide phone numbers.	Making appointments ensures follow-up care. The infant will need to be seen more frequently. Information and phone numbers help the family to provide care for the infant.

NIC: *Infection Prevention*

Evaluation

(Date/time of evaluation of goal)

(Has goal been met? not met? partially met?)

(Did infant receive appropriate prophylaxis? Specify drug, dose, route, and time. Is infant free of signs of infection? Describe temperature ranges, respiratory and abdominal status.)

(Revisions to care plan? D/C care plan? Continue care plan?)

RISK FOR IMBALANCED NUTRITION: LESS THAN BODY REQUIREMENTS

Related to: Feeding intolerance secondary to infectious processes. Inadequate absorption of nutrients secondary to diarrhea.

Defining Characteristics: None, as this is a potential diagnosis.

Goal: Infant will obtain adequate nutrition for body requirements by (date/time to evaluate).

Outcome Criteria

✔ Infant will lose no more than 10% of birth weight (specify for infant).

✔ Infant will ingest adequate formula to meet body needs (specify calories and ounces of formula needed each day).

NOC: *Nutritional Status*

INTERVENTIONS	RATIONALES
Weigh infant at birth and each day without diaper or clothing. Cover scale with blanket and zero before weighing. Protect from falls without touching infant. Compare to previous weights.	Daily weights provide information about infant's weight loss or gain.

INTERVENTIONS	RATIONALES
Assess infant's suck reflex during initial assessment. Inspect oral cavity for signs of thrush (white patches) and notify caregiver.	Assessment provides information about infant reflex needed for successful feeding. The HIV positive infant is at risk for opportunistic infection such as thrush.
Administer medications as ordered (specify: e.g., Nystatin for thrush).	(Specify action of drugs that are ordered.)
Assess infant for first stool and urine. Obtain specimens as needed. Label and notify lab of possible HIV status per agency protocol.	First stool and urine indicate normal GI and renal function. Specimens may be needed for lab tests. Lab personnel are alerted to potentially infected specimens.
Monitor all intake and output (weigh diapers, 1 gm = 1 cc).	Monitoring provides information about fluid balance and adequate caloric intake.
Provide sterile water for infant as ordered. Assess for swallowing, excessive gagging, choking, or vomiting and notify caregiver.	Sterile water allows assessment of infant's feeding ability with less risk for injury from aspiration than if formula were provided first.
If infant tolerated water feeding, assist mother to provide first formula feeding (specify formula type: e.g., 24-calorie and amount) as ordered.	Intervention promotes maternal–infant attachment and bonding. Infant is at risk for failure to thrive and may be started on high-calorie formula.
Monitor infant for signs of feeding intolerance: excessive spitting up, abdominal distention, test abnormal stools for occult blood. Notify caregiver.	Feeding intolerance may indicate presence of gastrointestinal infection.
Administer gavage feedings or TPN as ordered (specify). Check for residual before gavage feedings.	Gavage or TPN feedings provide optimal intake if the infant cannot tolerate oral feedings. Residual may indicate intolerance of gavage feedings.
Provide teaching to family as needed: hold infant close with head higher than stomach (do not prop the bottle); ensure nipple is full of formula; burp infant after each ounce or more frequently, and when finished; place infant on right side after eating.	Teaching promotes effective infant feeding and enhances family bonding with infant.
Teach parents that a small amount of regurgitated formula is normal after eating but to notify caregiver if infant vomits the whole feeding.	Teaching provides information the parents need to differentiate normal spitting up from vomiting that may signal GI infection.

INTERVENTIONS	RATIONALES
Inform mother of the schedule suggested by her caregiver (specify—may be frequent small feedings) and ensure that sterile formula is available for feedings.	Information helps the mother feed her baby effectively. Sterile formula for each feeding helps prevent gastrointestinal infection.
Praise parents for successful feeding of their new baby.	Praise promotes effective parenting.
Teach parents about the normal newborn's stools: meconium, transitional, and milk stools: color, consistency, smell, and frequency. Instruct them to notify caregiver for diarrhea or abnormal stools.	Teaching provides information the parents need to distinguish normal newborn bowel movements from signs of infection or diarrhea.
Teach parents that weight loss of up to 10% is normal after birth but then their baby should gain about an ounce per day after that for the first 6 months.	Teaching provides information that may allay parents' fears about normal neonatal weight loss.
Provide written and verbal instructions on infant feeding (and formula preparation) at discharge per infant's caregiver.	Written and verbal information provide reinforcement of caregiver's instructions after family has been discharged.

NIC: *Nutrition Management*

Evaluation

(Date/time of evaluation of goal)

(Has goal been met? not met? partially met?)

(What is infant's weight? What is percent of weight loss? Specify infant's caloric intake. Is this adequate?)

(Revisions to care plan? D/C care plan? Continue care plan?)

IMPAIRED PARENTING

Related to: Family at risk for developing parenting difficulties secondary to maternal terminal illness with a potential that infant has a terminal illness. Lack of knowledge, social isolation, and history of risk-taking behavior.

Defining Characteristics: Lack of parental attachment behaviors (specify: e.g., avoids eye contact with infant, doesn't talk to baby or explore with fingers). Parents avoid holding or caring for infant, make disparaging remarks about baby (specify with quotes).

Goal: Infant will experience appropriate parenting by (date/time to evaluate).

Outcome Criteria

✔ Parents will discuss their fears and the possibility of problems with parenting.

✔ Parents will exhibit appropriate bonding behaviors with newborn: seek eye contact, feed, hold, and talk appropriately to the baby.

NOC: *Parent–Infant Attachment*

INTERVENTIONS	RATIONALES
Review prenatal and labor records for information about maternal attitude towards pregnancy and birth of infant.	Review provides information about parenting risk behavior that was identified earlier.
Establish rapport and demonstrate respect for parents by providing privacy and dedicated time to discuss concerns.	Providing a safe and nonjudgmental environment assists the parents to feel comfortable discussing sensitive concerns.
Observe parent–infant bonding and attachment behaviors. Observe parents' caretaking activities. Provide feedback to parents about observations.	Observation provides information about the presence of expected parenting behaviors. Feedback gives the parents information they may be unaware of (e.g., that they avoid looking at the baby, etc.).
Encourage parents to identify and explore fears and concerns about parenting the infant now and in the future.	Encouragement helps the parents to begin to identify fears and concerns. Identification is necessary in order to plan coping strategies.
Assess parents' understanding of infant's condition and provide accurate information about the condition, treatment, and prognosis (specify: e.g., for HIV, hepatitis B, narcotic addiction, etc.).	Accurate information decreases unsubstantiated fears and provides anticipatory guidance to parents.
Provide information about infant's need for a safe nurturing environment to promote optimum growth and development.	Parenting is a learned skill. Information helps parents to provide for infant's growth and development needs.
Assist family to evaluate social and financial support systems. Discuss resources that may be available to the family.	The family may feel socially isolated, family members may avoid the infant, financial concerns may cause increased stress. Resources may help ease the financial burden and social isolation of parents.

(continues)

(continued)

INTERVENTIONS	RATIONALES
Help parents to make a plan for provision of appropriate care for their baby (specify: e.g., may include drug-treatment program for parents, foster care for baby, etc.).	Planning to provide for their infant's needs is part of effective parenting. Intervention empowers parents to make needed changes in lifestyle or decisions about infant care.
Initiate referrals as indicated (specify: e.g., social services, community resources, early-intervention programs, 12-step programs, counseling, etc.).	Referrals provide additional resources for the parents and infant.

NIC: *Attachment Promotion*

Evaluation

(Date/time of evaluation of goal)

(Has goal been met? not met? partially met?)

(Did parents discuss fears and risk of developing parenting problems? Describe parents' behaviors toward infant (e.g., eye contact, holding, talking to, and feeding the baby). Are they appropriate)

(Revisions to care plan? D/C care plan? Continue care plan?)

NEONATAL HIV/AIDS

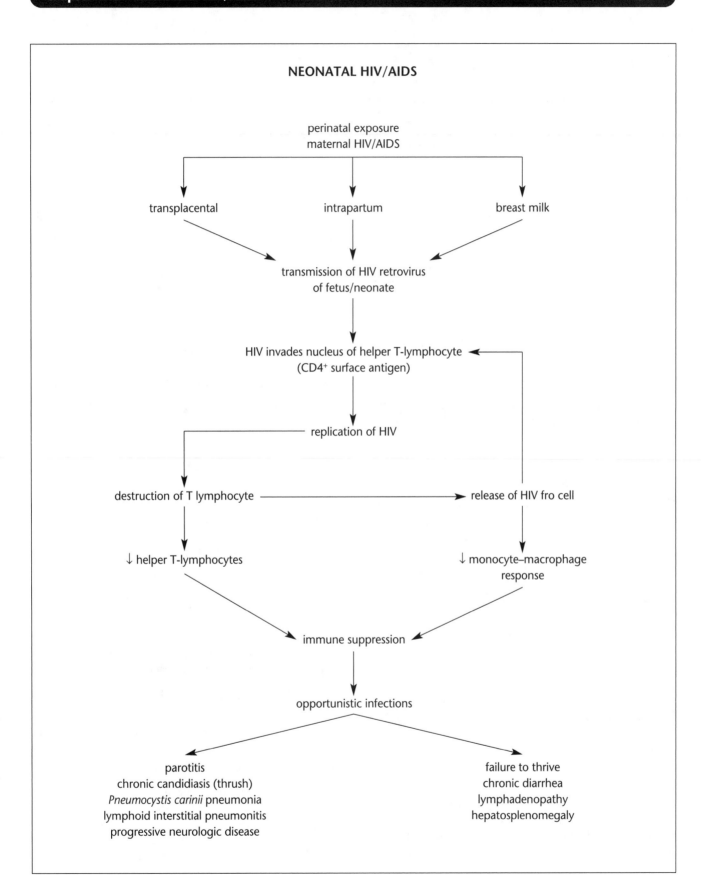

CHAPTER 4.13

INFANT OF SUBSTANCE-ABUSING MOTHER

Infants of mothers who use alcohol and/or illicit drugs during pregnancy are at risk for congenital defects, pregnancy complications, passive addiction, or a combination of these problems. Social or recreational alcohol and drug use is relatively common in women of childbearing age in the United States. Frequently the mother will use several substances including tobacco. Fear of reprisal may prevent the pregnant woman from seeking help or admitting substance abuse to caregivers.

SIGNS AND SYMPTOMS

- Pregnancy complications: placental abruption, IUGR, fetal distress, meconium aspiration
- SGA, LBW, or preterm infant usually without RDS
- Congenital defects: craniofacial anomalies, heart, brain defects
- Abnormal muscle tone: rigidity, arching, or hypotonia, lethargy
- Irritable, difficult to console, shrill cry, sleep disturbances
- Tremors, sneezing, yawning, seizures
- Uncoordinated suck/swallow reflex, poor feeding, vomiting, diarrhea
- Disorganized response to stimulation

MEDICAL CARE

- Heroin is replaced with methadone during pregnancy. Dose is gradually reduced but not discontinued to avoid fetal withdrawal
- Narcotic antagonists or agonist/antagonist drugs are avoided for mother/baby to prevent sudden narcotic withdrawal (e.g., Narcan, Stadol, Nubain)
- Toxicology screen of mother and infant to identify substances

- Positive drug screen for infant is reported to DCFS
- Labs: CBC, electrolytes, glucose monitoring, urine specific gravity, cultures as indicated
- Sedation: Phenobarbital, paregoric, diazepam in decreasing doses
- Decrease environmental stimulation, ↑ calorie formula

COMMON NURSING DIAGNOSES

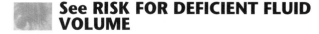 See RISK FOR INFECTION

Related to: Maternal risk behaviors

See RISK FOR DEFICIENT FLUID VOLUME

Related to: Insufficient intake secondary to poor suck and swallow. Excessive losses secondary to diarrhea.

See IMPAIRED PARENTING

Related to: Family at risk for ineffective parenting secondary to history of risk-taking behaviors and ineffective coping with stress.

ADDITIONAL NURSING DIAGNOSES

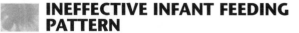 INEFFECTIVE INFANT FEEDING PATTERN

Related to: Muscle weakness/hypotonia secondary to neurologic impairment, maternal substance use, congenital defects, or lack of maternal skill (specify).

Defining Characteristics: Infant is unable to initiate or sustain an effective suck; unable to coordinate suck, swallow, and breathing. Infant vomits most of feedings (specify). Infant is unable to obtain adequate calories (specify intake/calories and calorie needs for this infant).

Goal: Infant will obtain needed nutrition by the oral route by (date/time to evaluate).

Outcome Criteria

✔ Infant ingests (specify ounces of formula/breast milk per feeding/day).

✔ Infant gains appropriate weight (specify).

✔ Infant shows increasing skill in oral feedings (specify for baby: e.g., obtains ½ of calories orally, etc.).

NOC: *Nutritional Status: Fluid Intake*

INTERVENTIONS	RATIONALES
Assess the mother's skill in feeding infant and infant's feeding pattern: suck, swallow, and coordination of swallowing with breathing.	Assessment provides information about the potential cause of ineffective feeding patterns.
Assess caloric intake compared with needs (specify). Monitor intake and output.	Assessment provides information about fluid balance and infant's additional caloric needs.
Support mother's attempts to feed baby and provide teaching as needed: promote a quiet, calm environment, upright positioning of infant, use of rooting reflex, support of infant's chin as needed.	Support and teaching assist the mother to feed her baby and promote maternal role attainment.
Offer praise for mother's attempts to feed her baby. Explain motor development delays and interventions to improve infant's feeding pattern.	The mother may be unsure of her skills and feel inadequate if the infant is a poor feeder. Support and explanation help the mother to understand the infant's needs.
Supplement oral feeding with gastric feeding to ensure caloric intake as ordered (specify formula type, amount/day: e.g., 150/250 kcal/kg/day may be ordered).	The infant needs adequate calories for growth and development of skills needed to obtain nutrients orally.
Encourage mother to hold and cuddle infant during gastric feedings (e.g., kangaroo care).	Kangaroo care during gastric feeding promotes maternal–infant attachment and bonding and calms infant to promote digestion.
Provide for nonnutritive sucking (pacifier, hands).	Nonnutritive sucking provides exercise to muscles needed for an effective feeding pattern.
Consult with occupational therapist as needed for interventions to improve oral muscle development and coordination.	Consult provides early interventions to promote optimum oral motor development.

NIC: *Nonnutritive Sucking*

Evaluation

(Date/time of evaluation of goal)

(Has goal been met? not met? partially met?)

(Specify infant's intake. Specify infant's weight and gain. Describe infant's skill in oral feedings: e.g., poor suck or sleepy)

DISTURBED SLEEP PATTERN

Related to: Parent–infant interaction.

Defining Characteristics: Infant is irritable, restless, and hyperresponsive to stimulation. Sleep pattern is short and easily interrupted (specify: e.g., sleeps lightly for 20 minutes and wakes with a shrill cry).

Goal: Infant will experience an improved sleep pattern by (date/time to evaluate).

Outcome Criteria

✔ Infant will sleep for (specify hours: e.g., 12–14 hours a day) without use of or gradual withdrawal of sedative medications.

NOC: *Sleep*

INTERVENTIONS	RATIONALES
Assess infant's sleep/wake pattern and response to environmental stimuli.	Assessment provides information about infant's current patterns and responses to stimulation.
Observe for signs of narcotic withdrawal: hyperactivity and irritability, muscle rigidity, shrill cry, sneezing, yawning. Notify caregiver.	Infants experiencing withdrawal may need sedative medications to promote adequate rest during acute phase.
Decrease environmental noise and light: cover isolette with blanket, dim nursery lights at night, move noisy equipment, avoid talking around infant's bed.	Interventions decrease environmental stimulation and infant's hyperactive responses.
Teach mother about her infant's sleep pattern disturbance and interventions to promote rest.	Share information and support mother's caretaking activities.
Wrap infant snugly and provide repetitive motion: rocking, walking, or patting back.	Wrapping, holding, and repetitive movements provide comfort, security, and promote behavioral organization.

(continues)

(continued)

INTERVENTIONS	RATIONALES
Play soft music or womb sounds and note infant's response.	Soft sounds may be comforting to infant or may be distracting.
Provide for nonnutritive sucking by using a pacifier or keeping hands free.	Pacifier or hand sucking provides comfort and promotes rest for infant.
Avoid waking infant for nonessential care activities. Cluster care while awake.	Interventions promote infant sleep periods. Most nursing care can be done during wakeful periods.
Teach breast-feeding mother to avoid caffeine, chocolate, gas-producing foods (e.g., cabbage) and highly spiced foods for a week. Foods may then be added one at a time and infant's response observed.	The specified foods have been reported by some breast-feeding mothers to cause GI upset in their babies.
Administer sedatives as ordered (specify: drug, route, time). Assist caregiver in decreasing dosage according to infant's responses.	(Specify action of particular drug.) Drugs interfere with REM and deep sleep stages and should be discontinued as soon as possible.

NIC: *Sleep Enhancement*

Evaluation

(Date/time of evaluation of goal)

(Has goal been met? not met? partially met?)

(Specify how long infant is sleeping. Specify dosage of sedative if being used and if dose has been decreased.)

(Revisions to care plan? D/C care plan? Continue care plan?)

 ## DISORGANIZED INFANT BEHAVIOR

Related to: Altered CNS response secondary to prenatal exposure to drugs/alcohol.

Defining Characteristics: Specify (e.g., irritability, tremors, seizures, tachycardia, tachypnea, apnea, sneezing, gagging, yawning, hypotonia, lethargy, shrill cry, difficult to console, etc.).

Goal: Infant will demonstrate increase in behavioral organization by (date/time to evaluate).

Outcome Criteria

✔ Infant demonstrates periods of calm, quiet alert state.

✔ Infant shows less motor instability (specify: e.g., tremors, rigidity, etc.). Holding can console infant, rocking, talking.

NOC: *Neurologic Status*

INTERVENTIONS	RATIONALES
Assess infant's behavioral responses to stimuli. Observe caretaking skills and emotional responses of parents.	Assessment provides information about individual infant's responses to particular stimuli. Parents who are substance abusers may also be at risk for neglect or abuse of their children.
Assist parents to identify behavioral cues of infant. Discuss infant's disorganized behavior with parents. Involve them in planning and implementing interventions to assist the baby.	Assisting parents to understand their infant promotes parent–infant attachment and facilitates effective parenting of the difficult infant.
Handle infant slowly and calmly. Maintain flexion when handling baby. Swaddle securely with hands free for sucking. Position in crib prone or on side with blanket rolls creating a nest.	Interventions provide external regulation of motor control promoting comfort and rest.
Decrease environmental stimulation as much as possible: cover isolette with a blanket, dim lights, decrease noise. Alert others to infant's needs by placing sign on isolette.	Excessive stimulation leads to increased behavioral disorganization and expenditure of energy needed for growth and development.
Maintain a calm routine for infant care. Cluster activity and avoid overstimulation or interruption of sleep.	Providing a consistent routine with clustered activity assists the infant to organize behavior.
Teach parents to provide kangaroo care holding infant securely in flexed position against skin of chest. Assess infant's response.	Kangaroo care may help calm the infant, or may be too stressful at first. Care is based on infant's response.
Gradually provide developmental stimulation (touch, talking, music, etc.) noting infant's response and increasing or decreasing stimulation based on infant's cues.	Developmental stimulation supports infant's growing abilities based on individual response.
Teach parents about growth and development milestones for infancy. Provide written materials if appropriate.	Anticipatory guidance helps parents to provide appropriate care for their baby.

INTERVENTIONS	RATIONALES
Teach parents to maintain a consistent routine for baby after discharge. Suggest trying an infant swing for baby.	The infant benefits from routine by developing patterns of organized behavior. Repetitive motion is calming for some infants.
Initiate home follow-up visit for infant. Provide phone number for parents to call with concerns.	Home visits provide information on infant's progress and parents' caretaking abilities. The infant may be at risk for neglect or abuse if parents become frustrated with caring for a difficult baby.
Refer parents as indicated (specify: e.g., early intervention programs, social service, counseling, etc.).	Referrals are initiated to provide continual support and surveillance.

NIC: *Environmental Management*

Evaluation

(Date/time of evaluation of goal)

(Has goal been met? not met? partially met?)

(Does infant exhibit periods of quiet alert state? Describe changes in motor excitability. How is infant consoled? Has this improved?)

(Revisions to care plan? D/C care plan? Continue care plan?)

INFANT OF SUBSTANCE-ABUSING MOTHER

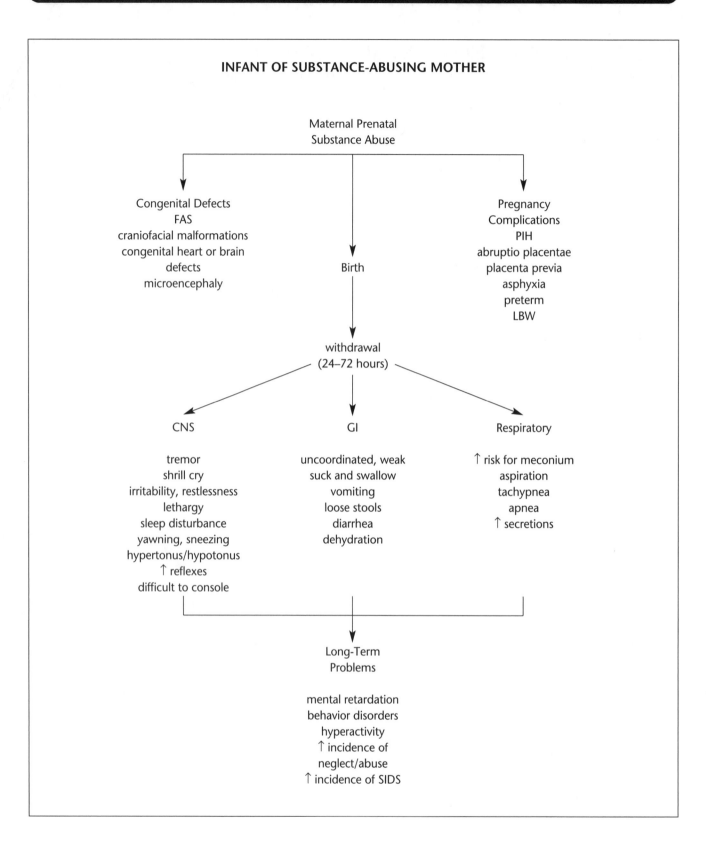

Maternal Prenatal
Substance Abuse

Congenital Defects
FAS
craniofacial malformations
congenital heart or brain
defects
microencephaly

Birth

Pregnancy
Complications
PIH
abruptio placentae
placenta previa
asphyxia
preterm
LBW

withdrawal
(24–72 hours)

CNS

tremor
shrill cry
irritability, restlessness
lethargy
sleep disturbance
yawning, sneezing
hypertonus/hypotonus
↑ reflexes
difficult to console

GI

uncoordinated, weak
suck and swallow
vomiting
loose stools
diarrhea
dehydration

Respiratory

↑ risk for meconium
aspiration
tachypnea
apnea
↑ secretions

Long-Term
Problems

mental retardation
behavior disorders
hyperactivity
↑ incidence of
neglect/abuse
↑ incidence of SIDS

UNIT 5

INFANT: BIRTH TO SIX WEEKS

CHAPTER 5.0

HEALTHY INFANT

During the first weeks of life, healthy infants complete the transition to extrauterine existence and move towards establishing individual patterns of eating, sleeping, and activity. The family adjusts to the demands of caring for a newborn and incorporates the new member into the family identity. New parents have many concerns and questions about caring for their infant. Minor conditions, such as colic or diaper rash, can take on major proportions when parental sleep patterns are disrupted. More serious conditions, such as congenital malformations, may necessitate surgical intervention during the first month.

Well-baby check-ups are usually scheduled to coincide with recommended immunizations. Infant growth and development is assessed and parental concerns addressed. The nurse uses anticipatory guidance and health promotion to assist the family to support optimal infant development.

TABLE 5.1   AAP Recommended Immunization Schedule

Hepatitis B vaccine: birth–2 months, 1–4 months, 6–18 months
DtaP vaccine: 2 months, 4 months, 6 months, 15–18 months, 4–6 years
Td vaccine: 11–16 months and boosters every 10 years after
H. influenzae type b (Hib): 2 or 3 doses at 2–6 months, booster at 12–15 months
Inactivated Polio vaccine (IPV): 2 months, 4 months, 6–18 months, 4–6 years
Pneumococcal conjugate vaccine: 2 months, 4 months, 6 months, 12–15 months
Measles, Mumps, Rubella vaccine (MMR): 12–15 months, 4–6 years
Varicella vaccine: 12–18 months

TABLE 5.2   Developmental Milestones in the First Year

0–1 month: gains 5–7 oz/week, turns head side-to-side when prone
2–3 months: holds head up, smiles, plays with hands, posterior fontanel closed
4–5 months: birth weight doubles, rolls over intentionally, reaches and grasps an object
6–7 months: teething, sits, transfer a toy from hand-to-hand, beginning object permanence
8–9 months: crude pincer grasp, sits alone, crawls → creeps, stranger anxiety, peek-a-boo
10–12 months: birth weight triples, height ↑ by 50%, stands alone, walks with help, patty-cake, has 4–5 word vocabulary

TABLE 5.3   Safety Teaching

Car seats:	Properly anchored in the middle back seat facing the rear of the vehicle.
Sleeping:	Place on back to sleep; firm, snug-fitted mattress and bumper pads with crib slats no further than 2⅜ inches apart; avoid pillows and keep crib away from curtain or blind cords.
Bathing:	Adjust home water heater to <120° F; always test bath water before putting baby in; never leave alone in water.
Eating:	Test warmed formula or food first; warm under hot water, not in microwave; don't give small pieces of food that could be aspirated.
Play:	Protect from falls—never leave alone on a raised surface; use gates for stairs and guards in front of heaters or fireplaces; check toys for small parts that could be aspirated; keep small objects out of reach; put all toxic substances out of reach.

TABLE 5.4   Infant Care Path Birth to Six Weeks

WEEK	FEEDING	SLEEPING	BATHING	PLAY	SAFETY	HEALTH CARE
1	Breast on-demand: 6 wet diapers/day or Iron-fortified formula: 2–3 oz q 3–4 hours; vitamins, iron, & fluoride supplements as prescribed	Sleeps between feedings Eats at 10 pm, 2 am, and 6 am	Sponge bath only until cord falls off Circumcision care as instructed	Rocking, talking, music, mobiles, human face is best Infant massage	Approved car seat properly placed & secured Crib slats maximum 2⅜ inches (width of a soup can) Mattress and pads fit snugly Do not leave alone on an unprotected surface	Call caregiver if T >100.4° F, spitting-up 2 feedings, inadequate intake, or signs of respiratory distress or illness
2	Gains 6 oz weekly			Promote sensorimotor learning		Retesting of metabolic screening (PKU) if indicated
4	Lactation schedule usually established Bottle-fed babies usually taking 2 to 3 oz each feeding	Try to stretch 2 am feeding	Bathing in an infant tub, sink, or tub if cord has fallen off	Provide variety of things to look at, listen to, and feel	Check bath temp before immersing infant Never leave alone in the water Hold securely	Well-baby visit Second dose of hepatitis B vaccine
6		Most infants will be able to sleep through the 2 am feeding		May begin social smiles		Mother's check-up

BASIC CARE PLAN: HEALTHY INFANT

COMMON NURSING DIAGNOSES

IMBALANCED NUTRITION: LESS THAN BODY REQUIREMENTS

Related to: Immature physiology.

Defining Characteristics: Infant weighs (specify for infant in either lb or kg). Infant needs (specify caloric needs of infant: 50 cal/lb/day or 108 cal/kg/day) and is obtaining (specify calories infant is currently ingesting per day). (Specify weight loss from birth weight; calculate percentage of birth weight lost.)

Goal: Infant will obtain adequate nutrition

Outcome Criteria

✔ Infant will ingest (specify intake of formula or breast milk needed to obtain sufficient calories for growth).

✔ Infant will gain 5–7 oz/ week.

NOC: *Nutritional Status: Nutrient Intake*

INTERVENTIONS	RATIONALES
Weigh infant as necessary (specify frequency: e.g., once a week, monthly, etc.).	Weight gain of 5–7 oz per week indicates adequate nutrition.
Assess current intake of formula per day or frequency and timing of breast-feeding.	Assessment provides information about current status.
Inform parents of the calories needed by their infant for growth (specify).	Parents may be unaware of caloric needs of the infant.
Assist parents to plan ways to ensure that their infant obtains adequate intake of calories. Suggest more frequent or longer feedings (if appropriate).	Empowers parents to make decisions regarding infant feeding.

INTERVENTIONS	RATIONALES
Teach formula-feeding parents to be sure to mix formula accurately as instructed.	Diluting the formula with too much water will result in inadequate calories.
Assist breast-feeding mother to develop pumping skills if mother plans to return to work and continue breast-feeding.	Developing pumping skill is less stressful before the mother returns to work.
Instruct parents to inform health care provider if infant spits up two or more feedings entirely or fails to wet 6 diapers a day.	Congenital defects may cause hyperemesis; fewer than six wet diapers a day may indicate dehydration.
Refer parents as needed to a lactation consultant, La Leche League, WIC, or support groups.	Specify reason for referral, e.g., parents can't afford formula or mother is having problems with breast-feeding.

NIC: *Nutrition Management*

Evaluation

(Date/time of evaluation of goal)

(Was goal met? Not met? Partially met?)

(Specify how much the infant is obtaining)

(Specify weight gain)

FATIGUE: PARENTAL

Related to: Effects of newborn care on sleep patterns and need for continuous attention.

Defining Characteristics: Parent(s) verbalize lack of energy and distress (specify using quotes). Parents indicate that they are not obtaining enough sleep (specify).

Goal: Parents will feel rested.

Outcome Criteria

✔ Parents will determine priorities of activities.

✔ Parents will verbalize three ways to obtain increased rest.

✔ Parents will state a decrease in feelings of fatigue.

NOC: *Energy Conservation*

INTERVENTIONS	RATIONALES
Assist parents to describe sleep and activity patterns and energy/fatigue levels.	Information can help parents to plan changes in activity patterns and assess if changes are working.
Teach parents that postpartum fatigue usually peaks during the second week and is decreased by 6 weeks.	Teaching reassures parents that fatigue will be short-lived.
Encourage parents to prioritize activities from those that are necessary to survival to those that are nice but not necessary.	Prioritization allows parents to identify what must be done and what isn't imperative.
Prompt parents to decide which activities they could delete for the time being; make suggestions as needed (e.g., cleaning house, gardening).	Prompting may imply permission, e.g., indicate that it is acceptable to not clean house when there is a newborn to care for.
Assist parents to plan ways to increase rest. Encourage napping and allowing others to help care for infant while parent sleeps.	Parents may feel they are lazy if they nap or allow others to help care for the infant while they rest.
Provide additional information on the benefits of nutrition and exercise in maintaining energy levels.	Parents may not be eating a balanced diet and may feel that exercise will be too tiring.
Initiate referrals if indicated.	Specify: e.g., mother of triplets may need a home health aid to help with feeding and bathing and allow her to rest.

NIC: *Energy Management*

Evaluation

(Date/time of evaluation of goal)

(Was goal met? Not met? Partially met?)

(Did parents prioritize activities? Did parents verbalize three ways to obtain increased rest? Did parents state a decrease in feelings of fatigue? Specify using quotes.)

RISK FOR SUFFOCATION

Related to: Infant lack of awareness of hazards and inability to control environment.

Defining Characteristics: None, as this is a potential diagnosis.

Goal: Infant will not suffocate.

Outcome Criteria

✔ Parents verbalize five important actions to prevent suffocation of their infant.

NOC: *Risk Control*

INTERVENTIONS	RATIONALES
Assess parent's understanding of the risk for suffocation for an infant.	Provides baseline information on which to prepare a teaching plan.
Instruct parents to be sure the infant's crib slats are no more than 2⅜ inches wide (no larger than a soup can).	Infants have caught their heads in wider crib slats and strangled.
Teach parents to ensure that mattress and bumper pads fit snugly against sides of crib.	Prevents infant being caught and suffocating between the mattress or pads and crib.
Advise parents to not place any soft pillows, toys, or thick blankets in the crib and to avoid letting infant sleep on soft mattresses.	Infant could suffocate on pillows, toys, or other soft surfaces.
Teach parents to keep crib away from drapery or blind cords and to never hang a pacifier around the infant's neck.	Prevents strangulation.
Teach parents to place their infant on his right side after eating and on his back for sleep. Teach parents to never prop a bottle and leave the infant unattended while eating.	Interventions prevent aspiration and provide a decreased risk for SIDS.

NIC: *Environmental Management: Safety*

Evaluation

(Date/time of evaluation of goal)

(Was goal met? Not met? Partially met?)

(List the five interventions the parents verbalized to prevent suffocation of their infant or specify if they were unable to do this.)

CHAPTER 5.2

COLIC

The infant with colic exhibits paroxysmal red-faced crying accompanied by indications of excessive gas. The baby screams and pulls up his arms and legs as if in severe abdominal pain. Some infants will have colicky periods at about the same time every afternoon or evening. Crying is often unrelieved by parental interventions and leads to frustration and feelings of helplessness.

The cause is not well-understood though around 20% of infants exhibit some form of colic. Overstimulation of the immature nervous system is one current theory. Cow's milk allergy is sometimes suspected with a change of formula or eliminating milk from the breast-feeding mother's diet being helpful. Other interventions are aimed at reducing the amount of air the infant may be swallowing. Usually colic is limited to the first three months of life and has no effect on weight gain.

MEDICAL CARE

- Change to a casein hydrolysate formula, e.g., Nutramingen, Pregestimil, or Alimentum
- Breast-feeding mothers are instructed to avoid milk products
- Medications: Simethicone (Mylicon) drops, phenobarbital, chloral hydrate

COMMON NURSING DIAGNOSES

See ANXIETY

Related to: Perceived threat to infant's well-being.

Defining Characteristics: Specify (e.g., parents state that they feel tense, nervous, and helpless when their baby is crying). Use quotes when possible.

See HEALTH-SEEKING BEHAVIORS

Related to: Lack of knowledge of infant health-promotion.

Defining Characteristics: Parent seeks information on health promotion for the infant (specify how the parent did this; use quotes whenever possible).

ADDITIONAL NURSING DIAGNOSES

PAIN

Related to: Abdominal cramps secondary to cow's milk sensitivity, overstimulation of immature central nervous system.

Defining Characteristics: (Provide specific data, e.g., parent reports that infant cries and expels gas for several hours after eating; infant's face turns red, pulls up his legs, abdomen is tense; infant has crying jags every afternoon; parents are unable to console the infant, etc.)

Goal: Infant will experience less pain by (date and time to evaluate).

Outcome Criteria

✔ Infant does not cry after feedings.
✔ Mother reports the infant expels less gas.
✔ Infant is consoled by parental actions.

NOC: *Comfort Level*

INTERVENTIONS	RATIONALES
Assess timing of the crying spells: relationship to eating or activity; what else is going on in the home at that time, and so forth.	Assessment helps to identify if the discomfort is related to food intake.

(continues)

(continued)

INTERVENTIONS	RATIONALES
Assess the infant's current diet: type of formula, times and amounts taken.	Some infants are sensitive or allergic to cow's milk protein found in regular formulas.
If breast-feeding (specify), assess mother's diet for foods that may be upsetting: gas-producing foods such as cabbage, beans, or broccoli; dairy products; caffeine and chocolate.	Some mothers believe that eating these foods cause their infants to produce excess gas and have colic.
Assist the mother to change her diet for a few days to see if this helps. If formula-fed, provide appropriate teaching (specify) if a change in formula is ordered by the caregiver.	Eliminating offending foods from the diet will help if allergy is the culprit.
Teach parent to carry the infant in a front-carrier or wrapped in a shawl held closely against the chest.	Being held securely with pressure on the abdomen combined with gentle movement seems to soothe some colicky infants.
Suggest other comfort methods for the parents to try: decreasing stimulation in the afternoons, playing soothing music, rocking, or using a baby-swing, swaddling the infant in a knitted blanket.	Some irritable infants are over-stimulated. Decreasing stimulation or replacing it with one repetitive movement is soothing for some colicky babies.
Inform parents about OTC drops that may decrease gas.	Specify action of preparation.
Instruct parents to consult the primary caregiver if these actions don't help or if the infant fails to gain weight, vomits excessively, or has other signs of illness.	Rules out more serious causes for crying. Colicky babies usually tolerate feedings and gain weight appropriately.

NIC: *Pain Management*

Evaluation

(Date/time of evaluation of goal)

(Was goal met? Not met? Partially met?)

(Does infant cry after feedings? What does parent say?)

(Does mother report that the infant expels less gas? Use quotes)

(Is the infant is consoled by parental actions? Provide data, e.g., what did the parents say?)

IMPAIRED PARENTING

Related to: Difficult-to-console infant; young, inexperienced parents.

Defining Characteristics: Parent exhibits nonnurturing behaviors towards infant; says infant is hard to console, parent is crying, frustrated, and so forth (describe behaviors, provide quotes if possible).

Goal: Parenting will be appropriate by (date and time to evaluate).

Outcome Criteria

✔ Parents will identify problems with parenting the difficult infant.

✔ Parents will identify resources to help them increase their parenting skills.

✔ Parents will agree to provide a safe environment for their infant.

NOC: *Family Coping*

INTERVENTIONS	RATIONALES
Assess parenting behaviors by observation and questioning. Observe for eye contact, physical touch, how the parent speaks to and tries to comfort the infant. Note reciprocal interactions between the parents and infant.	Observation provides objective data about parenting behaviors and infant–parent fit. Reciprocal interaction is necessary for the infant's needs to be met.
Ask parents to describe their baby and his behavior: e.g., who is he like? Is he easy to parent or difficult? Does he like to be held or prefer being wrapped tightly?	Questioning assists the parents to identify their infant as a unique person rather than an extension of themselves.
Encourage the family to explore problem infant behaviors: When does it happen? What is going on? What interventions have the parents tried and what has been the result?	Exploring the problem behaviors may indicate the source for solutions, e.g., if feeding elicits colic, perhaps the infant has a milk allergy.
Encourage parents to express their frustrations with the infant and the parent role. Indicate that they are not alone in feeling irritated and discouraged at times.	Expression acknowledges the legitimate feelings of the parents.
Teach family about normal infant development. Inform them that colic may be a result of too much stimulation and generally disappears by 3 months of age.	Parenting is a learned role. Teaching helps parents to understand their baby's behaviors in context.
Suggest changing the infant's schedule to decrease stimulation in the afternoons. Ask parents to identify how they might do this.	Decreasing stimulation may relieve some of the colicky behaviors that make parenting difficult.

INTERVENTIONS	RATIONALES
Discuss the infant's need for appropriate parenting in order to develop a sense of security and trust. Specify that the infant's needs should be met in a consistent and timely manner.	Information about infant needs help the parents to respond appropriately.
Discuss family beliefs about discipline. Stress that the infant is too young for any form of discipline. Ask family to verbalize understanding.	Parents may think they should discipline their infant to be good parents. A colicky baby can be very frustrating to parents and may elicit abuse.
Ask the family to identify their support system. Who takes care of the baby? Is there a trusted person who could care for the baby while the parents take a break?	Provides information about sources of help for the family.
Suggest that the parents plan some time away from the infant during his colicky periods. Ask a friend or relative to watch the baby while parents go for a walk or out to a movie. Explain that the baby may cry.	Removing themselves from the stressful situation occasionally will help parents maintain perspective.
Teach the parents that colic usually abates by 3 months of age without any harm to the infant.	Knowing that the uncomfortable situation will end helps parents cope.

INTERVENTIONS	RATIONALES
Offer praise for positive parenting that the parents exhibit. Reinforce the need to protect the infant and ask the parents to agree to provide safe care for their baby.	Reinforces positive parenting activity and provides a contract to protect the infant.
Refer parents to local parenting resources/classes (specify what is available in the parent's area) or on-line resources if applicable (specify).	Information and parenting classes can teach and reinforce positive parenting skills.

NIC: *Family Integrity Promotion*

Evaluation

(Date/time of evaluation of goal)

(Was goal met? Not met? Partially met?)

(Did parents identify problems with parenting the difficult infant? Specify)

(What resources did the parents identify to help increase parenting skills?)

(Did parents agree to provide a safe environment for their infant? Use quotes)

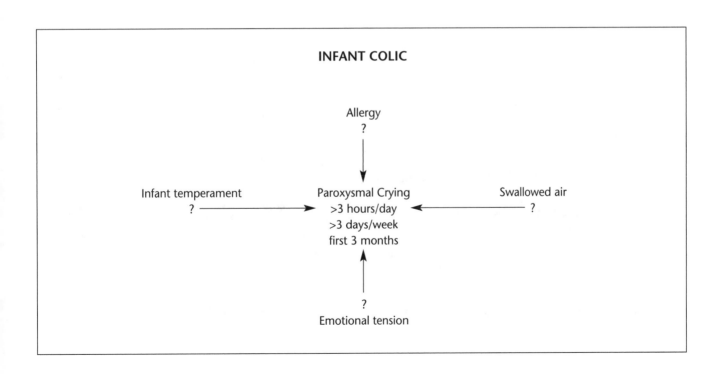

INFANT COLIC

Allergy
?

Infant temperament ? → Paroxysmal Crying >3 hours/day >3 days/week first 3 months ← ? Swallowed air

?
Emotional tension

CHAPTER 5.3

DERMATITIS

Several superficial inflammatory skin conditions are common in infancy. Diaper dermatitis, or diaper rash, is usually the result of irritation of the diaper area from friction and prolonged contact with urine and feces. Occasionally the cause is an inflammatory reaction to soaps, lotions, or chemicals used in disposable diapers. Seborrheic dermatitis produces characteristic thick, scaly, yellow patches of dried excess sebum on the scalp of young infants. The condition is known to mothers as cradle cap. Atopic dermatitis, or eczema, is a pruritic inflammation of the skin resulting in weepy inflamed lesions. It is associated with hereditary allergic reactions. Eczema is worse during winter when the air is very dry and the intense itching and scratching may lead to secondary infection. Infantile eczema usually subsides by 4 years of age.

MEDICAL CARE

- Avoid skin irritants
- Prevent over-drying of skin
- Evaluate for allergens, avoid cow's milk or soy formulas (eczema)
- Medications: antihistamines, topical steroid ointments, possible mild sedatives (eczema), medicated shampoo (seborrheic dermatitis), topical nystatin (*Candida albicans* diaper dermatitis)

COMMON NURSING DIAGNOSES

 ### See HEALTH-SEEKING BEHAVIORS

Related to: Lack of understanding about infant skin care.

Defining Characteristics: Parent seeks information about the skin condition and how to care for the infant (specify; use quotes whenever possible).

 ### See INEFFECTIVE HEALTH MAINTENANCE

Related to: Ineffective infant care practices.

Defining Characteristics: Parent demonstrates lack of appropriate infant care (specify: e.g., severe diaper dermatitis: describe lesions). Parent identifies inability to solve the problem and requests help (specify, using quotes).

ADDITIONAL NURSING DIAGNOSES

 ### PAIN

Related to: Skin inflammation and pruritus.

Defining Characteristics: Specify, e.g., infant wakes and cries; scratches/rubs body against surfaces; skin is reddened, weepy, and so forth (describe).

Goal: Infant will experience less discomfort.

Outcome Criteria

✔ Skin exhibits less inflammation (define here, e.g., if lesion is 4 cm, expect it to reduce to 2 cm; if red, expect it to decrease to pink, etc.).

✔ Infant sleeps comfortably and wakes without crying. Infant doesn't scratch/rub lesions.

NOC: *Pain Control*

INTERVENTIONS	RATIONALES
Assess skin for inflammation, types and location of lesions, character and amount of any drainage. Observe for signs of secondary infection: ↑ edema, prurulent drainage, and report to caregiver.	Assessment provides information about the source of discomfort and possible complications.

INTERVENTIONS	RATIONALES
Observe infant for signs of discomfort: waking up crying, rubbing face against the bed, and so forth.	Indication of pruritus helps with diagnosis of the condition.
Ask parent to describe usual infant care regimen: type of formula, bathing, soap and other products used on the skin, type of diapers and how many used per day, fabric in clothing, and soaps used for washing.	Assessment provides clues to the source of the discomfort: allergies, diaper dermatitis.
Assess family history of allergies and report findings to caregiver.	Eczema is associated with heredity and allergies. A change in formula to avoid cow's milk and soy protein may relieve allergic reactions.
Teach parent to administer medications correctly as ordered, e.g., antihistamines, topical steroids. (Specify drug, dose, route, and times with additional considerations as needed, i.e., to apply thin layers of ointments rather than thick) and observe for desired results.	Specify action of drug, reason for additional teaching.
Instruct parent to wash infant's linens and clothing in mild soap and rinse twice.	Decreases the infant's exposure to chemical irritants.
Teach parent to use soft knitted cotton crib sheets and clothing for the infant. Avoid overdressing.	Teaching helps the parent to avoid friction and allergic irritation of the skin. Increased warmth aggravates pruritus.
Suggest bathing the baby in tepid water with cornstarch before bedtime. Apply moisturizer to keep skin moist.	Cornstarch may be soothing and added moisture will ↓ skin irritation and itching.
Apply cool wet compresses to inflamed areas followed by glycerin-based lubricants to retain moisture.	Cool moisture is soothing to the skin and decreases pruritus. Lubricants are applied to retain moisture of skin.
Refer clients as indicated for allergy testing or dietary modification (specify).	Referrals provide additional expertise to diagnose the cause of the problem and help the family adapt care of the infant.

NIC: *Pain Management*

Evaluation

(Date/time of evaluation of goal)

(Was goal met? Not met? Partially met?)

(Describe skin lesions)

(Does infant sleep comfortably without waking crying?)

(Does infant rub/scratch lesions?)

IMPAIRED SKIN INTEGRITY

Related to: (Specify: e.g., mechanical factors, lack of moisture, allergic reactions, overactive sebaceous glands.)

Defining Characteristics: Disruption of epidermis (describe lesions).

Goal: Infant will demonstrate healing of impaired skin by (date and time to evaluate).

Outcome Criteria

✔ Progressive healing of impaired skin (specify expected changes for client: e.g., diaper area will be pink not red; eczema will ↓ in size from 3 to 1 cm patch; scalp will be free of any scales).

NOC: *Tissue Integrity: Skin*

INTERVENTIONS	RATIONALES
Assess infant's skin and scalp for signs of impaired skin integrity: redness, edema, lesions, patches or scales (specify frequency of assessments).	Assessment provides information about extent of impairment.
Encourage breast-feeding for infants with a family history of allergies.	Breast milk is less allergenic than formulas.
Assist parent to identify cause or contributing factors of impairment. Explore diapering practices, family history of allergies or eczema, bathing, shampooing, and skin care regimens and products.	Identification of possible causes will provide direction for treatment.
Instruct parents in measures to reduce skin irritation in the diaper area: keep area dry, change diapers frequently.	Avoiding skin contact with irritants helps improve skin integrity.
Administer medications and apply ointments as instructed by caregiver (specify: e.g., Benadryl [dose, route, times]; topical zinc oxide, A & D, nystatin for *Candida*).	Specify action of medications.

(continues)

(continued)

INTERVENTIONS	RATIONALES
Discourage use of baby powders. If parent insists on powder, teach to use cornstarch shaken into the hand and then applied to the skin.	Inhaling talcum powder may cause serious pulmonary irritation. Cornstarch is safer but measures should still be taken to prevent inhalation.
Teach parents to wash the infant's skin with warm water and mild soap or cold cream only. Avoid friction, perfumed soaps and presaturated wipes.	Soap is drying to the skin, commercial wipes and perfumed soaps may be irritating, and friction can cause trauma to infant's skin.
Demonstrate to the parent how to shampoo the infant's head and while still wet, use a fine-toothed comb to gently lift and comb away the scales of cradle cap. If patches are very thick, suggest application of glycerin or baby oil for several minutes before shampooing and combing.	The patchy scales of seborrheic dermatitis are easily removed once softened. Parents may benefit from demonstration of how to clean the infant's scalp.

INTERVENTIONS	RATIONALES
Provide positive reinforcement for parent's attempts to improve skin integrity of their infant. Reassure that many skin conditions of infancy will be outgrown.	Parent's may be frustrated and discouraged by their infant's impaired skin. Reinforcement and reassurance empower the parents to provide good infant care.

NIC: *Wound Care*

Evaluation

(Date/time of evaluation of goal)

(Was goal met? Not met? Partially met?)

(Describe expected changes for client—is the diaper area pink?)

(Did the eczema ↓ in size to 1 cm patch?—describe.)

(Is scalp free of any scales? Describe scalp.)

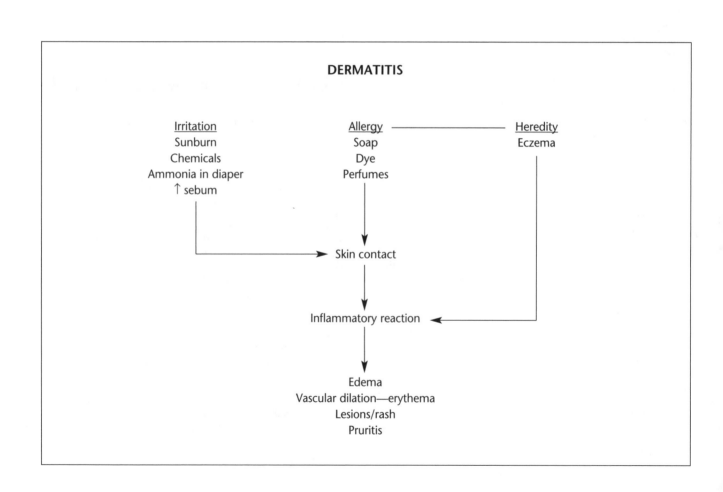

DERMATITIS

Irritation
Sunburn
Chemicals
Ammonia in diaper
↑ sebum

Allergy ——————— Heredity
Soap   Eczema
Dye
Perfumes

Skin contact

Inflammatory reaction

Edema
Vascular dilation—erythema
Lesions/rash
Pruritis

CHAPTER 5.4

SIBLING RIVALRY

The addition of a new member of a family creates some degree of change in all the relationships and dynamics in the family. Each member must make some adjustments whether it is waking up for night feedings, giving up a crib, or having to share a parent's lap with the new baby. The small child who is very dependent on the mother is frequently thought to be the one most affected by sibling rivalry, but adolescents may have equally strong reactions to sharing family time and affection with a new rival. Jealousy towards the new baby may be expressed by regression, bids for attention, and acting-out behaviors including hitting the baby.

Lenient visitation policies in hospitals help families to feel connected to the new addition. Sibling classes are offered at many hospitals to introduce children to the new experiences they will encounter as older brothers and sisters. Some children, who have been prepared for seeing a birth, will be present when their new baby is born. Most siblings will be able to visit their mother and see, even hold, the new brother or sister on the day of birth.

Historically there have been many ideas on ways to minimize the negative feelings a child might have towards a new sibling while enhancing the growth and development of the older child. Some suggestions are:

- Prepare the child during pregnancy by encouraging him to feel the fetus move and help with preparations
- If the child is to move out of the crib, this should be done well in advance of the birth
- Bake a birthday cake and put it in the freezer to be thawed and eaten by the siblings on the day of the new baby's birth
- Gather and wrap a selection of small toys and gifts and give one of these to the older child whenever the baby gets a present
- Encourage grandparents and others to say hello to the older child before showing how much they enjoy the baby

- Give the older child a present of a life-like baby doll to care for as the mother cares for the new baby. A teddy bear may be substituted if parents are uncomfortable with a boy having a baby doll
- Allow the child to "help" at whatever level is appropriate—bringing diapers or feeding a bottle. Offer lots of praise
- Plan time for parents to give full attention to the older child without interruptions from the newborn. Perhaps doing something that only "big" boys and girls can do
- For older children, allow uninterrupted time to talk and explore their feelings—they may feel that they are being replaced by this cute new baby who never does anything wrong
- Expect regression as a means of coping and provide increased reassurance and love as the child works through this challenging time

COMMON NURSING DIAGNOSES

 ### See INEFFECTIVE COPING

Related to: Changes in family composition.

Defining Characteristics: Since the birth of a sibling, (describe), child has regressed (describe), is acting out (specify behavior), or exhibiting anger towards the new baby (describe behavior).

 ### See RISK FOR IMPAIRED PARENTING

Related to: Ineffective adaptation to stressors of having a new baby.

Defining Characteristics: Parents exhibit nonnurturing behavior towards older sibling (describe behavior); parents verbalize frustration or misunderstanding of the needs of the older sibling (specify).

See FATIGUE

Related to: Care of a newborn in addition to older children.

Defining Characteristics: Parent verbalizes decreased energy (specify, use quotes), Older children demand care or appear unkempt (specify and describe)

 READINESS FOR ENHANCED FAMILY COPING

Related to: Parental acknowledgment of sibling rivalry.

Defining Characteristics: Parent seeks information to diminish the effects of sibling rivalry and enhance family coping (specify what parents said, use quotes). Parents exhibit behaviors designed to limit sibling rivalry (describe).

Goal: Positive family coping will continue.

Outcome Criteria

✔ Parents will identify sibling's needs.
✔ Parents will verbalize plans to meets the children's needs.
✔ Parents will identify resources to assist in family coping.

NOC: *Family Coping*

INTERVENTIONS	RATIONALES
Assess family perceptions about current coping situation with newborn and siblings.	Assessment data provides the basis for care.
Offer praise and support for current effective coping behaviors of family (specify).	Supports the family coping; provides information.
Assist parents to identify the dependency needs of each sibling.	Helps parents to focus on individual needs of children.
Ask parents to verbalize how they plan to meet the needs of each child.	Verbalization of plans helps parents to commit to implementation.
Provide information about additional methods to diminish sibling rivalry (specify).	Provides additional information and options to family.
Encourage family to identify additional resources available to help support family coping (e.g., grandparents, friends, etc.).	Additional resources can help support positive coping.
Support family decisions regarding ways to cope with sibling rivalry.	Support promotes family unity.

NIC: *Family Support*

Evaluation

(Date/time of evaluation of goal)

(Was goal met? Not met? Partially met?)

(Did parents identify sibling's needs? Specify plans parents verbalized to meet the children's needs. Specify resources the family identified to assist in family coping.)

SIBLING RIVALRY

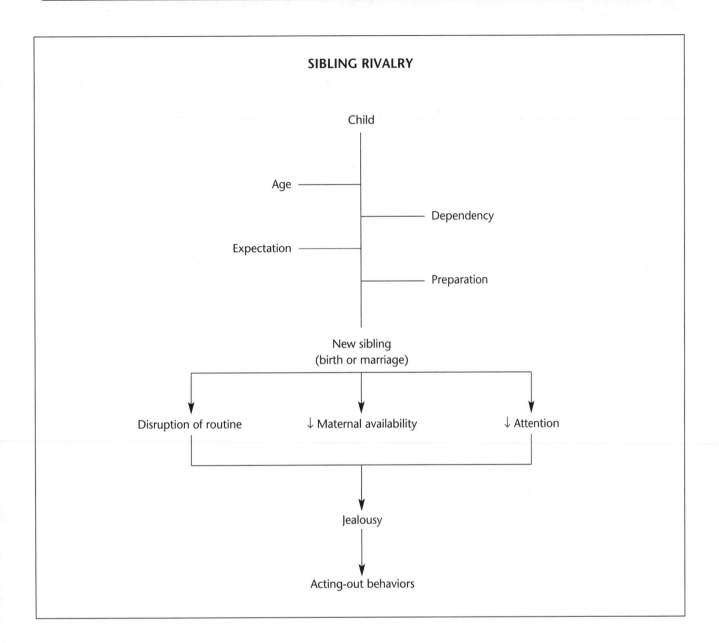

CHAPTER 5.5

CONGENITAL ANOMALIES

Congenital abnormalities range from mild, familial traits such as polydactyly or umbilical hernia to serious, life-threatening malformations of the CNS, heart, or GI tract and include chronic physical and mental deficits. Many syndromes characterized by multiple congenital anomalies have been identified with Down's syndrome being one of the most familiar. Cognitive and developmental defects may be implied as part of a syndrome recognized at birth, or not diagnosed until the infant fails to meet expected developmental milestones as in the child with cerebral palsy. Heredity, teratogenic insult, and environmental conditions have been implicated in congenital malformations and deformities. Chromosomal defects may result from heredity, insult, or random errors in cell division and translocation of genetic material.

The family presented with a newborn with a physical abnormality faces the sometimes monumental task of relinquishing their desired, imagined child and learning to care for and love a physical stranger. The appearance of an infant with bilateral cleft lip may be shocking to parents who have never seen this condition. Infants with congenital anomalies may be at high risk emotionally as well as physically. Holistic nursing care includes measures to facilitate parental grieving and promote bonding. The nurse coordinates and collaborates with the health care team to stabilize or correct the abnormality. The family is educated about the infant's particular needs, often becoming experts about the condition or syndrome. Referrals are made for continuing therapeutic and supportive measures for the infant and family.

COMMON NURSING DIAGNOSES

 See ANXIETY

Related to: Perceived threat to well-being of newborn.

Defining Characteristics: Parent exhibits anxious behaviors (specify: e.g., shaking, tremulous voice, diaphore-sis, etc.); verbalizes anxiety (specify, using quotes: e.g., "I am so nervous." "I can't sleep or eat." Etc.).

 See RISK FOR IMPAIRED PARENT/INFANT ATTACHMENT

Related to: Birth of infant with physical defect.

 See ANTICIPATORY GRIEVING

Related to: Birth of newborn with congenital abnormality.

Defining Characteristics: (Specify, e.g., newborn has a life-threatening congenital anomaly, newborn with congenital defect that may result in chronic illness or developmental delays.) Parents exhibit signs of grief: denial, sorrow, anger, bargaining (specify and describe parental behaviors or verbalizations to support the diagnosis).

 See DELAYED GROWTH AND DEVELOPMENT

Related to: Congenital abnormality (specify).

Defining Characteristics: (Specify for client, e.g., failure of neural tube to close, failure of fusion of palate, abnormal enervation will prevent ambulation, signs of Down's syndrome.)

ADDITIONAL NURSING DIAGNOSES

 DEFICIENT KNOWLEDGE (SPECIFY)

Related to: Lack of exposure to congenital defect (specify).

Defining Characteristics: Parents verbalize that they have no knowledge about (specify the condition and what the parents said). Parents demonstrate incorrect care of the infant (specify).

Goal: Parents will demonstrate knowledge related to (specify: congenital abnormality) by (date/time to evaluate).

Outcome Criteria

✔ Parents will verbalize understanding of the etiology, effects and treatment options for (specify anomaly).

✔ Parents will demonstrate understanding of infant care by providing correct care (specify what skills parents need to care for a child with the anomaly).

NOC: *Knowledge: Disease Process*

INTERVENTIONS	RATIONALES
Explore parent's current knowledge base about congenital abnormality (specify). Assist them to identify any similar/related familial conditions.	Teaching should build on a base of current level of understanding.
Evaluate readiness to learn.	High anxiety or denial may interfere with ability to understand and use new information.
Provide privacy and a supportive, comfortable environment.	Discomfort or distraction may interfere with learning.
Begin with simple explanations of the abnormality, the suspected etiology, and usual course of treatment. Use visual aids to improve understanding.	Simple explanations are more likely to be understood by the beginner. Many people are visual learners. The before and after photos of cleft lip are powerful sources of hope for parents.
Divide learning sessions into logical segments. (Specify, e.g., teach about feeding the infant with cleft palate first, then pre-op teaching followed by postoperative and continuing care). Note parent cues of exhaustion or being overwhelmed.	Information is best learned in short sessions that are related to what is happening.
Allow ample time for parent's questions and responses to information.	Information may be overwhelming or confusing at first.
Demonstrate how to care for the infant (specify: e.g., to feed the infant with cleft palate, position upright, use a long, soft lambs nipple or syringe feeder; proceed slowly and burp frequently.)	Demonstration provides a role model for the parent to imitate.

INTERVENTIONS	RATIONALES
Assist the parent to return–demonstrate the skill (specify what the parent will do: e.g., application of the Pavlik harness.)	Return–demonstration allows the parent to practice a new skill under supervision.
Offer praise and support for parental efforts. Reassure that they will gain skill over time.	Positive reinforcement enhances learning.
Provide written (if literate) information about the infant's condition. (Specify).	Parents may learn additional information at their own pace by reading additional information.
Refer the parents to local, state, and national resources (identify what is available for the specific congenital abnormality). Provide addresses, phone numbers and web site information to reliable information.	Provides additional information and support to parents of children with congenital anomalies. The nurse can help the client find reliable sources on-line.
Provide follow-up care or contacts (specify).	Caring for a child with a congenital abnormality is a long-term process.

NIC: *Teaching, Disease Process*

Evaluation

(Date/time of evaluation of goal)

(Was goal met? Not met? Partially met?)

(Can parents verbalize understanding of the etiology, effects and treatment options? Provide data.)

(What skills did the parents demonstrate?)

PARENTAL ROLE CONFLICT

Related to: Birth of a child with a congenital defect.

Defining Characteristics: Parents express concerns about caring for their baby. Parents express concern about caring for other children, feeling inadequate, and so forth (specify for parents; provide data).

Goal: The parent(s) will demonstrate appropriate parenting skills by (date/time to evaluate).

Outcome Criteria

✔ Parents will participate in caring for their child (specify activity: i.e., feeding, bathing).

✔ Parents will identify and contact available support (specify for parents: e.g., family, church, foundations, etc.).

NOC: *Role Performance*

INTERVENTIONS	RATIONALES
Establish a therapeutic relationship with parents. Ensure continuity of caregivers for infant whenever possible.	Parents may feel overwhelmed by multiple caregivers telling them different things.
Demonstrate respect for the parent's concerns about caring for the infant. Allow expression of fears and feelings of inadequacy about parenting the ill infant.	Respect and validation of feelings allow parents to explore their fears openly.
Assist the parents to assess their family's strengths and stressors. Observe interactions between family members.	Provides information about family member's ability to adapt and support each other.
Assist family to identify additional sources of support. Provide suggestions if needed (chaplain, social services, etc.). Ask family to agree to contact at least one additional source.	Agreement acts as a contract to encourage parents to seek additional support.
Provide information about the infant's need for parenting even in the hospital setting.	Information helps the parent value their contributions to the care of the infant.

INTERVENTIONS	RATIONALES
Provide opportunities for parents to assist in caring for their infant (specify: e.g., talking/singing to infant; pumping breasts; etc.). Offer support and praise efforts.	Providing care with supervision and support facilitates confidence in the parent role.
Encourage parents to participate in decision-making about their infant's care. Provide simple explanations and allow time for questions.	Making decisions about the care of a child is integral to the parental role. The parents may feel inadequate at first.
Refer parents to additional resources as appropriate (specify: e.g., national support groups, counseling, etc.).	

NIC: *Crisis Intervention*

Evaluation

(Date/time of evaluation of goal)

(Was goal met? Not met? Partially met?)

(Did parents participate in caring for their child? Describe.)

(Will parents identify and contact available support? Specify.)

TABLE 5.5 Selected Congenital Malformations

CONDITION	ABNORMALITY	SYMPTOMS	TREATMENT	NURSING CARE
Cleft lip & palate	Failure of fusion of the soft palate and maxilla	Varies from just partial palate defect to bilateral palate and lift defects	Surgical repair: lip at 10 weeks, palate between 1–3 years. Ongoing dental and speech tx, ↑ risk for URI & otitis media	Feed upright with long soft nipple or syringe. Prevent crying or tension on suture line. Promote bonding: show before & after repair photos
Tracheoesophageal fistula (TEF)	Esophagus ends in an abnormal connection to the trachea	Excessive oral secretions. Three C's: crying, choking, cyanosis	Surgical repair with gastrostomy tube for feedings until healed	Assess all newborns for TEF before feeding. Maintain airway, keep NPO
Imperforate anus	Varies from a thin membrane obstructing the anus to the rectum ending in a blind pouch	Failure to pass meconium	Surgical repair with possible temporary colostomy	Evaluate all newborns for passage of meconium. Do not attempt to take rectal temps
Hirschsprung's disease (congenital aganglionic megacolon)	Lack of ganglionic enervation to a segment of the large intestine	Failure to pass meconium, thin, ribbon-like stools, distended abdomen	Surgical removal of affected segment. Temporary colostomy, TPN	Evaluate all newborns for passage of meconium or ribbon-like stools
Congenital heart defects	Varies: PDA, ASD, VSD, aortic & pulm. stenosis, TGV, tetrology of Fallot, coarctation of the aorta	Varies: none to murmurs, unequal pulses, dyspnea, tachypnea, CHF, cyanosis, "tet spells"	Cardiac cath, surgical repair, medications: digoxin, furosemide, Prostaglandin E, indomethacin, antibiotics	Decrease oxygen demands, prevent infection, monitor HR, I&O & potassium levels, prepare for cardiac cath and surgery. Provide post-cath & post-op care
Hypospadius & epispadius	Abnormal opening of the male urethra on the ventral (hypo-) or dorsal (epi-)surface of the penis	Urine is expelled from an abnormal site on the penis or at an abnormal angle from the tip. ↑ risk of UTI & infertility	No circumcision for infants with hypospadius. Surgical reconstruction	Assess all newborns for conditions. Keep area clean to prevent infection. Provide pre- and post-surgical care. Monitor I&O
Myelomeningocele	NTD with meninges and spinal cord protruding from the back. Associated with ↓ prenatal folic acid	Obvious spinal deformity, motor paralysis, abnormal bowel & bladder function, hydrocephalus	Surgical repair of defect within 24–48 hours. Monitoring for hydrocephalus with V P shunt	Protect the sac, position on side or abdomen, keep clean & moist, observe for leakage of CSF, observe motor, bowel, & bladder function, measure OFC
Congenital hip dysplasia	Abnormal development of acetabulum & head of femur	Head of femur slips out of acetabulum, Ortolani's click, uneven buttock folds & leg length	Abduction devices × 3 months to deepen the acetabulum: double-triple diapering, Pavlik harness	Assess all newborns for condition. Teach parents to maintain abduction of the hip and to monitor skin integrity under the harness.

CONGENITAL ANOMALIES

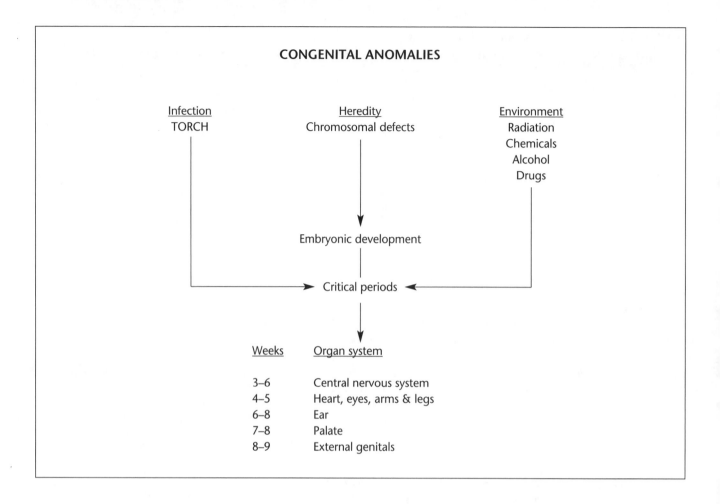

Infection
TORCH

Heredity
Chromosomal defects

Environment
Radiation
Chemicals
Alcohol
Drugs

Embryonic development

Critical periods

Weeks	Organ system
3–6	Central nervous system
4–5	Heart, eyes, arms & legs
6–8	Ear
7–8	Palate
8–9	External genitals

BIBLIOGRAPHY

BOOKS

Alfaro-LaFevre, R. (2004). *Critical thinking in nursing: A practical approach* (3rd ed.). Philadelphia: W.B. Saunders Co.

American Psychiatric Association (APA). (2000). *Diagnostic and statistical manual of mental disorders* (4th ed., Rev.). Washington DC: Author.

Barnum, B.S. (1999). *Teaching nursing in the era of managed care*. New York: Springer Publishing.

Carpenito, L.J. (2004). *Handbook of nursing diagnosis* (10th ed.). Philadelphia: Lippincott.

Carpenito, L. J. (2004). *Nursing diagnosis: Application to clinical practice* (10th ed.). Philadelphia: J. B. Lippincott.

Cunningham, G. F., Gant, N. F., Leveno, K. J., Gilstrap, L. C., Hauth, J. C., Wenstrom, K. D., & Cox, S. M. (2001). *Williams Obstetrics* (21st ed.). Norwalk, CT: Appleton & Lange.

DeLaune, S.C. & Ladner, P.K. (2002). *Fundamentals of nursing: Standards and practice* (2nd ed.). Clifton Park, NY: Thomson Delmar Learning.

Dochterman, J.M., & Bulechek, G.M. (2004). *Nursing Interventions Classificaton (NIC)* (4th ed.). St. Louis: Mosby, Inc.

Doenges, M. E., Geissler, A. C., & Moorhouse, M. F. (2002). *Nursing care plans: Guidelines for individualizing patient care,* (5th ed.). Philadelphia: F. A. Davis.

Fischbach, F. T. (2004). *A manual of laboratory and diagnostic tests,* (7th ed.). Philadelphia: J. B. Lippincott.

Gardner, P. (2003). *Nursing process in action*. Clifton Park, NY: Thomson Delmar Learning.

Harkreader, H. (2004). *Fundamentals of nursing: Caring and clinical judgment* (2nd ed.). Philadelphia: W.B. Saunders Co.

Hatcher, R. A., Trussell, J., Stewart, F., Cates, W., Stewart, G. K., Guest, F., & Kowal, D. (1998). *Contraceptive technology* (17th ed.). New York: Ardent Media, Inc.

Kelly-Heidenthal, P. (2003). *Nursing leadership and management*. Clifton Park, NY: Thomson Delmar Learning.

Klaus, M. H., Kennell, J. H., & Klaus, P. H. (1993). *Mothering the mother*. Cambridge, MA: Perseus Books.

Kozier, B., Erb, G., Blais, K., & Wilkinson, J. (2004). *Fundamentals of nursing: Concepts, process, and practice*. Upper Saddle River, NJ: Pearson Education.

Littleton, L., & Engebretson, J. (2002). *Maternal, neonatal, and women's health nursing*. Clifton Park, NY: Thomson Delmar Learning.

Lowdermilk, D. L, Perry, S. E., & Bobak, I. M. (2004). *Maternity and women's health care* (8th ed.). St. Louis, MO: Mosby-Yearbook.

Masten, Y. (1997). *The Skidmore–Roth outline series: Obstetric nursing* (2nd ed.). Englewood, CO: Skidmore–Roth Publishing, Inc.

McCance, K. L., & Huether, S. (2002). *Pathophysiology: The biologic basis for disease in adults and children* (4th ed.). St. Louis, MO: Mosby-Yearbook.

Moorhead, S., Johnson, M., & Maas, M. (2004). *Nursing Outcomes Classification (NOC)* (3rd ed.). St. Louis: Mosby, Inc.

Murray, M. L. (1997). *Antepartal and intrapartal fetal monitoring* (2nd ed.). Albuquerque, NM: Learning Resources International.

Murray, M. (1989). *Essentials of electronic fetal monitoring: Antepartal and intrapartal fetal monitoring*. Washington, DC: NAACOG Educational Resource.

Murray, S., McKinney, E., & Gorrie, E. (2002). *Foundations of maternal-newborn nursing* (3rd ed.). Philadelphia: W.B. Saunders Co.

Nettina, S. (2001). *The Lippincott manual of nursing practice* (7th ed.). Philadelphia: Lippincott, Williams & Wilkins.

North American Nursing Diagnosis Association (NANDA) (2003). *Nursing diagnoses: Definitions & classification 2003–2004*. Philadelphia: North American Nursing Diagnosis Association.

Olds, S. B., London, M. L., & Ladewig, P. W. (2000). *Maternal newborn nursing: A family and community-based approach* (6th ed.). Upper Saddle River, NJ: Prentice-Hall.

Perez, P. & Snedeker, C. (2000). *Special women*. Johnson, VT: Cutting Edge Press.

Pryor, G. (1997). *Nursing mother: Working mother*. Boston: The Harvard Common Press.

Riordan, J. & Auerbach, K. (1999). *Breastfeeding and human lactation* (2nd ed.). Boston: James & Bartlett.

Rudolph, A. M., Kamei, R. K., & Overby, K. J. (Eds.). (2002). *Rudolph's pediatrics* (21st ed.). Stamford, CT: Appleton & Lange.

Simkin, P. (2001). *The birth partner*. Boston: The Harvard Common Press.

Simkin, P., Whalley, J., & Keppler, A. (2001). *Pregnancy, childbirth, and the newborn*. New York: Simon & Schuster.

Smeltzer, S., & Bare, B. (2004). *Brunner and Suddarth's textbook of medical-surgical nursing* (10th ed.). Philadelphia: Lippincott, Williams & Wilkins.

Spratto, G., & Woods, A. (2004). *2004 PDR Nurse's drug handbook*. Clifton Park, NY: Delmar Learning.

Ulrich, S., & Canale, W. (2001). *Nursing care planning guides: For adults in acute, extended and home care settings* (5th ed.). Philadelphia: W. B. Saunders Co.

White, L. (2003). Documentation and the Nursing Process. Clifton Park N.Y. Delmar Learning.

Wilkinson, J. M. (2000). *Nursing diagnosis handbook with NIC Interventions and NOC Outcomes* (7th ed.). Upper Saddle River, NJ: Prentice Hall Health.

Wong, D., Hockenberry-Eaton, M., Wilson, D., Winkelstein, M., & Schwartz, P. (2001). *Wong's essentials of pediatric nursing* (6th ed.). St. Louis: Mosby.

Wong, D., Perry, S., & Hockenberry-Eaton, M. (2002). *Maternal child nursing care* (2nd ed.). St. Louis: Mosby.

PERIODICALS

American Academy of Pediatrics. AAP. (1997). *Guidelines for perinatal care* (4th ed.). Chicago: Author.

American Academy of Pediatrics. AAP. (1999). *Circumcision policy statement*. Chicago: Author.

American Academy of Pediatrics. AAP. (2001). *Combined immunization schedule*. Chicago: Author.

American College of Obstetric Gynecology (ACOG). (2002). Prevention of early-onset group B streptococcal disease in newborns. *Obstetrics & Gynecology, 100*(6), 1405–1412.

Association of Women's Health, Obstetric, and Neonatal Nurses (AWHONN). (1993). *Cervical ripening and induction and augmentation of labor*. Washington DC: Author.

Association of Women's Health, Obstetric, & Neonatal Nurses (AWHONN). (2000). *Nursing management of the second stage of labor*. Washington, DC: Author.

Beck, C. T. (1998). A checklist to identify women at risk for developing postpartum depression. *Journal of Obstetric Gynecologic and Neonatal Nursing, 27*(1), 39–46.

Drake, P. (1996). Addressing developmental needs of pregnant adolescents. *Journal of Obstetric Gynecologic and Neonatal Nursing, 25*(6), 518–524.

Findlay, R. D., et al. (1996). Surfactant therapy for meconium aspiration syndrome. *Pediatrics, 90*(1), 48–52.

Fishwick, N. J. (1998). Assessment of women for partner abuse. *Journal of Obstetric Gynecologic and Neonatal Nursing, 27*(6), 661–670.

Gebauer, C. L., & Lowe, N. K. (1993). The biophysical profile: Antepartal assessment of fetal well-being. *Journal of Obstetric Gynecologic and Neonatal Nursing, 22*(2), 115–124.

Griffin, T., Kavanaugh, K., Soto, C. F., & White, M. (1997). Parental evaluation of a tour of the neonatal intensive care unit during a high-risk pregnancy. *Journal of Obstetric Gynecologic and Neonatal Nursing, 26*(1), 59–65.

Haggerty, L. A., Kelly, U., Hawkins, J., Pearce, C., & Kearney, M. H. (2001). Pregnant women's perceptions of abuse. *Journal of Obstetric Gynecologic and Neonatal Nursing, 30*(3), 283–290.

Hutti, M. H. (1988). A quick reference table of interventions to assist families to cope with pregnancy loss or neonatal death. *Birth, 15*(1), 33–35.

Keleher, K. C. (1991). Occupational health: How work environments can affect reproductive capacity and outcome. *Nurse Practitioner, 16*(1), 23–33.

Kenner, C., & D'Apolito, K. (1997). Outcomes for children exposed to drugs in utero. *Journal of Obstetric Gynecologic and Neonatal Nursing, 26*(5), 595–603.

Lowe, N. K., & Reiss, R. (1996). Parturition and fetal adaptation. *Journal of Obstetric Gynecologic and Neonatal Nursing, 25*(4), 339–349.

Ludington-Hoe, S. M., & Swinth, J. Y. (1996). Developmental aspects of kangaroo care. *Journal of Obstetric Gynecologic and Neonatal Nursing, 25*(8), 691–703.

Maloni, J. A., & Ponder, M. B. (1997). Father's experience of their partners' antepartum bed rest. *IMAGE, 29*(2), 183–188.

Maloni, J. A. (1992). Bed rest during pregnancy: Implications for nursing. *Journal of Obstetric Gynecologic and Neonatal Nursing, 22*(5), 422–426.

Mandelbrot, L., Le Chenadec, J., Berribi, A., et al. (1998). Perinatal HIB-1 transmission: Interaction between zidovudine prophylaxis and mode of delivery in the French perinatal cohort. *Journal of the American Medical Association, 280*(1), 55–60.

Miles, M. S. Maternal concerns about parenting prematurely born children. *Maternal Child Nursing, 23*(2), 70–75.

Obstetric epidural analgesia and the role of the professional registered nurse. (1996). *AWHONN Clinical Commentary*. The Association of Women's Health, Obstetric, and Neonatal Nurses.

Penny-MacGillivray, T. (1996). A newborn's first bath: When? *Journal of Obstetric Gynecologic and Neonatal Nursing, 25*(6), 481–487.

Perinatal Group B Streptococcal Disease. (1996). *AWHONN Clinical Commentary*. The Association of Women's Health, Obstetric, and Neonatal Nurses.

Schmidt, J. V. (1995). Intrapartum care of the adolescent. *Capsules & Comments in Perinatal and Women's Health Nursing, 1*(2), 132–138.

Schroeder, C. A. (1996). Women's experience of bed rest in high-risk pregnancy. *IMAGE, 28*(3), 253–258.

Swanson, S. C., & Naber, M. M. (1997). Neonatal integrated home care: Nursing without walls. *Neonatal Network, 16*(7), 33–38.

Weber, S. E. (1996). Cultural aspects of pain in childbearing women. *Journal of Obstetric Gynecologic and Neonatal Nursing, 25*(1), 67–72.

Williams, L. R., & Cooper, M. K. (1993). Nurse-managed postpartum home care. *Journal of Obstetric Gynecologic and Neonatal Nursing, 22*(1), 25–31.

APPENDIX A

NANDA NURSING DIAGNOSES

Activity Intolerance
Acute Confusion
Acute Pain
Adult Failure To Thrive
Anticipatory Grieving
Anxiety
Autonomic Dysreflexia

Bathing/Hygiene Self-Care Deficit
Bowel Incontinence

Caregiver Role Strain
Chronic Confusion
Chronic Low Self-Esteem
Chronic Pain
Chronic Sorrow
Compromised Family Coping
Constipation

Death Anxiety
Decisional Conflict (specify)
Decreased Cardiac Output
Decreased Intracranial Adaptive Capacity
Defensive Coping
Deficient Diversional Activity
Deficient Fluid Volume
Deficient Knowledge (specify)
Delayed Growth And Development
Delayed Surgical Recovery
Diarrhea
Disabled Family Coping
Disorganized Infant Behavior
Disturbed Body Image
Disturbed Energy Field
Disturbed Personal Identity
Disturbed Sensory Perception (specify: visual, auditory,
    kinesthetic, gustatory, tactile, olfactory)
Disturbed Sleep Pattern
Disturbed Thought Processes
Dressing/Grooming Self-Care Deficit
Dysfunctional Family Processes: Alcoholism
Dysfunctional Grieving
Dysfunctional Ventilatory Weaning Response

Effective Breast-Feeding
Effective Therapeutic Regimen Management
Excess Fluid Volume

Fatigue
Fear
Feeding Self-Care Deficit
Functional Urinary Incontinence

Health-Seeking Behaviors (specify)
Hopelessness
Hyperthermia
Hypothermia

Imbalanced Nutrition: Less Than Body Requirements
Imbalanced Nutrition: More Than Body Requirements
Impaired Adjustment
Impaired Bed Mobility
Impaired Dentition
Impaired Environmental Interpretation Syndrome
Impaired Gas Exchange
Impaired Home Maintenance
Impaired Memory
Impaired Oral Mucous Membrane
Impaired Parenting
Impaired Physical Mobility
Impaired Skin Integrity
Impaired Social Interaction
Impaired Spontaneous Ventilation
Impaired Swallowing
Impaired Tissue Integrity
Impaired Transfer Ability
Impaired Urinary Elimination
Impaired Verbal Communication
Impaired Walking
Impaired Wheelchair Mobility
Ineffective Airway Clearance
Ineffective Breast-Feeding
Ineffective Breathing Pattern
Ineffective Community Coping
Ineffective Community Therapeutic Regimen
    Management
Ineffective Coping

Ineffective Denial
Ineffective Family Therapeutic Regimen Management
Ineffective Health Maintenance
Ineffective Infant Feeding Pattern
Ineffective Protection
Ineffective Role Performance
Ineffective Sexuality Patterns
Ineffective Therapeutic Regimen Management
Ineffective Thermoregulation
Ineffective Tissue Perfusion (specify type: renal, cerebral, cardiopulmonary, gastrointestinal, peripheral)
Interrupted Breast-Feeding
Interrupted Family Processes

Latex Allergy Response

Nausea
Noncompliance (specify)

Parental Role Conflict
Perceived Constipation
Post-Trauma Syndrome
Powerlessness

Rape-Trauma Syndrome
Rape-Trauma Syndrome: Compound Reaction
Rape-Trauma Syndrome: Silent Reaction
Readiness for Enhanced Communicaton
Readiness for Enhanced Community Coping
Readiness for Enhanced Coping
Readiness for Enhanced Family Coping
Readiness for Enhanced Family Processes
Readiness for Enhanced Fluid Balance
Readiness for Enhanced Knowledge (specify)
Readiness for Enhanced Nutrition
Readiness for Enhanced Organized Infant Behavior
Readiness for Enhanced Parenting
Readiness for Enhanced Self-Concept
Readiness for Enhanced Sleep
Readiness for Enhanced Spiritual Well-Being
Readiness for Enhanced Therapeutic Regimen Management
Readiness for Enhanced Urinary Elimination
Reflex Urinary Incontinence
Relocation Stress Syndrome
Risk for Activity Intolerance
Risk for Aspiration
Risk for Autonomic Dysreflexia
Risk for Caregiver Role Strain
Risk for Constipation

Risk for Deficient Fluid Volume
Risk for Delayed Development
Risk for Disorganized Infant Behavior
Risk for Disproportionate Growth
Risk for Disuse Syndrome
Risk for Falls
Risk for Imbalanced Body Temperature
Risk for Imbalanced Fluid Volume
Risk for Imbalanced Nutrition: More Than Body Requirements
Risk for Impaired Parent/Infant/Child Attachment
Risk for Impaired Parenting
Risk for Impaired Skin Integrity
Risk for Infection
Risk for Injury
Risk for Latex Allergy Response
Risk for Loneliness
Risk for Other-Directed Violence
Risk for Perioperative-Positioning Injury
Risk for Peripheral Neurovascular Dysfunction
Risk for Poisoning
Risk for Post-Trauma Syndrome
Risk for Powerlessness
Risk for Relocation Stress Syndrome
Risk for Self-Directed Violence
Risk for Self-Mutilation
Risk for Situational Low Self-Esteem
Risk for Spiritual Distress
Risk for Sudden Infant Death Syndrome
Risk for Suffocation
Risk for Suicide
Risk for Trauma
Risk for Urge Urinary Incontinence

Self-Mutilation
Sexual Dysfunction
Situational Low Self-Esteem
Sleep Deprivation
Social Isolation
Spiritual Distress
Stress Urinary Incontinence

Toileting Self-Care Deficit
Total Urinary Incontinence

Unilateral Neglect
Urinary Retention
Urge Urinary Incontenance

Wandering

APPENDIX B

NURSING OUTCOMES CLASSIFICATIONS (NOC)

Abuse Cessation
Abuse Protection
Abuse Recovery Status
Abuse Recovery: Emotional
Abuse Recovery: Financial
Abuse Recovery: Physical
Abuse Recovery: Sexual
Abusive Behavior Self-Restraint
Acceptance: Health Status
Activity Tolerance
Adaptation to Physical Disability
Adherence Behavior
Aggression Self-Control
Allergic Response: Localized
Allergic Response: Systemic
Ambulation
Ambulation: Wheelchair
Anxiety Level
Anxiety Self-Control
Appetite
Aspiration Prevention
Asthma Self-Management

Balance
Blood Coagulation
Blood-Glucose Level
Blood Loss Severity
Blood Transfusion Reaction
Body Image
Body Mechanics Performance
Body Positioning: Self-Initiated
Bone Healing
Bowel Continence
Bowel Elimination
Breastfeeding Establishment: Infant
Breastfeeding Establishment: Maternal
Breastfeeding: Maintenance
Breastfeeding: Weaning

Cardiac Disease Self-Management
Cardiac Pump Effectiveness
Caregiver Adaptation to Patient Institutionalization

Caregiver Emotional Health
Caregiver Home Care Readiness
Caregiver Lifestyle Disruption
Caregiver-Patient Relationship
Caregiver Performance: Direct Care
Caregiver Performance: Indirect Care
Caregiver Physical Health
Caregiver Stressors
Caregiver Well-Being
Caregiving Endurance Potential
Child Adaptation to Hospitalization
Child Development: 1 Month
Child Development: 2 Months
Child Development: 4 Months
Child Development: 6 Months
Child Development: 12 Months
Child Development: 2 Years
Child Development: 3 Years
Child Development: 4 Years
Child Development: Middle Childhood
Child Development: Adolescence
Circulation Status
Client Satisfaction: Access to Care Resources
Client Satisfaction: Caring
Client Satisfaction: Communication
Client Satisfaction: Continuity of Care
Client Satisfaction: Cultural Needs Fulfillment
Client Satisfaction: Functional Assistance
Client Satisfaction: Physical Care
Client Satisfaction: Physical Environment
Client Satisfaction: Protection of Rights
Client Satisfaction: Psychological Care
Client Satisfaction: Safety
Client Satisfaction: Symptom Control
Client Satisfaction: Teaching
Client Satisfaction: Technical Aspects of Care
Cognition
Cognitive Orientation
Comfort Level
Comfortable Death
Communication
Communication: Expressive

Communication: Receptive
Community Competence
Community Disaster Readiness
Community Health Status
Community Health Status: Immunity
Community Risk Control: Chronic Disease
Community Risk Control: Communicable Disease
Community Risk Control: Lead Exposure
Community Risk Control: Violence
Community Violence Level
Compliance Behavior
Concentration
Coordinated Movement
Coping

Decision Making
Depression Level
Depression Self-Control
Diabetes Self-Management
Dignified Life Closure
Discharge Readiness: Independent Living
Discharge Readiness: Supported Living
Distorted Thought Self-Control

Electrolyte and Acid/Base Balance
Endurance
Energy Conservation

Fall Prevention Behavior
Falls Occurrence
Family Coping
Family Functioning
Family Health Status
Family Integrity
Family Normalization
Family Participation in Professional Care
Family Physical Environment
Family Resiliency
Family Social Climate
Family Support During Treatment
Fear Level
Fear Level: Child
Fear Self-Control
Fetal Status: Antepartum
Fetal Status: Intrapartum
Fluid Balance
Fluid Overload Severity

Grief Resolution
Growth

Health Beliefs
Health Beliefs: Perceived Ability to Perform
Health Beliefs: Perceived Control
Health Beliefs: Perceived Resources
Health Beliefs: Perceived Threat

Health Orientation
Health-Promoting Behavior
Health-Seeking Behavior
Hearing Compensation Behavior
Hemodialysis Access
Hope
Hydration
Hyperactivity Level

Identity
Immobility Consequences: Physiological
Immobility Consequences: Psycho-Cognitive
Immune Hypersensitivity Response
Immune Status
Immunization Behavior
Impulse Self-Control
Infection Severity
Infection Severity: Newborn
Information Processing

Joint Movement: Ankle
Joint Movement: Elbow
Joint Movement: Fingers
Joint Movement: Hip
Joint Movement: Knee
Joint Movement: Neck
Joint Movement: Passive
Joint Movement: Shoulder
Joint Movement: Spine
Joint Movement: Wrist

Kidney Function
Knowledge: Body Mechanics
Knowledge: Breastfeeding
Knowledge: Cardiac Disease Management
Knowledge: Child Physical Safety
Knowledge: Conception Prevention
Knowledge: Diabetes Management
Knowledge: Diet
Knowledge: Disease Process
Knowledge: Energy Conservation
Knowledge: Fall Prevention
Knowledge: Fertility Promotion
Knowledge: Health Behavior
Knowledge: Health Promotion
Knowledge: Health Resources
Knowledge: Illness Care
Knowledge: Infant Care
Knowledge: Infection Control
Knowledge: Labor and Delivery
Knowledge: Medication
Knowledge: Ostomy Care
Knowledge: Parenting
Knowledge: Personal Safety
Knowledge: Postpartum Maternal Health
Knowledge: Preconception Maternal Health

Knowledge: Pregnancy
Knowledge: Prescribed Activity
Knowledge: Sexual Functioning
Knowledge: Substance Abuse Control
Knowledge: Treatment Procedure(s)
Knowledge: Treatment Regimen

Leisure Participation
Loneliness Severity

Maternal Status: Antepartum
Maternal Status: Intrapartum
Maternal Status: Postpartum
Mechanical Ventilation Response: Adult
Mechanical Ventilation Weaning Response: Adult
Medication Response
Memory
Mobility
Mood Equilibrium
Motivation

Nausea & Vomiting Control
Nausea & Vomiting: Disruptive Effects
Nausea & Vomiting Severity
Neglect Cessation
Neglect Recovery
Neurological Status
Neurological Status: Autonomic
Neurological Status: Central Motor Control
Neurological Status: Consciousness
Neurological Status: Cranial Sensory/Motor Function
Neurological Status: Spinal Sensory/Motor Function
Newborn Adaptation
Nutritional Status
Nutritional Status: Biochemical Measures
Nutritional Status: Energy
Nutritional Status: Food and Fluid Intake
Nutritional Status: Nutrient Intake

Oral Health
Ostomy Self-Care

Pain: Adverse Psychological Response
Pain Control
Pain: Disruptive Effects
Pain Level
Parent-Infant Attachment
Parenting: Adolescent Physical Safety
Parenting: Early/Middle Childhood Physical Safety
Parenting: Infant/Toddler Physical Safety
Parenting Performance
Parenting: Psychosocial Safety
Participation in Health Care Decisions
Personal Autonomy
Personal Health Status
Personal Safety Behavior

Personal Well-Being
Physical Aging
Physical Fitness
Physical Injury Severity
Physical Maturation: Female
Physical Maturation: Male
Play Participation
Post Procedure Recovery Status
Prenatal Health Behavior
Preterm Infant Organization
Psychomotor Energy
Psychosocial Adjustment: Life Change

Quality of Life

Respiratory Status: Airway Patency
Respiratory Status: Gas Exchange
Respiratory Status: Ventilation
Rest
Risk Control
Risk Control: Alcohol Use
Risk Control: Cancer
Risk Control: Cardiovascular Health
Risk Control: Drug Use
Risk Control: Hearing Impairment
Risk Control: Sexually Transmitted Diseases (STDs)
Risk Control: Tobacco Use
Risk Control: Unintended Pregnancy
Risk Control: Visual Impairment
Risk Detection
Role Performance

Safe Home Environment
Seizure Control
Self-Care Status
Self-Care: Activities of Daily Living (ADL)
Self-Care: Bathing
Self-Care: Dressing
Self-Care: Eating
Self-Care: Hygiene
Self-Care: Instrumental Activities of Daily Living (IADL)
Self-Care: Nonparenteral Medication
Self-Care: Oral Hygiene
Self-Care: Parenteral Medication
Self-Care: Toileting
Self-Direction of Care
Self-Esteem
Self-Mutilation Restraint
Sensory Function Status
Sensory Function: Cutaneous
Sensory Function: Hearing
Sensory Function: Proprioception
Sensory Function: Taste and Smell
Sensory Function: Vision
Sexual Functioning
Sexual Identity

Skeletal Function
Sleep
Social Interaction Skills
Social Involvement
Social Support
Spiritual Health
Stress Level
Student Health Status
Substance Addiction Consequences
Suffering Severity
Suicide Self-Restraint
Swallowing Status
Swallowing Status: Esophageal Phase
Swallowing Status: Oral Phrase
Swallowing Status: Pharyngeal Phase
Symptom Control
Symptom Severity
Symptom Severity: Perimenopause
Symptom Severity: Premenstrual Syndrome (PMS)
Systemic Toxin Clearance: Dialysis

Thermoregulation
Thermoregulation: Neonate

Tissue Integrity: Skin and Mucous Membranes
Tissue Perfusion: Abdominal Organs
Tissue Perfusion: Cardiac
Tissue Perfusion: Cerebral
Tissue Perfusion: Peripheral
Tissue Perfusion: Pulmonary
Transfer Performance
Treatment Behavior: Illness or Injury

Urinary Continence
Urinary Elimination

Vision Compensation Behavior
Vital Signs

Weight: Body Mass
Weight Control
Will to Live
Wound Healing: Primary Intention
Wound Healing: Primary Intention

Reprinted from Moorhead, S., Johnson, M., & Maas, M., *Nursing Outcomes Classifications*, 3rd edition, © 2004. Copyright 2004, with permission from Elsevier Science.

APPENDIX C

NURSING INTERVENTIONS CLASSIFICATIONS (NIC)

Abuse Protection Support
Abuse Protection Support: Child
Abuse Protection Support: Domestic Partner
Abuse Protection Support: Elder
Abuse Protection Support: Religious
Acid-Base Management
Acid-Base Management: Metabolic Acidosis
Acid-Base Management: Metabolic Alkalosis
Acid-Base Management: Respiratory Acidosis
Acid-Base Management: Respiratory Alkalosis
Acid-Base Monitoring
Active Listening
Activity Therapy
Acupressure
Admission Care
Airway Insertion And Stabilization
Airway Management
Airway Suctioning
Allergy Management
Amnioinfusion
Amputation Care
Analgesic Administration
Analgesic Administration: Intraspinal
Anaphylaxis Management
Anesthesia Administration
Anger Control Assistance
Animal-Assisted Therapy
Anticipatory Guidance
Anxiety Reduction
Area Restriction
Aromatherapy
Art Therapy
Artificial Airway Management
Aspiration Precautions
Assertiveness Training
Asthma Management
Attachment Promotion
Autogenic Training
Autotransfusion

Bathing
Bed Rest Care
Bedside Laboratory Testing
Behavior Management
Behavior Management: Overactivity/Inattention
Behavior Management: Self-Harm
Behavior Management: Sexual
Behavior Modification
Behavior Modification: Social Skills
Bibliotherapy
Biofeedback
Bioterrorism Preparedness
Birthing
Bladder Irrigation
Bleeding Precautions
Bleeding Reduction
Bleeding Reduction: Antepartum Uterus
Bleeding Reduction: Gastrointestinal
Bleeding Reduction: Nasal
Bleeding Reduction: Postpartum Uterus
Bleeding Reduction: Wound
Blood Products Administration
Body Image Enhancement
Body Mechanics Promotion
Bottle Feeding
Bowel Incontinence Care
Bowel Incontinence Care: Encopresis
Bowel Irrigation
Bowel Management
Bowel Training
Breast Examination
Breastfeeding Assistance

Calming Technique
Capillary Blood Sample
Cardiac Care
Cardiac Care: Acute
Cardiac Care: Rehabilitative
Cardiac Precautions

Caregiver Support
Care Management
Cast Care: Maintenance
Cast Care, Wet
Cerebral Edema Management
Cerebral Perfusion Promotion
Cesarean Section Care
Chemical Restraint
Chemotherapy Management
Chest Physiotherapy
Childbirth Preparation
Circulatory Care: Arterial Insufficiency
Circulatory Care: Mechanical Assist Device
Circulatory Care: Venous Insufficiency
Circulatory Precautions
Circumcision Care
Code Management
Cognitive Restructuring
Cognitive Stimulation
Communicable Disease Management
Communication Enhancement: Hearing Deficit
Communication Enhancement: Speech Deficit
Communication Enhancement: Visual Deficit
Community Disaster Preparedness
Community Health Development
Complex Relationship Building
Conflict Mediation
Constipation/Impaction Management
Consultation
Contact Lens Care
Controlled Substance Checking
Coping Enhancement
Cost Containment
Cough Enhancement
Counseling
Crisis Intervention
Critical Path Development
Culture Brokerage
Cutaneous Stimulation

Decision-Making Support
Delegation
Delirium Management
Delusion Management
Dementia Management
Dementia Management: Bathing
Deposition/Testimony
Developmental Care
Developmental Enhancement: Adolescent
Developmental Enhancement: Child
Dialysis Access Maintenance
Diarrhea Management
Diet Staging
Discharge Planning
Distraction

Documentation
Dressing
Dying Care
Dysreflexia Management
Dysrhythmia Management

Ear Care
Eating Disorders Management
Electroconvulsive Therapy (ECT) Management
Electrolyte Management
Electrolyte Management: Hypercalcemia
Electrolyte Management: Hyperkalemia
Electrolyte Management: Hypermagnesemia
Electrolyte Management: Hypernatremia
Electrolyte Management: Hyperphosphatemia
Electrolyte Management: Hypocalcemia
Electrolyte Management: Hypokalemia
Electrolyte Management: Hypomagnesemia
Electrolyte Management: Hyponatremia
Electrolyte Management: Hypophosphatemia
Electrolyte Monitoring
Electronic Fetal Monitoring: Antepartum
Electronic Fetal Monitoring: Intrapartum
Elopement Precautions
Embolus Care: Peripheral
Embolus Care: Pulmonary
Embolus Precautions
Emergency Care
Emergency Cart Checking
Emotional Support
Endotracheal Extubation
Energy Management
Enteral Tube Feeding
Environmental Management
Environmental Management: Attachment Process
Environmental Management: Comfort
Environmental Management: Community
Environmental Management: Home Preparation
Environmental Management: Safety
Environmental Management: Violence Prevention
Environmental Management: Worker Safety
Environmental Risk Protection
Examination Assistance
Exercise Promotion
Exercise Promotion: Strength Training
Exercise Promotion: Stretching
Exercise Therapy: Ambulation
Exercise Therapy: Balance
Exercise Therapy: Joint Mobility
Exercise Therapy: Muscle Control
Eye Care

Fall Prevention
Family Integrity Promotion
Family Integrity Promotion: Childbearing Family

Family Involvement Promotion
Family Mobilization
Family Planning: Contraception
Family Planning: Infertility
Family Planning: Unplanned Pregnancy
Family Presence Facilitation
Family Process Maintenance
Family Support
Family Therapy
Feeding
Fertility Preservation
Fever Treatment
Financial Resource Assistance
Fire-Setting Precautions
First Aid
Fiscal Resource Management
Flatulence Reduction
Fluid/Electrolyte Management
Fluid Management
Fluid Monitoring
Fluid Resuscitation
Foot Care
Forgiveness Facilitation

Gastrointestinal Intubation
Genetic Counseling
Grief Work Facilitation
Grief Work Facilitation: Perinatal Death
Guilt Work Facilitation

Hair Care
Hallucination Management
Health Care Information Exchange
Health Education
Health Policy Monitoring
Health Screening
Health System Guidance
Heat/Cold Application
Heat Exposure Treatment
Hemodialysis Therapy
Hemodynamic Regulation
Hemofiltration Therapy
Hemorrhage Control
High-Risk Pregnancy Care
Home Maintenance Assistance
Hope Instillation
Hormone Replacement Therapy
Humor
Hyperglycemia Management
Hypervolemia Management
Hypnosis
Hypoglycemia Management
Hypothermia Treatment
Hypovolemia Management

Immunization/Vaccination Administration
Impulse Control Training
Incident Reporting
Incision Site Care
Infant Care
Infection Control
Infection Control: Intraoperative
Infection Protection
Insurance Authorization
Intracranial Pressure (ICP) Monitoring
Intrapartal Care
Intrapartal Care: High-Risk Delivery
Intravenous (IV) Insertion
Intravenous (IV) Therapy
Invasive Hemodynamic Monitoring

Kangaroo Care

Labor Induction
Labor Suppression
Laboratory Data Interpretation
Lactation Counseling
Lactation Suppression
Laser Precautions
Latex Precautions
Learning Facilitation
Learning Readiness Enhancement
Leech Therapy
Limit Setting
Lower Extremity Monitoring

Malignant Hyperthermia Precautions
Mechanical Ventilation
Mechanical Ventilatory Weaning
Medication Administration
Medication Administration: Ear
Medication Administration: Enteral
Medication Administration: Eye
Medication Administration: Inhalation
Medication Administration: Interpleural
Medication Administration: Intradermal
Medication Administration: Intramuscular (IM)
Medication Administration: Intraosseous
Medication Administration: Intraspinal
Medication Administration: Intravenous (IV)
Medication Administration: Nasal
Medication Administration: Oral
Medication Administration: Rectal
Medication Administration: Skin
Medication Administration: Subcutaneous
Medication Administration: Vaginal
Medication Administration: Ventricular Reservoir
Medication Management
Medication Prescribing

Meditation Facilitation
Memory Training
Milieu Therapy
Mood Management
Multidisciplinary Care Conference
Music Therapy
Mutual Goal Setting

Nail Care
Nausea Management
Neurologic Monitoring
Newborn Care
Newborn Monitoring
Nonnutritive Sucking
Normalization Promotion
Nutrition Management
Nutrition Therapy
Nutritional Counseling
Nutritional Monitoring

Oral Health Maintenance
Oral Health Promotion
Oral Health Restoration
Order Transcription
Organ Procurement
Ostomy Care
Oxygen Therapy

Pain Management
Parent Education: Adolescent
Parent Education: Childrearing Family
Parent Education: Infant
Parenting Promotion
Pass Facilitation
Patient Contracting
Patient Controlled Analgesia (PCA) Assistance
Patient Rights Protection
Peer Review
Pelvic Muscle Exercise
Perineal Care
Peripheral Sensation Management
Peripherally Inserted Central (PIC) Catheter Care
Peritoneal Dialysis Therapy
Pessary Management
Phlebotomy: Arterial Blood Sample
Phlebotomy: Blood Unit Acquisition
Phlebotomy: Cannulated Vessel
Phlebotomy: Venous Blood Sample
Phototherapy: Mood/Sleep Regulation
Phototherapy: Neonate
Physical Restraint
Physician Support
Pneumatic Tourniquet Precautions
Positioning
Positioning: Intraoperative

Positioning: Neurologic
Positioning: Wheelchair
Postanesthesia Care
Postmortem Care
Postpartal Care
Preceptor: Employee
Preceptor: Student
Preconception Counseling
Pregnancy Termination Care
Premenstrual Syndrome (PMS) Management
Prenatal Care
Preoperative Coordination
Preparatory Sensory Information
Presence
Pressure Management
Pressure Ulcer Care
Pressure Ulcer Prevention
Product Evaluation
Program Development
Progressive Muscle Relaxation
Prompted Voiding
Prosthesis Care
Pruritus Management

Quality Monitoring

Radiation Therapy Management
Rape-Trauma Treatment
Reality Orientation
Recreation Therapy
Rectal Prolapse Management
Referral
Religious Addiction Prevention
Religious Ritual Enhancement
Relocation Stress Reduction
Reminiscence Therapy
Reproductive Technology Management
Research Data Collection
Resiliency Promotion
Respiratory Monitoring
Respite Care
Resuscitation
Resuscitation: Fetus
Resuscitation: Neonate
Risk Identification
Risk Identification: Childbearing Family
Risk Identification: Genetic
Role Enhancement

Seclusion
Security Enhancement
Sedation Management
Seizure Management
Seizure Precautions
Self-Awareness Enhancement

Self-Care Assistance
Self-Care Assistance: Bathing/Hygiene
Self-Care Assistance: Dressing/Grooming
Self-Care Assistance: Feeding
Self-Care Assistance: IADL
Self-Care Assistance: Toileting
Self-Care Assistance: Transfer
Self-Esteem Enhancement
Self-Hypnosis Facilitation
Self-Modification Assistance
Self-Responsibility Facilitation
Sexual Counseling
Shift Report
Shock Management
Shock Management: Cardiac
Shock Management: Vasogenic
Shock Management: Volume
Shock Prevention
Sibling Support
Simple Guided Imagery
Simple Massage
Simple Relaxation Therapy
Skin Care: Donor Site
Skin Care: Graft Site
Skin Care: Topical Treatments
Skin Surveillance
Sleep Enhancement
Smoking Cessation Assistance
Socialization Enhancement
Specimen Management
Spiritual Growth Facilitation
Spiritual Support
Splinting
Sports-Injury Prevention: Youth
Staff Development
Staff Supervision
Subarachnoid Hemorrhage Precautions
Substance Use Prevention
Substance Use Treatment
Substance Use Treatment: Alcohol Withdrawal
Substance Use Treatment: Drug Withdrawal
Substance Use Treatment: Overdose
Suicide Prevention
Supply Management
Support Group
Support System Enhancement
Surgical Assistance
Surgical Precautions
Surgical Preparation
Surveillance
Surveillance: Community
Surveillance: Late Pregnancy
Surveillance: Remote Electronic
Surveillance: Safety
Sustenance Support

Suturing
Swallowing Therapy

Teaching: Disease Process
Teaching: Foot Care
Teaching: Group
Teaching: Individual
Teaching: Infant Nutrition
Teaching: Infant Safety
Teaching: Infant Stimulation
Teaching: Preoperative
Teaching: Prescribed Activity/Exercise
Teaching: Prescribed Diet
Teaching: Prescribed Medication
Teaching: Procedure/Treatment
Teaching: Psychomotor Skill
Teaching: Safe Sex
Teaching: Sexuality
Teaching: Toddler Nutrition
Teaching: Toddler Safety
Teaching: Toilet Training
Technology Management
Telephone Consultation
Telephone Follow-Up
Temperature Regulation
Temperature Regulation: Intraoperative
Temporary Pacemaker Management
Therapeutic Play
Therapeutic Touch
Therapy Group
Total Parenteral Nutrition (TPN) Administration
Touch
Traction/Immobilization Care
Transcutaneous Electrical Nerve Stimulation (TENS)
Transport
Trauma Therapy: Child
Triage: Disaster
Triage: Emergency Center
Triage: Telephone
Truth Telling
Tube Care
Tube Care: Chest
Tube Care: Gastrointestinal
Tube Care: Umbilical Line
Tube Care: Urinary
Tube Care: Ventriculostomy/Lumbar Drain

Ultrasonography: Limited Obstetric
Unilateral Neglect Management
Urinary Bladder Training
Urinary Catheterization
Urinary Catheterization: Intermittent
Urinary Elimination Management
Urinary Habit Training
Urinary Incontinence Care

Urinary Incontinence Care: Enuresis
Urinary Retention Care

Values Clarification
Vehicle Safety Promotion
Venous Access Device (VAD) Maintenance
Ventilation Assistance
Visitation Facilitation
Vital Signs Monitoring
Vomiting Management

Weight Gain Assistance
Weight Management
Weight Reduction Assistance
Wound Care
Wound Care: Closed Drainage
Wound Irrigation

APPENDIX D

ABBREVIATIONS

↑: increase

↓: decrease

→: leads to

>: greater than

<: less than

": minutes

°: degree

AAP: American Academy of Pediatrics

ABO: refers to the blood types A, B, or O

ABG: arterial blood gas

ADHD: attention deficit hyperactivity disorder

AFDC: Aid to Families with Dependent Children

AFI: amniotic fluid index

AFV: amniotic fluid volume

AGA: average for gestational age

AIDS: acquired immunodeficiency syndrome

ALT: alanine aminotransferase (also SGPT)

APTT: activated partial thromboplastin time

ARDS: adult respiratory distress syndrome

AROM: artificial rupture of membranes

ASD: atrial septal defect

AST: aspartate aminotransferase (also SGOT)

BBT: basal body temperature

BM: bowel movement

BP: blood pressure

BPP: biophysical profile

BRP: bathroom privileges

BUN: blood urea nitrogen

C: centigrade

cal: calories

CBC: complete blood count

cc: cubic centimeters

CD & I: clean, dry, and intact

CHF: congestive heart failure

Cl: clear

CMV: cytomegalovirus

CNM: certified nurse midwife

CNS: central nervous system

c/o: complains of

CO: cardiac output

CO_2: carbon dioxide

CPAP: continuous positive airway pressure

CPD: cephalopelvic disproportion

CPT: chest physiotherapy

CRP: C-reactive protein

CSF: cerebral spinal fluid

CST: contraction stress test

CT: computerized axial tomography

ctx: contractions

CVP: central venous pressure

CVA: cerebral vascular accident

CVS: chorionic villi sampling

DAT: diet as tolerated

D/C: discharge; discontinue

DCFS: Department of Children and Family Services

DES: diethylstilbestrol

DIC: disseminating intravascular coagulation

dL: deciliter

DNA: deoxyribonucleic acid

dsg: dressing

DtaP: diptheria, tetanus, activated pertussis

DTR: deep tendon reflexes

DVT: deep vein thrombosis

EBL: estimated blood loss

ECMO: extracorporeal membrane oxygenation

ECT: electroconvulsive therapy

EEG: electroencephalogram

EFM: electronic fetal monitor

e.g.: for example

EGA: estimated gestational age

ELBW: excessively low birth weight

ELISA: enzyme-linked immunosorbent assay

F: Fahrenheit

FAS: fetal alcohol syndrome

FDP: fibrin degradation products

FFP: fresh frozen plasma

FHT: fetal heart tones

FHR: fetal heart rate

FiO$_2$: fraction of inspired oxygen

FSH: follicle-stimulating hormone

FSP: fibrin split products

FVE: fluid volume excess

FVD: fluid volume deficit

GBS: group B streptococcus

GC: gonorrhea

GFR: glomerular filtration rate

GI: gastrointestinal

GIFT: gamete intrafallopian transfer

gm: gram

GTT: glucose tolerance test

GU: genitourinary

H$^+$: hydrogen ion

HBsAg: hepatitis B surface antigen

hCG: human chorionic gonadotropin

hCS: human chorionic somatomammotropin (hPL)

Hct: hematocrit

HELLP: hemolysis, elevated liver enzymes, and low
   platelets

HFV: high-frequency ventilation

Hgb: hemoglobin

Hib: *Haemophilus influenzae*, type b

HIE: hypoxic–ischemic encephalopathy

HIV: human immunodeficiency virus

H$_2$O: water

HOB: head of bed

hPL: human placental lactogen (hCS)

hr: hour

HR: heart rate

Ht: height

hx: history

I&O: intake & output

ICP: intracranial pressure

ID: identification

IDDM: insulin-dependent diabetes mellitus

IDM: infant of diabetic mother

Ig: immune globulin

IM: intramuscular

IMV: intermittent mechanical ventilation

IPPB: intermittent positive pressure breathing

IPV: inactivated poliovirus vaccine

IUFD: intrauterine fetal demise

IUGR: intrauterine growth restriction

IUPC: intrauterine pressure catheter

IV: intravenous

IVF: in vitro fertilization

IVH: intraventricular hemorrhage

IVP: intravenous push

K$^+$: potassium

KVO: keep vein open

kcal: kilocalories

kg: kilogram

L: liter

LBW: low birth weight

L&D: labor and delivery

LGA: large for gestational age

LH: luteinizing hormone

LMP: last menstrual period

LNMP: last normal menstrual period

LOA: left occiput anterior

LOP: left occiput posterior

LOC: level of consciousness

LR: lactated Ringer's

L/S: lecithin to sphingomyelin

LSA: left sacrum anterior

LSP: left sacrum posterior

LTV: long-term variability

MAE: moves all extremities

MAS: meconium aspiration syndrome

mEq: milliequivalent

mg: milligram

ml: milliliter

mm Hg: millimeters of mercury

MRI: magnetic resonance imaging

$MgSO_4$: magnesium sulfate

MMR: measles, mumps, rubella vaccine

MsAFP: maternal serum alpha fetoprotein

mOsm: milliosmol

mU: milliunits

Na^+: sodium

NEC: necrotizing enterocolitis

NIC: nursing interventions classification

NICU: neonatal intensive care unit

NPO: nothing by mouth

NST: nonstress test

NTD: neural tube defect

N&V: nausea & vomiting

O_2: oxygen

OA: occiput anterior

OB: obstetrics

OCT: oxytocin challenge test

OG: orogastric

OP: occiput posterior

OFC: occipital–frontal circumference

OTC: over-the-counter

OR: operating room

oz: ounce

P: pulse

$PaCO_2$: arterial carbon dioxide pressure

PaO_2: arterial oxygen pressure

PCA: patient-controlled analgesia

PEEP: positive end expiratory pressure

PDA: patent ductus arteriosus

PG: phosphatidylglycerol

PGE_2: prostaglandin

PIH: pregnancy-induced hypertension

PKU: phenylketonuria

PNC: prenatal care

PNV: prenatal vitamins

po: by mouth

PO_2: partial pressure of oxygen

PP: postpartum

PPHN: persistent pulmonary hypertension of the newborn

PPV: positive pressure ventilation

PROM: premature rupture of membranes

PPROM: prolonged premature rupture of membranes

prn: as needed

PT: prothrombin time

PTL: preterm labor

PTT: partial thromboplastin time

PUBS: percutaneous umbilical blood sampling

PVC: premature ventricular contraction

PVR: pulmonary vascular resistance

q: every

R: respirations

RBC: red blood cell

RDS: respiratory distress syndrome

REEDA: redness, edema, echymosis, approximation

RN: registered nurse

ROA: right occiput anterior

ROM: rupture of membranes

ROP: right occiput posterior

RSA: right sacrum anterior

RSP: right sacrum posterior

SaO_2: oxygen saturation

SA: sacrum anterior

SC: subcutaneous

SGA: small for gestational age

SGOT: serum glutamic-oxaloacetic transaminase (AST)

SGPT: serum glutamic-pyruvic transaminase (ALT)

SIDS: sudden infant death syndrome

S/O: significant other

SP: sacrum posterior

sp. gr: specific gravity

SR: side rails

SROM: spontaneous rupture of membranes

s/s: signs and symptoms

STD: sexually transmitted disease

STV: short-term variability

SVR: systemic vascular resistance

SVT: superficial vein thrombosis

T: temperature

TCDB: turn, cough, and deep breathe

TcPaO$_2$: transcutaneous partial pressure of oxygen

TcPaCO$_2$: transcutaneous partial pressure of carbon dioxide

Td: tetanus toxid vaccine

TEF: tracheoesophageal fistula

TGV: transposition of the great vessels

TORCH: toxoplasmosis, other, rubella, cytomegalovirus, hepatitis B

TPN: total parenteral nutrition

TPR: temperature, pulse, respirations

TSH: thyroid stimulating hormone

U: unit

UA: urinalysis

UAC: umbilical artery catheter

URI: upper respiratory infection

UTI: urinary tract infection

VBAC: vaginal birth after cesarean

VDRL: venereal disease research laboratories

VLBW: very low birth weight

VP: venticuloperitoneal

VS: vital signs

VSD: ventricular septal defect

WBC: white blood cell

WIC: women, infants, and children program

WNL: within normal limits

Wt: weight

w/o: without

ZDT: zidovudine

ZIFT: zygote intrafallopian transfer

INDEX

Note: **Bold** type indicates main entries which are nursing diagnoses.

NOTES

License Agreement for Delmar Cengage Learning, Inc.

Educational Software/Data

You the customer, and Delmar Cengage Learning, Inc. incur certain benefits, rights, and obligations to each other when you open this package and use the software/data it contains. BE SURE YOU READ THE LICENSE AGREEMENT CAREFULLY, SINCE BY USING THE SOFTWARE/DATA YOU INDICATE YOU HAVE READ, UNDERSTOOD, AND ACCEPTED THE TERMS OF THIS AGREEMENT.

Your rights:

1. You enjoy a non-exclusive license to use the software/data on a single microcomputer in consideration for payment of the required license fee, (which may be included in the purchase price of an accompanying print component), or receipt of this software/data, and your acceptance of the terms and conditions of this agreement.

2. You acknowledge that you do not own the aforesaid software/data. You also acknowledge that the software/data is furnished "as is," and contains copyrighted and/or proprietary and confidential information of Delmar Cengage Learning, Inc. or its licensors.

There are limitations on your rights:

1. You may not copy or print the software/data for any reason whatsoever, except to install it on a hard drive on a single microcomputer and to make one archival copy, unless copying or printing is expressly permitted in writing or statements recorded on the diskette(s).

2. You may not revise, translate, convert, disassemble or otherwise reverse engineer the software/data except that you may add to or rearrange any data recorded on the media as part of the normal use of thesoftware/data.

3. You may not sell, license, lease, rent, loan or otherwise distribute or network the software/data except that you may give the software/data to a student or an instructor for use at school or, temporarily at home.

Should you fail to abide by the Copyright Law of the United States as it applies to this software/data your license to use it will become invalid. You agree to erase or otherwise destroy the software/data immediately after receiving note of termination of this agreement for violation of its provisions from Delmar Learning.

Delmar Learning, a division of Thomson Learning, Inc. gives you a LIMITED WARRANTY covering the enclosed software/data. The LIMITED WARRANTY follows this License.

This license is the entire agreement between you and Delmar Cengage Learning, Inc. interpreted and enforced under New York law.

LIMITED WARRANTY

Delmar Learning, a division of Thomson Learning, Inc. warrants to the original licensee/purchaser of this copy of microcomputer software/data and the media on which it is recorded that the media will be free from defects in material and workmanship for ninety (90) days from the date of original purchase. All implied warranties are limited in duration to this ninety (90) day period. THEREAFTER, ANY IMPLIED WARRANTIES, INCLUDING IMPLIED WARRANTIES OF MERCHANTABILITY AND FITNESS FOR A PARTICULAR PURPOSE, ARE EXCLUDED. THIS WARRANTY IS IN LIEU OF ALL OTHER WARRANTIES, WHETHER ORAL OR WRITTEN, EXPRESS OR IMPLIED.

If you believe the media is defective please return it during the ninety (90) day period to the address shown below. Defective media will be replaced without charge provided that it has not been subjected to misuse or damage.

This warranty does not extend to the software or information recorded on the media. The software and information are provided "AS IS." Any statements made about the utility of the software or information are not to be considered as express or implied warranties.

Limitation of liability: Our liability to you for any losses shall be limited to direct damages, and shall not exceed the amount you paid for the software. In no event will we be liable to you for any indirect, special, incidental, or consequential damages (including loss of profits) even if we have been advised of the possibility of such damages.

Some states do not allow the exclusion or limitation of incidental or consequential damages, or limitations on the duration of implied warranties, so the above limitation or exclusion may not apply to you. This warranty gives you specific legal rights, and you may also have other rights which vary from state to state. Address all correspondence to: Delmar Cengage Learning, Inc., 5 Maxwell Drive, P.O. Box 8007, Clifton Park, NY 12065-8007. Attention: Technology Department.

SYSTEM REQUIREMENTS

The CD-ROM version will be developed to run on client systems with the following minimum configuration:

- Operating System: Microsoft Windows 98 SE, Windows 2000, Windows XP
- Processor: Pentium PC 120 MHz or higher
- RAM: 64 MB of RAM or better
- Free Drive Space: 25 MB free disk space
- CD-ROM Drive—necessary for installation only
- Internet Connection Speed: 56K or better in order to view web links provided in program but is not required.
- Screen Resolution: 800 × 600 pixels or better
- Color Depth: 16-bit color (thousands of colors) or 24-bit color (millions of colors)
- Sound card: N/A

SET UP INSTRUCTIONS

To install the program, simply run the "X:\setup.exe", where X is the drive letter of you CD-ROM drive. Follow the on screen prompts to complete the installation. You may also:

1. Double click My Computer
2. Double click the Control Panel icon
3. Double click Add/Remove Programs
4. Click the Install button and follow the on screen prompts from there.